Web-Based Behavioral Therapies for Mental Disorders

Sitwat Usman Langrial
Sur University College, Oman

A volume in the Advances in Psychology, Mental Health, and Behavioral Studies (APMHBS) Book Series

IGI Global
DISSEMINATOR OF KNOWLEDGE

Published in the United States of America by
IGI Global
Medical Information Science Reference (an imprint of IGI Global)
701 E. Chocolate Avenue
Hershey PA, USA 17033
Tel: 717-533-8845
Fax: 717-533-8661
E-mail: cust@igi-global.com
Web site: http://www.igi-global.com

Library of Congress Cataloging-in-Publication Data

Names: Langrial, Sitwat Usman, 1975- editor.
Title: Web-based behavioral therapies for mental disorders / Sitwat Usman Langrial, editor.
Description: Hershey PA : Medical Information Science Reference, [2018] | Includes bibliographical references.
Identifiers: LCCN 2017013741| ISBN 9781522532415 (hardcover) | ISBN 9781522532422 (ebook)
Subjects: | MESH: Mental Disorders--therapy | Therapy, Computer-Assisted--methods | Telemedicine--methods | Counseling--methods | Remote Consultation--ethics
Classification: LCC RC489.B4 | NLM WM 400 | DDC 616.89/14200285--dc23 LC record available at https://lccn.loc.gov/2017013741

This book is published in the IGI Global book series Advances in Psychology, Mental Health, and Behavioral Studies (APMHBS) (ISSN: 2475-6660; eISSN: 2475-6679)

British Cataloguing in Publication Data
A Cataloguing in Publication record for this book is available from the British Library.

Advances in Psychology, Mental Health, and Behavioral Studies (APMHBS) Book Series

ISSN:2475-6660
EISSN:2475-6679

Editor-in-Chief: Bryan Christiansen, PryMarke, LLC, USA

MISSION

The complexity of the human mind has puzzled researchers and physicians for centuries. While widely studied, the brain still remains largely misunderstood.

The **Advances in Psychology, Mental Health, and Behavioral Studies (APMHBS)** book series presents comprehensive research publications focusing on topics relating to the human psyche, cognition, psychiatric care, mental and developmental disorders, as well as human behavior and interaction. Featuring diverse and innovative research, publications within APMHBS are ideally designed for use by mental health professionals, academicians, researchers, and upper-level students.

COVERAGE

- Treatment & Care
- Personality Disorders
- Human Behavior
- Addiction
- Mental Health & Disorders
- Human Interaction
- Neurological Disorders
- Developmental Disorders
- Eating Disorders
- Trauma & Stress

IGI Global is currently accepting manuscripts for publication within this series. To submit a proposal for a volume in this series, please contact our Acquisition Editors at Acquisitions@igi-global.com or visit: http://www.igi-global.com/publish/.

The Advances in Psychology, Mental Health, and Behavioral Studies (APMHBS) Book Series (ISSN 2475-6660) is published by IGI Global, 701 E. Chocolate Avenue, Hershey, PA 17033-1240, USA, www.igi-global.com. This series is composed of titles available for purchase individually; each title is edited to be contextually exclusive from any other title within the series. For pricing and ordering information please visit http://www.igi-global.com/book-series/advances-psychology-mental-health-behavioral/110200. Postmaster: Send all address changes to above address.

Titles in this Series

For a list of additional titles in this series, please visit:
http://www.igi-global.com/book-series/advances-psychology-mental-health-behavioral/110200

Measuring the Psychological and Electrophysiological Attributes of Human Personality ...
Sanja Tatalović Vorkapić (University of Rijeka, Croatia)
Information Science Reference • ©2017 • 242pp • H/C (ISBN: 9781522522836) • US $130.00

Emerging Research in Play Therapy, Child Counseling, and Consultation
Rheta LeAnne Steen (Loyola University New Orleans, USA)
Information Science Reference • ©2017 • 436pp • H/C (ISBN: 9781522522249) • US $205.00

Workforce Development Theory and Practice in the Mental Health Sector
Mark Smith (Te Pou o te Whakaaro Nui: National Workforce Center for Adult Mental Health, Addiction and Disability, New Zealand) and Angela F. Jury (Te Pou o te Whakaaro Nui: National Workforce Center for Adult Mental Health, Addiction and Disability, New Zealand)
Information Science Reference • ©2017 • 378pp • H/C (ISBN: 9781522518747) • US $190.00

Improving the Quality of Life for Dementia Patients through Progressive Detection, ...
Jinglong Wu (Okayama University, Japan)
Med Info Science Reference • ©2017 • 353pp • H/C (ISBN: 9781522509257) • US $205.00

Police Psychology and Its Growing Impact on Modern Law Enforcement
Cary L. Mitchell (Pepperdine University, USA) and Edrick H. Dorian (Los Angeles Police Department, USA)
Information Science Reference • ©2017 • 345pp • H/C (ISBN: 9781522508137) • US $190.00

Seduction in Popular Culture, Psychology, and Philosophy
Constantino Martins (Nova University of Lisbon, Portugal) and Manuel Damásio (Lusófona University, Portugal)
Information Science Reference • ©2017 • 332pp • H/C (ISBN: 9781522505259) • US $175.00

For an enitre list of titles in this series, please visit:
http://www.igi-global.com/book-series/advances-psychology-mental-health-behavioral/110200

IGI Global
DISSEMINATOR OF KNOWLEDGE

701 East Chocolate Avenue, Hershey, PA 17033, USA
Tel: 717-533-8845 x100 • Fax: 717-533-8661
E-Mail: cust@igi-global.com • www.igi-global.com

Table of Contents

Preface xii

Chapter 1
Mental Health and Cognitive Behavioral Therapy: Advanced Issues and Approaches 1
Kijpokin Kasemsap, Suan Sunandha Rajabhat University, Thailand

Chapter 2
User Experiences and Perceptions of Internet Interventions for Depression 27
Filip Drozd, National Network for Infant Mental Health, Norway
Caroline Emilie Andersen, University of Oslo, Norway
Silje Marie Haga, National Network of Infant Mental Health, Norway
Kari Slinning, National Network for Infant Mental Health, Norway
Cato Alexander Bjørkli, University of Oslo, Norway

Chapter 3
Treating Sleep Disorders with an ACT-Based Behavior Change Support System 53
Sitwat Usman Langrial, Sur University College, Oman
Harri Oinas-Kukkonen, University of Oulu, Finland
Päivi Lappalainen, University of Jyväskylä, Finland
Raimo Lappalainen, University of Jyväskylä, Finland

Chapter 4
From Science to Practice: Implementation and Clinical Guidelines for an Internet Intervention for Postpartum Depression 79
Filip Drozd, National Network for Infant Mental Health, Norway
Silje Marie Haga, National Network of Infant Mental Health, Norway
Kari Slinning, National Network for Infant Mental Health, Norway

Chapter 5
EHealth Interventions for People Suffering From Sleep Problems and Depressive Symptoms: Qualitative Findings and Future Research Directions 111
Sitwat Usman Langrial, Sur University College, Oman
Päivi Lappalainen, University of Jyväskylä, Finland

Chapter 6
An Internet-Based Quantum Biofeedback and Neurotechnology Cybertherapy System for the Support of Transpersonal Psychology 139
Raul Valverde, Concordia University, Canada

Chapter 7
Neurotechnology in the Development of Cyber-Psychotherapy Systems for Inducing and Measuring Altered States of Consciousness in Transpersonal Psychotherapy 185
Raul Valverde, Concordia University, USA

Chapter 8
The Development of Ethical Guidelines for Online Counselling and Psychotherapy 212
Stephen Goss, Metanoia Institute, UK
Kate Elizabeth Anthony, Online Therapy Institute, UK

Chapter 9
Revisiting the Issue of Trust in E-Health 241
Elizabeth Sillence, Northumbria University, UK
Pam Briggs, Northumbria University, UK
Peter R. Harris, University of Sussex, UK

Compilation of References 260

About the Contributors 304

Index 308

Detailed Table of Contents

Preface xii

Chapter 1
Mental Health and Cognitive Behavioral Therapy: Advanced Issues and Approaches..1
Kijpokin Kasemsap, Suan Sunandha Rajabhat University, Thailand

This chapter reveals the important perspectives on mental health, mental illness, and technology utilization; mental health education and mental health nursing; the overview of Cognitive Behavioral Therapy (CBT); CBT, depression, anxiety, and insomnia; CBT and Obsessive-Compulsive Disorder (OCD); and CBT and heart failure. Mental health strengthens the individuals' ability to have healthy relationships; make good life choices; maintain physical health and well-being; handle the natural ups and downs of life; and grow toward individuals' potential. Mental health is associated with higher productivity, better performance, more consistent work attendance, and fewer workplace accidents. CBT is a goal-oriented psychotherapy treatment that takes a practical approach to problem-solving skills. CBT involves recognizing the unhelpful or destructive patterns of thinking and reacting, thus modifying or replacing these patterns with more realistic or helpful ones.

Chapter 2
User Experiences and Perceptions of Internet Interventions for Depression.......27
Filip Drozd, National Network for Infant Mental Health, Norway
Caroline Emilie Andersen, University of Oslo, Norway
Silje Marie Haga, National Network of Infant Mental Health, Norway
Kari Slinning, National Network for Infant Mental Health, Norway
Cato Alexander Bjørkli, University of Oslo, Norway

The purpose of this chapter is to review qualitative research on user experiences with internet interventions for depression and present original results from in-depth interviews from a preventive unguided intervention for postpartum depression. The first part reviews the literature on qualitative studies of client experiences and perceptions of internet interventions for depression. The next part describes original data from a study investigating participants' experiences using semi-structured interviews, following the modified SWOT-format (i.e., strengths, weakness, opportunities, and threats). In total, 10 pregnant and postpartum women aged 28 to 41 were interviewed. Insights from the current review and study are used as a point of departure for discussing future directions in research on internet interventions for depression. This chapter should be valuable for clinicians, researchers, and other health professionals interested in the applicability of internet interventions for their clients, design of future studies, and development of internet interventions.

Chapter 3
Treating Sleep Disorders with an ACT-Based Behavior Change Support System....53
Sitwat Usman Langrial, Sur University College, Oman
Harri Oinas-Kukkonen, University of Oulu, Finland
Päivi Lappalainen, University of Jyväskylä, Finland
Raimo Lappalainen, University of Jyväskylä, Finland

Suitable duration and appropriate quality of sleep are essential for mental and cognitive wellbeing. Sleep disorders, whether mild or severe, have proven to have adverse effects on general wellbeing. One's quality of life could be disturbed as a consequence of various mental conditions, sleep disorders being one of them. Researchers have started paying attention to designing, implementing and evaluating eHealth interventions to address sleep disorders. In this chapter, we highlight findings from a field study that was conducted to evaluate effect of software features on a Web-based intervention for sleep disorders. Tyyne is a Web-based eHealth intervention that will be repeatedly mentioned as Behavior Change Support Systsm (BCSS). Tynne offered weekly modules that were drawn from Acceptance and Commitment Therapy (ACT). From an Information system's perspective, the modules were identified and applied as a persuasive software feature that is promoted by the Persuasive Systems Design Model (PSD Model). The duration of the Web-based intervention was 6 weeks. Upon completion of the intervention, about one third (37.2%) of the participants reported that they could better manage their sleep problems. We argue that a relatively low percentage is still highly encouraging, as treatment of sleep-related disorders is a complicated and understudied area. Manifestly, longitudinal studies would help determine the effect of ACT-incorporated Web-based interventions. However, the chapter underscores the effect of persuasive software features incorporated with ACT-based components as a step towards managing sleep disorders.

Chapter 4
From Science to Practice: Implementation and Clinical Guidelines for an Internet Intervention for Postpartum Depression...79
Filip Drozd, National Network for Infant Mental Health, Norway
Silje Marie Haga, National Network of Infant Mental Health, Norway
Kari Slinning, National Network for Infant Mental Health, Norway

This chapter provides a practical hands-on blueprint needed to design and plan the implementation of internet interventions, addressing all the important aspects of the implementation process. The guidelines are based on the active implementation framework by Fixsen and colleagues (2005) and provide readers with a case example of an internet intervention in Norwegian primary care. They describe the "how-to" of implementation from presenting the background of the intervention, the theory behind implementation, actual implementation planning, evaluation, and clinical work. This serves to give stakeholders a common framework for understanding the requirements for implementing an intervention in practice, the activities and resources needed, and may guide an organization through the implementation process. The case example also shows that implementation and clinical guidelines are mutually affected by each other, and should be developed and viewed together.

Chapter 5
EHealth Interventions for People Suffering From Sleep Problems and Depressive Symptoms: Qualitative Findings and Future Research Directions...111
Sitwat Usman Langrial, Sur University College, Oman
Päivi Lappalainen, University of Jyväskylä, Finland

This chapter highlights qualitative findings from two field studies that focused on supporting people with sleeplessness (Study 1) and moderate depression (Study II). Both the studies were designed to examine the prospective impact of reminders and rehearsal on the effectiveness of web- based eHealth interventions. The interventions were incorporated with Acceptance and Commitment Therapy. In this chapter, qualitative findings are reported with an aim to highlight issues that are at times overlooked. Further, the findings are expected to help researchers better understand eHealth interventions for mental health care. Results from the two studies uncover interesting contrasts. While the participants of the Study I (Sleeplessness) generally did not find reminders to be helpful, on the contrary, the participants of study II (Moderate Depression) largely approved reminders especially in terms of task completion. In terms of rehearsal, participants from both the studies approved the virtual exercises in terms of learning desirable self-help behaviors. Finally, the chapter highlights some of the grey areas in the field of eHealth interventions for mental health care. The identified grey areas are expected to create opportunities for further research and advances in the field of mental health care.

Chapter 6
An Internet-Based Quantum Biofeedback and Neurotechnology Cybertherapy System for the Support of Transpersonal Psychology 139
Raul Valverde, Concordia University, Canada

Transpersonal psychology is the study of human nature and proceeds on the assumption that human beings possess potentials that exceed the limits of their ego and integrate the spiritual experience within a broader understanding of the human psyche and consciousness. Altered states of consciousness have been used as psychotherapy in transpersonal psychology for decades. A Cyberpsychotherapy system is proposed to support transpersonal psychotherapy. The system can be used to induce non-ordinary state of consciousness that can be used by transpersonal psychologists as a healing tool to cure his patients with psychological problems such as psychosis at a distance location with the help of Internet technologies. The Cyberpsychotherapy system uses quantum signal generator for the induction of altered states of consciousness based on the God's helmet of Persinger (1983). The Cyberpsychotherapy has integrated an EEG that serves as a biofeedback device in order to assess if the patient has reached the desired level of consciousness and can be used it to adjust the frequencies of the signal generator in order to improve the psychotherapy experience of the patient if necessary. A sample of 10 patients was used to test the Cybertherapy system based on Neurotechnology and quantum biofeedback, data was collected and analyzed. Although the results show that the patients were not able to reach the desired level of consciousness for the psychotherapy, there is statistical significant evidence that the proposed system can help to raise the level of consciousness; this can help with future designs that will eventually assist to reach the desired level for the psychotherapy.

Chapter 7
Neurotechnology in the Development of Cyber-Psychotherapy Systems for Inducing and Measuring Altered States of Consciousness in Transpersonal Psychotherapy 185
Raul Valverde, Concordia University, USA

Transpersonal psychotherapy is based on transpersonal psychology and considers that the psyche is multidimensional and that there are several "levels of consciousness" and each has different characteristics and is governed by different laws. Transpersonal psychology is the study of human nature and proceeds on the assumption that human beings possess potentials that exceed the limits of their ego and integrate the spiritual experience within a broader understanding of the human psyche and consciousness. Altered states of consciousness have been used as psychotherapy in transpersonal psychology for decades. Although there are very well known techniques to induce altered state of consciousness as holotropic breathwork, Neurotechnology offers an alternative way not only to induce these states for transpersonal therapy but also to measure the level of a state of consciousness. The objective of this chapter is to provide a review of the main concepts of Neurotechnology and the main technologies that can be used to induce and measure altered state of consciousness for transpersonal psychotherapy and propose an architecture for a Cyber psychotherapy system that uses these technologies.

Chapter 8
The Development of Ethical Guidelines for Online Counselling and Psychotherapy 212
Stephen Goss, Metanoia Institute, UK
Kate Elizabeth Anthony, Online Therapy Institute, UK

The history and development of guidelines on the ethics of providing online counselling and guidance are considered. Some issues the authors have found to be of particular importance are highlighted with reference to particular publications as exemplars of the ongoing development of ethical practice in this field. Changes in ethical guidelines produced by the British Association for Counselling and Psychotherapy (BACP) are examined to elucidate the evolution in ethical thinking and practice that has been necessitated by the continual rapid development of technological applications relevant to mental health care that have typified the field and led to the current approach which defines competencies required. The article ends with a look to the advent of web 2.0 philosophies and the need for practitioners to remain constantly vigilant with regard to their work.

Chapter 9
Revisiting the Issue of Trust in E-Health..241
Elizabeth Sillence, Northumbria University, UK
Pam Briggs, Northumbria University, UK
Peter R. Harris, University of Sussex, UK

As people continue to go online for their health information needs we revisit the issue of trust in relation to e-health. This chapter begins by briefly presenting an overview of e-health and describing current ways in which people are using the Internet for health advice and information. Models of trust are revisited and we then explore two emerging areas within the e-health field: peer resources and mobile health applications. Finally, we revisit and update our guidelines and point to further sources of information in this field.

Compilation of References 260

About the Contributors 304

Index 308

Preface

Mental health disorders are conditions that negatively affect individuals' approach towards life and cognitive abilities. These conditions may reduce people's capacities to relate with others and accomplish everyday errands. While people suffering from mental disorders are generally diagnosed with the similar conditions, yet, their individual experiences often differ. One in five adults experience a mental health condition each year. One in seventeen people suffer from serious mental illnesses such as schizophrenia or bipolar disorder. Mental disorders not only distress the patients but also at the same time affect families, friends and communities at large[1]. A greater number of populations are experiencing mental disabilities. These disabilities or disorders range from psychological health to physical impairment resulting in poor life quality, low self-esteem, seclusion and social stigma.

There is a range of mental disorders that include but are not limited to Anxiety, Stress, Autism, Bipolar Disorder, Borderline Personality Disorder, Depressive Thoughts, Depression, Psychosis, Schizophrenia, Obsessive-compulsive Disorder, Posttraumatic Stress Disorder and Insomnia. It has been frequently emphasized that mortality rates among people suffering from mental disorders is on the rise. Several studies on the global burden of disease demonstrate that there is a mounting problem of mental disorders (Walker et al. 2015). While there is a debate about the relationship between mental disorders and consequent deaths, it is generally believed that mental conditions are contributing factors to, for example, heart diseases, stigma and suicides (Whiteford et al., 2010). Yet another perplexing and problematic issue is the positive correlation between mental disorders and higher rates of adverse health behaviors such as substance abuse, lack of physical activity, social isolation, restlessness and unhealthy or poor diet. As a consequence of these adverse health behaviors, chronic health conditions are more commonly found in people with mental disorders (Laursen et al., 2014).

Over the past decade, technology-mediated eHealth interventions have shown promising results that highlight the potential role of Information Technology as a platform to deliver cost effective and innovative interventions for people suffering from different mental conditions and disorders. It is the need of the hour that we abstract and implement proactive and innovative eHealth interventions that can support people with cognitive disabilities. Technology-based interventions grounded on latest psychological expertise are an achievable solution that target people suffering from mental disorders. Use of the Internet and pervasive computing technologies can help us reach a large number of users and provide them with innovative eHealth interventions. Moreover, use of computing technologies ensures continuous access to such interventions. These interventions can be used and applied at individual or group level.

Available research suggests that Internet-based psychological interventions are effective, and generally well accepted (Lappalainen et al., 2015; Langrial et al., 2014; Mohr et al., 2011; Strecher, 2008). Despite the fact that several eHealth interventions have been developed and examined for mental disorders, the results indicate that these interventions have somewhat similar outcomes when compared with more traditional face-to-face therapies (Andersson & Titov, 2014). Other challenges in the area of eHealth intervention include lack of clarity, lack of consistency and a unified understanding on the part of system developers as well as eHealth researchers (Barak et al. 2009). In recent years, most of the studies in the area of mental health care have focused on issues related with task adherence (Kelders et al., 2012), high dropout rates, perceived benefits (Drozd et al., 2012) and persuasiveness of eHealth interventions. Further, the overlap in terminologies as well as vague descriptions (Langrial et al., 2012) have caused the field to become rather diffused and unnecessarily over-complicated. Yet another issue in the area of mental health care is extra focuses on technological aspects while designing the interventions and somewhat overlooking the significance of psychological content.

Psychological eHealth interventions for mental health care are a relatively new area of research that builds on doctrines and substantiations founded by technology-mediated solutions (Marks et al., 2007). Literature provides convincing evidence that eHealth interventions are an effective tool for guided as well as self-help therapies. Self-help therapies have shown the potential of being effective in reducing mental health issues (Cuijpers, 1997). Technology-delivered eHealth interventions may be more effective when compared with traditional therapies as they offer cost effective alternatives especially for a high majority of people with mental conditions (an estimated 65%) that do not receive professional mental health care services (Andrews et al. 2002). Currently available self-help therapies are generally disorder-specific such as depression, panic disorder, anxiety, posttraumatic disorder and insomnia. These therapies are mostly grounded on Cognitive Behavioral Therapy (CBT). CBT- based interventions help people identify their problems and offer methods to regain control over them. Both face-to-face and web- based therapies have shown decent effect in dealing with depression and other mental health problems (van Straten et al., 2008).

Emerging technologies, advances in Information and Communication Technologies and ever-growing acceptance and adoption of eHealth interventions for mental health care create several opportunities but at the same time pose a number of challenges for maintaining good health care practice. For one instance, there is lack of knowledge about tailored eHealth interventions and services targeting individual needs. Similarly, the effectiveness of Web-based eHealth interventions promoting mental health highlight mixed outcomes. It is critical that eHealth solutions promoting mental health are adapted according to the needs of the patients. eHealth interventions offer varying solutions for mental health care for achieving and sustaining mental well-being and improved quality of life. Such interventions are designed for people with a range of mental disorders and largely speaking, the interventions are incorporated with carefully selected software. While some eHealth interventions are designed and evaluated to assist people in overcoming a specific mental condition, others are designed for more of a prolonged interaction embedded with a fusion of therapeutic elements and technologies.

The aim of the current interdisciplinary book is to collect individual data of emotional, psychophysiological and subjective responses from Web-based eHealth interventions for improving mental disorders, and to enhance knowledge base that would help develop individually effective eHealth interventions for people suffering from mental health conditions. The book aims to introduce new approaches for understanding, designing and creating innovative eHealth interventions for mental disorders.

THE CHALLENGES

It goes without saying that, Internet-based eHealth interventions for mental health care are plagued with challenges such as poor implementation of persuasive techniques (Baumel et al., 2017), high dropout rates (Thabrew et al., 2017), high rates of attrition (Andersson & Cuijpers, 2009; Eysenbach, 2005), vague description of measured effects (Ritterband et al., 2009), lack of trust (Vedder et al., 2014) and relatively short periods of interventions (Langrial et al., 2014). Any attempt to overcome the said challenges calls for an adequate understanding of the highlighted issues. It becomes ever so important to overcome the challenges as Web-based eHealth interventions have become a focal point in the research area of health psychology (Kraft & Yardley, 2009). Such challenges can be categorized as follows:

- The challenge of appropriate selection and implementation of persuasive software features while designing eHealth interventions for mental health.

- The challenge of finding out core reasons behind high dropout rates in Internet- based interventions for health and general well-being.
- The challenge of finding the causes behind high rates of attrition.
- The challenge of measuring the actual effect of a given intervention on the mental well being of patients.
- The challenge of designing longitudinal studies to examine the effect of eHealth interventions.
- The challenge of establishing security and privacy policies and procedures that help develop Soft Trust in eHealth interventions.

ORGANIZATION OF THE BOOK

The book is organized into nine chapters. A brief description of the chapters is given below:

Chapter 1 underlines the important viewpoints on mental health, mental illness, and technology utilization; mental health education and mental health nursing; the overview of Cognitive Behavioral Therapy (CBT); CBT, depression, anxiety, and insomnia; CBT and Obsessive- Compulsive Disorder (OCD); and CBT and heart failure. The chapter highlights the significance of mental health and its positive impact of an individual's inability to have healthy relationships; make good life choices; maintain physical health and well-being; handle the natural ups and downs of life; and grow toward individuals' potential.

Chapter 2 reviews qualitative research on user experiences (UX) with internet interventions for depression and present original results from in- depth interviews from a preventive unguided intervention for postpartum depression. The first part reviews the literature on qualitative studies of client experiences and perceptions of internet interventions for depression. The next part describes original data from a study investigating participants' experiences using semi-structured interviews, following the modified SWOT-format (i.e., Strengths, Weakness, Opportunities, and Threats). The chapter provides valuable information for clinicians, researchers, and other health professionals interested in the applicability of internet interventions for their clients, design of future studies, and development of Internet interventions.

Chapter 3 highlights findings from a field study that was conducted to evaluate influence of selected persuasive software features on a Web-based intervention for sleep deprivation. The Web-based intervention named *Tynne* in Finnish language can also be categorized as a Behavior Change Support System (BCSS). Tynne offered weekly modules that were drawn from Acceptance and Commitment Therapy (ACT). From the Information Systems' perspectives, the modules were identified and applied as a persuasive software feature that is promoted by the Persuasive

Systems Design Model (PSD Model) proposed by Oinas-Kukkonen and Harjumaa (2009). The duration of the Web-based intervention was 6 weeks. Upon completion of the intervention, about one third (37.2%) of the participants reported that they could better manage their sleep disorder. We argue that a relatively low percentage is still highly encouraging as treatment of sleep-related disorders is a complicated and understudied phenomenon. Manifestly, longitudinal studies would help determine the effect of ACT-incorporated Web-based interventions. However, the chapter underscores the prospective influence of persuasive software features incorporated with Acceptance and Commitment Therapy components as a step towards managing chronic sleep disorders.

Chapter 4 provides a practical hands-on blueprint needed to design and plan the implementation of internet interventions, addressing all the important aspects of the implementation process. The chapter discusses an implementation framework proposed by Fixen et al. (2005) and discusses a case example of an Internet-based intervention in Norwegian primary care. It describes the 'how-to' of implementation from presenting the background of the intervention, the theory behind implementation, actual implementation planning, evaluation, and clinical work. The chapter aims to serve stakeholders with a common framework for understanding the requirements for implementing an intervention in practice, the activities and resources needed, and may guide an organization through the implementation process.

Chapter 5 highlights qualitative findings from two field studies that focused on supporting people with sleeplessness and moderate depression. Both studies were designed to examine the prospective impact of reminders and rehearsal on the effectiveness of web- based eHealth interventions. The interventions were incorporated with Acceptance and Commitment Therapy (ACT). In this chapter, qualitative findings are reported with an aim to highlight issues that are at times overlooked. The findings are expected to help researchers better understand eHealth interventions for mental health care. Finally, the chapter highlights some of the grey areas in the field of eHealth interventions for mental health care. The identified grey areas are expected to create opportunities for further research and advances in the field of mental health care.

Chapter 6 introduces transpersonal psychology as the study of human nature and proceeds on the assumption that human beings possess potentials that exceed the limits of their ego and integrate the spiritual experience within a broader understanding of the human psyche and consciousness. Altered states of consciousness have been used as psychotherapy in transpersonal psychology for decades. The chapter proposes a Cyberpsychotherapy system to support transpersonal psychotherapy. The system can be used to induce non-ordinary state of consciousness that can be used by transpersonal psychologists as a healing tool to cure his patients with psychological problems such as psychosis at a distance location with the help of Internet technologies. The

Cyberpsychotherapy system is integrated an EEG that serves as a biofeedback device in order to assess if the patient has reached the desired level of consciousness and can be used it to adjust the frequencies of the signal generator in order to improve the psychotherapy experience of the patient if necessary.

Chapter 7 reviews transpersonal psychology and considers that psyche is multidimensional and that there are several "levels of consciousness" and each has different characteristics and is governed by different laws. Transpersonal psychology is the study of human nature and proceeds on the assumption that human beings possess potentials that exceed the limits of their ego and integrate the spiritual experience within a broader understanding of the human psyche and consciousness. The chapter highlights some of the main concepts of Neuro-technology and technologies that can be used to induce and measure altered state of consciousness for transpersonal psychotherapy and propose architecture for a cyber-psychotherapy system that uses these technologies.

Chapter 8 highlights the history and development of guidelines on the ethics of providing online counseling and guidance is considered. Some issues the authors have found to be of particular importance are highlighted with reference to particular publications as exemplars of the on-going development of ethical practice in this field. Changes in ethical guidelines produced by the British Association for Counseling and Psychotherapy (BACP) are examined to elucidate the evolution in ethical thinking and practice that has been necessitated by the continual rapid development of technological applications relevant to mental health care that have typified the field and led to the current approach which defines competencies required. The article ends with a look to the advent of web 2.0 philosophies and the need for practitioners to remain constantly vigilant with regard to their work. The chapter concludes with a look to the advent of web 2.0 philosophies and the need for practitioners to remain constantly vigilant with regard to their work.

Chapter 9 addresses the issue of trust in relation to e-health. It begins by briefly presenting an overview of e-health and describing current ways in which people are using the Internet for health advice and information. Models of trust are revisited and we then explore two emerging areas within the e-health field: peer resources and mobile health applications. Finally, the chapter revisits and updates guidelines and point to further sources of information in this field.

This book is intended for healthcare professionals, healthcare educators, researchers, system designers, clinical psychologists and anyone who is interested in learning about Web-Based Behavioral Therapies for mental disorders. We hope that this book will create opportunities for further research in the area of mental health care where both researchers and practitioners will be able to design effective interventions.

Finally, we would like to thank all the authors for their valuable contribution. We would extend our gratitude for all the reviewers (who preferred to remain anonymous) for their effort in reviewing and giving constructive feedback.

Sitwat Usman Langrial
Sur University College, Oman

REFERENCES

Andersson, G., & Cuijpers, P. (2009). Internet-based and other computerized psychological treatments for adult depression: A meta-analysis. *Cognitive Behaviour Therapy*, *38*(4), 196–205. doi:10.1080/16506070903318960 PMID:20183695

Andersson, G., & Titov, N. (2014). Advantages and limitations of Internet-based interventions for common mental disorders. *World Psychiatry; Official Journal of the World Psychiatric Association (WPA)*, *13*(1), 4–11. doi:10.1002/wps.20083 PMID:24497236

Andrews, G., Henderson, S., & Hall, W. (2002). Prevalence, comorbidity, disability and service utilisation: Overview of the Australian National Mental Health Survey. *Yearbook of Psychiatry and Applied Mental Health, 2002*(1), 230-231.

Baumel, A., Faber, K., Mathur, N., Kane, J. M., & Muench, F. (2017). Enlight: A Comprehensive Quality and Therapeutic Potential Evaluation Tool for Mobile and Web-Based eHealth Interventions. *Journal of Medical Internet Research*, *19*(3), e82. doi:10.2196/jmir.7270 PMID:28325712

Cuijpers, P. (1997, June). Bibliotherapy in unipolar depression: A meta-analysis. *Journal of Behavior Therapy and Experimental Psychiatry*, *28*(2), 139–147. doi:10.1016/S0005-7916(97)00005-0 PMID:9194011

Eysenbach, G. (2005). The law of attrition. *Journal of Medical Internet Research*, *7*(1), e11. doi:10.2196/jmir.7.1.e11 PMID:15829473

Fixsen, D. L., Naoom, S. F., Blase, K. A., Friedman, R. M., & Wallace, F. (2005). *Implementation research: A synthesis of the literature*. Tampa, FL: National Implementation Research Network, University of Florida.

Kraft, P., & Yardley, L. (2009). Current issues and new directions in Psychology and Health: What is the future of digital interventions for health behaviour change?

Langrial, S., Oinas-Kukkonen, H., Lappalainen, P., & Lappalainen, R. (2014, May). Managing depression through a behavior change support system without face-to-face therapy. *Proceedings of the International Conference on Persuasive Technology* (pp. 155-166). Springer International Publishing.

Lappalainen, P., Langrial, S., Oinas-Kukkonen, H., Tolvanen, A., & Lappalainen, R. (2015). Web-based acceptance and commitment therapy for depressive symptoms with minimal support: A randomized controlled trial. *Behavior Modification, 39*(6), 805–834. doi:10.1177/0145445515598142 PMID:26253644

Laursen, T. M., Nordentoft, M., & Mortensen, P. B. (2014). Excess early mortality in schizophrenia. *Annual Review of Clinical Psychology, 10*(1), 425–448. doi:10.1146/annurev-clinpsy-032813-153657 PMID:24313570

Marks, I. M., Cavanagh, K., & Gega, L. (2007). *Hands-on help: Computer-aided psychotherapy*. Psychology Press.

Mohr, D., Cuijpers, P., & Lehman, K. (2011). Supportive accountability: A model for providing human support to enhance adherence to eHealth interventions. *Journal of Medical Internet Research, 13*(1), e30. doi:10.2196/jmir.1602 PMID:21393123

Ritterband, L. M., Thorndike, F. P., Gonder-Frederick, L. A., Magee, J. C., Bailey, E. T., Saylor, D. K., & Morin, C. M. (2009). Efficacy of an Internet-based behavioral intervention for adults with insomnia. *Archives of General Psychiatry, 66*(7), 692–698. doi:10.1001/archgenpsychiatry.2009.66 PMID:19581560

Strecher, V. (2007). Internet methods for delivering behavioral and health-related interventions (eHealth). *Annual Review of Clinical Psychology, 3*(1), 53–76. doi:10.1146/annurev.clinpsy.3.022806.091428 PMID:17716048

Thabrew, H., Stasiak, K., Hetrick, S. E., Wong, S., Huss, J. H., & Merry, S. N. (2017). eHealth interventions for anxiety and depression in children and adolescents with long-term physical conditions. *The Cochrane Library*.

Vedder, A., Cuijpers, C., Vantsiouri, P., & Ferrari, M. Z. (2014). The law as a 'catalyst and facilitatorfor trust in e-health: Challenges and opportunities. *Law. Innovation and Technology, 6*(2), 305–325. doi:10.5235/17579961.6.2.305

Walker, E. R., McGee, R. E., & Druss, B. G. (2015). Mortality in mental disorders and global disease burden implications: A systematic review and meta-analysis. *JAMA Psychiatry, 72*(4), 334–341. doi:10.1001/jamapsychiatry.2014.2502 PMID:25671328

Whiteford, H. A., Degenhardt, L., Rehm, J., Baxter, A. J., Ferrari, A. J., Erskine, H. E., & Vos, T. et al. (2013). Global burden of disease attributable to mental and substance use disorders: Findings from the Global Burden of Disease Study 2010. *Lancet*, *382*(9904), 1575–1586. doi:10.1016/S0140-6736(13)61611-6 PMID:23993280

ENDNOTE

1 http://www.nami.org/Learn-More/Mental-Health-Conditions

Chapter 1
Mental Health and Cognitive Behavioral Therapy:
Advanced Issues and Approaches

Kijpokin Kasemsap
Suan Sunandha Rajabhat University, Thailand

ABSTRACT

This chapter reveals the important perspectives on mental health, mental illness, and technology utilization; mental health education and mental health nursing; the overview of Cognitive Behavioral Therapy (CBT); CBT, depression, anxiety, and insomnia; CBT and Obsessive-Compulsive Disorder (OCD); and CBT and heart failure. Mental health strengthens the individuals' ability to have healthy relationships; make good life choices; maintain physical health and well-being; handle the natural ups and downs of life; and grow toward individuals' potential. Mental health is associated with higher productivity, better performance, more consistent work attendance, and fewer workplace accidents. CBT is a goal-oriented psychotherapy treatment that takes a practical approach to problem-solving skills. CBT involves recognizing the unhelpful or destructive patterns of thinking and reacting, thus modifying or replacing these patterns with more realistic or helpful ones.

INTRODUCTION

The severity and high levels of disability associated with mental illness have led to the increased global efforts to address the mental health problems, in particular those targeted at prevention (Martin & McKay, 2014). Health problems often track from youth to adulthood, indicating the requirement to effectively understand the overall

DOI: 10.4018/978-1-5225-3241-5.ch001

health of young people with mental illness (McCloughen, Foster, Huws-Thomas, & Delgado, 2012). The emerging mental illness increases the existing stress and contradicts the expectations of this stage, as many young adults encounter physical and emotional weakness for the first time and divert from intended plans (Cameron, 2014). As health information becomes available through the Internet and the Web 2.0, mental health professionals are able to develop the strategic plans for taking care of their patients (Prasad, 2017).

With the advent of the Internet and the Web 2.0, mental health services have led to an increase in the presentation and care of mental health patients in generalist health settings (Brunero, Jeon, & Foster, 2012). There is an abundance of research available about the utilization of information and communication technology (ICT) in mental health (Namle, Ghapanchi, & Amrollahi, 2016). The rapid application of technology offers the potentially innovative approaches to promoting mental health among young people, addressing a significant public health challenge (Burns, Blanchard, & Metcalf, 2013). Technology designed specifically for health has proved useful as a complementary form of providing the mental health services (Marks & Bowers, 2015). Mental health patients need to be able to reintegrate in the community to achieve the full normality (Cooper, 2010).

The advances in modern technology have created a diverse field of applications for the care of people with cognitive impairment (Georgakopoulos, Chatzidimitriou, & Tsolaki, 2015). The web-based CBT has several benefits compared to the face-to-face treatment, including high treatment reliability, increased convenience, reduced cost, and scalability (Newby, Twomey, Li, & Andrews, 2016). CBT is a relatively efficacious intervention for a range of psychological disorders when delivered in the well-controlled research trials (Levita, Duhne, Girling, & Waller, 2016) and refers to a collection of therapeutic techniques and strategies that are used to alter behavior by teaching individuals to actively participate in understanding their own thoughts and behaviors (Cajanding, 2016).

This chapter is based on a literature review of mental health and CBT. The extensive literature of mental health and CBT provides a contribution to practitioners and researchers by revealing the advanced issues and approaches of mental health and CBT in the health care industry.

Background

Research into mental health has resulted in a wide range of information and publications covering different aspects of mental health and addressing a variety of problems (Hadzic & Dillon, 2010). In the health care industry, the contemporary models of mental health care emphasize the importance of multidisciplinary approaches in supporting the recovery for individuals (Rosenberg & McDermott, 2016). There is an important relationship between physical activity and mental health (Happell, Platania-Phung, & Scott, 2011). It is essential to have a fundamental shift in the context of the provider–service user relationship to effectively facilitate service users' engagement in their mental health care (Newman, O'Reilly, Lee, & Kennedy, 2015).

Mental health is the successful performance of mental function that results in productive activities, fulfilling relationships, the ability to adapt to change, and the ability to cope with adversity (Matthews, Doherty, Coyle, & Sharry, 2008). Mental health issues often become obvious as adolescents emerge into young adulthood (Albritton, Angley, Gibson, Sipsma, & Kershaw, 2015). Mental health promotion is concerned with achieving the positive mental health and well-being in the general population as well as addressing the needs of those at risk from mental health problems (Wand, 2011). The number of children experiencing mental health issues is underreported, as children, especially younger ones, are often below the threshold for diagnosis because they do not yet meet the criteria (Graham, Killoran, & Parekh, 2016).

CBT is an integration of two theories that were separately born to respond to psychological disorders (i.e., behavioral theory and cognitive theory) (Selene, Omar, & Silvia, 2016). Behavioral theory in its strictest form, focuses only on observable and measurable behavior and ignores all mental events. Cognitive therapy focuses on the role they play and how these cognitions determine feelings and behaviors (Ledley, Marx, & Heimberg, 2010). That is why cognitive behavioral approach aims to understand all knowledge, skills, and psychological techniques that are able to solve all those psychological complications that arise in the course and treatment of the disease.

CBT is based on the premise that since cognitions can be intentionally modified through a process called cognitive restructuring, it is possible to transform the negative and irrational thinking into the rational and balanced thoughts (Deacon, Fawzy, Lickel, & Wolitzky-Taylor, 2011) toward leading to more productive behaviors, healthy emotional responses, more positive appraisals, and the relief of feelings of anxiety and depression (Dimidjian & Davis, 2009). CBT intends to encourage thinking focused on positivism and hope in how patients perceive their disease process until the end of their lives (Selene et al., 2016).

ASPECTS OF MENTAL HEALTH AND COGNITIVE BEHAVIORAL THERAPY

This section provides the important perspectives on mental health, mental illness, and technology utilization; mental health education and mental health nursing; the overview of CBT; CBT, depression, anxiety, and insomnia; CBT and OCD; and CBT and heart failure.

Important Perspectives on Mental Health, Mental Illness, and Technology Utilization

Mental health is one of the leading causes of morbidity worldwide (Fleury et al., 2012). Mental health services for children and adolescents in low-income and middle-income countries are extremely scarce and greatly limit access to the appropriate mental health care (Morris et al., 2011). In recent years, policymakers in high-income countries have placed an increasing concern on the value of maintaining good mental health toward improving the quality of life (McDaid, Knapp, & Raja, 2008). In practice, people managing mental health difficulties struggle to improve their quality of life (Kidd, Kenny, & McKinstry, 2015). Medications lessen or attempt to control the symptoms of mental illness (Bathory, 2015).

In the Western world, there is an increasing concern regarding the ability of health care professionals to meet the physical health care needs of those diagnosed with mental illness (Walker & McAndrew, 2015). Supporting both mental health and well-being is an important aspect of primary care (McKinlay et al., 2011). Public mental health deals with the promotion of mental health, the prevention of mental disorders, the reduction of mental health inequalities, and the organization of mental health service provision (Wahlbeck, 2015). Public mental health efforts are needed to raise caregiver mental health literacy in health care settings (Mendenhall & Frauenholtz, 2015).

Adolescence is the period of highest risk for the development of mental illness (Plaistow et al., 2014). The relationship between childhood maltreatment and adolescent aggression is well-documented (Hoeve et al., 2015). People with serious mental ill health suffer the excessive physical illness (Collins, Tranter, & Irvine, 2012) and have increased the rates of physical ill-health and reduced the contact with primary care services (Happell, Platania-Phung, & Scott, 2013). They often prematurely die from the common physical illnesses, such as cardiovascular disease and diabetes (Happell, Scott, & Platania-Phung, 2013).

Mental intelligence of an individual is important to all humans (Hashim, Kaur, Bahar, & Ismail, 2016). People with intellectual disability (ID) experience higher rates of major mental disorders than their non-ID peers, but in many countries have difficulty accessing the appropriate mental health services (Evans et al., 2012). A positive relationship between the mental health consultant (MHC) and early care and education staff is important for achieving the positive early childhood mental health consultation outcomes (Allen & Green, 2012). Infant and early childhood mental health consultation has emerged as one of the most effective strategies for supporting young children's socioemotional development (DeNatale, 2013). Mental health consultation can increase individuals' competence in specific areas related to children's socioemotional development (Heller et al., 2011).

The Internet allows mental health organizations to provide the mental health services to more people through the new models of care (Calvo et al., 2016). The rapid growth of information technology (IT), such as the Internet, smartphones, and videoconferencing, has improved the access to mindfulness therapies, which focus on enhancing individual's awareness of the present moment toward improving mental health (Krolikowski, 2013). Mobile tracking is the latest burgeoning area in the field of technology in mental health care with mobile apps, SMS protocols, and new devices used to track mood and behavior in order to improve both mental health and well-being (Kauer & Reid, 2015).

Mental Health Education and Mental Health Nursing

Education is an important approach to attracting students to the field of mental health nursing (Happell et al., 2014). Professional education and policy strategies increasingly emphasize the need for service users to be involved in the education of all nursing students, including students undertaking mental health field programs (O'Donnell & Gormley, 2013). The educational preparation of mental health nursing students in higher education must address the philosophical, conceptual, social and ethical dimensions of contemporary mental health care practice (McKie & Naysmith, 2014).

Collaboration between school-based and community-employed professionals is critical to the success of school mental health (SMH) programs (Weist et al., 2012). However, the changes to the educational preparation of the nursing workforce in mental health continue to have the profound effects on the availability of sufficient numbers of skilled graduates willing to work in this field (Happell & McAllister, 2014). Nurses working in mental health settings are placed to provide the exercise advice for people with mental illness (Stanton, Reaburn, & Happell, 2015). Accessing mental health services is a critical step toward reducing the burden of mental illness (Dardas & Simmons, 2015).

The nursing profession must have a responsibility to the global community to ensure that registered nurses are educated to meet the health challenges and the needs of the health consumer in the 21st century (Wynaden, 2010). Hamdan-Mansour et al. (2011) stated that the changes in mental health services have an impact on the practice of mental health nurses. Clinical placements in mental health are the significant preparation for undergraduate students to maximize the improvement in the positive attitudes to the care of people diagnosed with a mental illness and to mental health nursing (Happell & Platania-Phung, 2012).

Mental health nurses have a significant role in improving the physical health of people with a serious mental illness (Robson, Haddad, Gray, & Gournay, 2013). An approach focusing on reducing underinsurance for all mental health services among rural residents may help reduce the unmet mental health needs among the rural residents privately insured (Ziller, Anderson, & Coburn, 2010). Rural nurses represent the skilled mental health toward helping the capital in their local communities and providing the early mental health services in the rural communities (Wilson & Usher, 2015).

School nurses play a critical role in the provision of mental health services in the school environment and are the significant members of the coordinated student mental health team (Bohnenkamp, Stephan, & Bobo, 2015). Mental health nurses have the potential to make a significant contribution to enhancing the access to mental health care through the flexible and innovative approaches (Happell, Palmer, & Tennent, 2010). Mental health nurses who are older, have more clinical experiences in mental health care, and demonstrate the greater empathy expressed more positive attitudes toward people with mental illness (Hsiao, Lu, & Tsai, 2015).

Negative attitudes of mental health professionals have been identified as a major barrier to achieving the effective mental health service delivery (Byrne, Happell, Welch, & Moxham, 2013). Through recovery-focused support aimed at avoiding deteriorating physical health, mental health nurses can significantly contribute to improving the current rate of premature death experienced by people with enduring mental illness (Hardy & Thomas, 2012).

Overview of Cognitive Behavioral Therapy

Cognitive behavioral therapy (CBT) is a type of psychotherapy that helps individuals identify and teaches skills to modify the unhelpful thinking patterns, feelings, and behaviors (Eapen & Walter, 2016). CBT interventions include many behavioral interventions and incorporate various cognitive strategies toward identifying, challenging, and altering the counterproductive thoughts (Cassin et al., 2016). The individuals' cognitive processes play an essential role in the development and maintenance of their emotional and behavioral responses to them (González-Prendes & Resko, 2012). Freedland et al. (2015) indicated that CBT is effective in improving mood and reducing anxiety.

Research on process factors in psychotherapy can be divided into two perspectives: one emphasizing specific and unique factors for the specific treatment orientation, and other emphasizing trans-theoretical mechanisms, frequently termed common factors (Messer & Wampold, 2002). Researchers emphasizing the specific factors in the treatment hypothesize that the therapist's adherence to and competence in delivering treatment in accordance with the specified theoretical and technical model are important in explaining psychotherapy outcomes (Haug et al., 2016). Higher therapist competence is related to the better treatment outcomes in the CBT of depression (Kuyken & Tsivrikos, 2009).

CBT can improve the outcomes for youths with chronic pain in research trials (Kashikar-Zuck et al., 2012) and in clinical settings (Lynch-Jordan et al., 2014). CBT is of importance in the pediatric chronic pain populations given the potential risks and side effects of pharmacotherapy for pain (Cunningham et al., 2016). CBT for chronic pain typically utilized the combination of cognitive strategies (e.g., distraction, thought modification, and problem solving) and behavioral approaches (e.g., activity pacing and relaxation training) to improve the functioning and reduce the pain symptoms in youths.

Cognitive Behavioral Therapy, Depression, Anxiety, and Insomnia

CBT is viewed as the first-line treatment for both depression and anxiety disorders, as a stand-alone intervention for the mild-to-moderate cases, or in combination with pharmacological treatments for more complex cases and those with comorbidities. Depression and anxiety disorders represent two of the top five leading causes of disability worldwide and have high comorbidity rates, share many similar symptoms, features, latent structure, and vulnerability factors (Goldberg, Krueger, Andrews, & Hobbs, 2009). Tully et al. (2014) suggested that CBT may have the significant impact on alleviating the cognitive symptoms among HF patients with a depressive comorbidity.

Understanding the nature of the anxiety facets that are relevant to the delivery of CBT elements is important for two primary reasons: the identification of clinicians who will need the additional support to deliver the specific elements of the therapy and the planning of interventions to support those clinicians (Farrell, Deacon, Dixon, & Lickel, 2013). The therapist competence/adherence and the working alliance have contributions to the outcome from CBT for anxiety disorders (Haug et al., 2016).

Insomnia is a common clinical condition with an annual prevalence of 10-20 percent (Buysse, 2013) and approximately 6 percent with a chronic trajectory, such as persisting for more than 3 months (Ohayon, 2002). Chronic insomnia is associated with a number of negative health outcomes (e.g., obesity and metabolic dysregulation) and increases the risk of myocardial infarction (Palagini et al., 2013), susceptibility to infections (Patel et al., 2012), and depression (Staner, 2010). Sleep-specific CBT appears to be efficacious and feasible in treating posttraumatic stress disorder (PTSD) symptoms (Ho, Chan, & Tang, 2016).

Cognitive behavioral therapy for insomnia (CBT-I) has been found efficacious in improving sleep outcomes (Okajima, Komada, & Inoue, 2011) with acute effects comparable or superior to those found for pharmacotherapy (Smith et al., 2002) and these effects have been maintained for up to 3 years. While CBT-I is desired by many patients preferring non-pharmacological approaches (Espie, Barrie, &

Forgan, 2012), the challenge remains to make it accessible to meet population needs regarding the limited availability of trained therapists (Perils & Smith, 2008). The web-based CBT-I can improve insomnia severity, sleep efficiency, subjective sleep quality, wake after sleep onset, sleep onset latency, and total sleep time (Zachariae, Lyby, Ritterband, & O'Toole, 2016).

Cognitive Behavioral Therapy and Obsessive-Compulsive Disorder

Obsessive-compulsive disorder (OCD) is the highly debilitating disorder, in which many patients inadequately respond to the standard outpatient care (Dowling et al., 2016). CBT, consisting of exposure and response prevention (EX/RP), remains the most prominent psychological treatment for OCD with substantial empirical support (Abramowitz, Taylor, & McKay, 2009). Specialized EX/RP alone, or in combination with serotonin reuptake inhibitors (SRIs), can be equally effective for improving OCD symptoms (Foa et al., 2005), and is more effective than placebo, stress management training (SMT), antidepressant monotherapy (Simpson et al., 2008), or antipsychotic augmentation (Simpson et al., 2013).

Patient scan experience the significant improvements to OCD symptoms and psycho-social functioning with large effect sizes (Veale et al., 2016). Knopp et al. (2013) indicated that while factors associated with treatment outcomes within these settings are highly varied, OCD symptom severity, marital status, hoarding pathology, and alcohol misuse are recognized as the predictors (Veale et al., 2016). The intensive doses of EX/RP serve as an opportunity to address the previous difficulties and optimize the response to CBT (Dowling et al., 2016).

Cognitive Behavioral Therapy and Heart Failure

The diagnosis and complications associated with heart failure have been well-established to adversely impact an individual's physical and psychosocial well-being, and interventions (e.g., CBT) have demonstrated positive benefits among patients with HF (Cajanding, 2016). Heart failure significantly impacts an individual's physical and emotional functioning (Burke, Jones, Ho, & Bekelman, 2014), increases psychological distress and negatively affects mood (Moser et al., 2010), disrupts psychosocial adjustment (Carels et al., 2004), and leads to the significant impairment in an individual's quality of life (Samartzis, Dimopoulos, Tziongourou, & Nanas, 2013).

Cardiac rehabilitation and disease management programs appear to be useful in improving the functional capacity, exercise tolerance, quality of life, and mortality among patients with heart failure (Austin, Williams, Ross, & Hutchison 2008).

Cardiac rehabilitation programs targeting psychosocial factors in the form of CBT has been previously shown to improve the outcomes among patients with cardiovascular diseases, including those with coronary heart diseases (Gulliksson et al., 2011) and heart failure (Freedland et al., 2015).

FUTURE RESEARCH DIRECTIONS

The classification of the extensive literature in the domains of mental health and CBT will provide the potential opportunities for future research. Health information technology (health IT) makes it possible for health care providers to better manage patient care through the secure use and sharing of health information (Kasemsap, 2017a). Health literacy is about how patients understand health information about health and health care, and how they apply that health information to their daily lives, utilize it to make health-related decisions, and act on it (Kasemsap, 2017b). Health professionals must commit to promoting for improved health literacy in health care organizations and should establish the specific health care goals toward improving health literacy in strategic plans, performance plans, programs, and educational initiatives (Kasemsap, 2017c). Critical thinking is the unbiased examination of assumptions underlying current beliefs to assess their correctness and legitimacy, and thus to validate or invalidate the beliefs (Kasemsap, 2017d). Problem solving is the process of working through the details of a problem to reach a solution (Kasemsap, 2017e). An examination of linkages among mental health, CBT, health IT, health literacy, critical thinking, and problem solving would seem to be viable for future research efforts.

Neuroscience is the field of study encompassing the various scientific disciplines dealing with the structure, development, function, chemistry, pharmacology, and pathology of the nervous system (Kasemsap, 2017f). Cognitive neuroscience is the study of higher cognitive functions in humans and its neural foundations (Kasemsap, 2017g). Considering the associations among mental health, CBT, neuroscience, and cognitive neuroscience should be further studied.

CONCLUSION

This chapter explained the important perspectives on mental health, mental illness, and technology utilization; mental health education and mental health nursing; the overview of CBT; CBT, depression, anxiety, and insomnia; CBT and OCD; and CBT and heart failure. Mental health strengthens the individuals' ability to have healthy relationships; make good life choices; maintain physical health and well-being; handle the natural ups and downs of life; and grow toward individuals' potential. Mental health is associated with higher productivity, better performance, more consistent work attendance, and fewer workplace accidents. Employers can strengthen and safeguard their businesses by choosing employee health plans with strong mental health benefits.

CBT is a goal-oriented psychotherapy treatment that takes a practical approach to problem-solving skills. Its goal is to change patterns of thinking or behavior that are behind people's difficulties, and so change the way they feel. CBT involves recognizing the unhelpful or destructive patterns of thinking and reacting, thus modifying or replacing these patterns with more realistic or helpful ones. CBT works by changing people's attitudes and their behavior by focusing on the thoughts, images, beliefs, and attitudes that are held and how these processes relate to the way a person behaves, as a way of dealing with emotional problems. During CBT, patients learn the specific skills that they can use for the rest of their lives. These skills involve identifying distorted thinking, modifying beliefs, relating to others in different ways, and changing behaviors.

REFERENCES

Abramowitz, J. S., Taylor, S., & McKay, D. (2009). Obsessive-compulsive disorder. *Lancet*, *374*(9688), 491–499. doi:10.1016/S0140-6736(09)60240-3 PMID:19665647

Albritton, T., Angley, M., Gibson, C., Sipsma, H., & Kershaw, T. (2015). Mental health utilization among diverse parenting young couples. *American Journal of Community Psychology*, *56*(1/2), 89–100. doi:10.1007/s10464-015-9738-7 PMID:26163272

Allen, M. D., & Green, B. L. (2012). A multilevel analysis of consultant attributes that contribute to effective mental health consultation services. *Infant Mental Health Journal*, *33*(3), 234–245. doi:10.1002/imhj.21333

Austin, J., Williams, W., Ross, L., & Hutchison, S. (2008). Five-year follow-up findings from a randomized controlled trial of cardiac rehabilitation for heart failure. *European Journal of Cardiovascular Prevention and Rehabilitation*, *15*(2), 162–167. doi:10.1097/HJR.0b013e3282f10e87 PMID:18391642

Bathory, D. S. (2015). Behavioral health and relational dynamics. *International Journal of Applied Behavioral Economics*, *4*(2), 36–52. doi:10.4018/ijabe.2015040103

Bohnenkamp, J. H., Stephan, S. H., & Bobo, N. (2015). Supporting student mental health: The role of the school nurse in coordinated school mental health care. *Psychology in the Schools*, *52*(7), 714–727. doi:10.1002/pits.21851

Brunero, S., Jeon, Y. H., & Foster, K. (2012). Mental health education programmes for generalist health professionals: An integrative review. *International Journal of Mental Health Nursing, 21*(5), 428–444. doi:10.1111/j.1447-0349.2011.00802.x PMID:22500589

Burke, R., Jones, J., Ho, P., & Bekelman, D. (2014). Caregivers' perceived roles in caring for patients with heart failure: What do clinicians need to know? *Journal of Cardiac Failure, 20*(10), 731–738. doi:10.1016/j.cardfail.2014.07.011 PMID:25084216

Burns, J., Blanchard, M., & Metcalf, A. (2013). Bridging the digital divide in Australia: The potential implications for the mental health of young people experiencing marginalisation. In *Digital literacy: Concepts, methodologies, tools, and applications* (pp. 772–793). Hershey, PA: IGI Global. doi:10.4018/978-1-4666-1852-7.ch040

Buysse, D. J. (2013). Insomnia. *Journal of the American Medical Association, 309*(7), 706–716. doi:10.1001/jama.2013.193 PMID:23423416

Byrne, L., Happell, B., Welch, T., & Moxham, L. J. (2013). "Things you can't learn from books": Teaching recovery from a lived experience perspective. *International Journal of Mental Health Nursing, 22*(3), 195–204. doi:10.1111/j.1447-0349.2012.00875.x PMID:23020070

Cajanding, R. J. M. (2016). The effectiveness of a nurse-led cognitive–behavioral therapy on the quality of life, self-esteem and mood among Filipino patients living with heart failure: A randomized controlled trial. *Applied Nursing Research, 31*, 86–93. doi:10.1016/j.apnr.2016.01.002 PMID:27397824

Calvo, R. A., Hussain, M. S., Milne, D., Nordbo, K., Hickie, I., & Danckwerts, P. (2016). Augmenting online mental health support services. In D. Villani, P. Cipresso, A. Gaggioli, & G. Riva (Eds.), *Integrating technology in positive psychology practice* (pp. 82–103). Hershey, PA: IGI Global. doi:10.4018/978-1-4666-9986-1.ch004

Cameron, P. S. (2014). Learning with a curve: Young women's "depression" as transformative learning. In V. Wang (Ed.), *Handbook of research on adult and community health education: Tools, trends, and methodologies* (pp. 100–122). Hershey, PA: IGI Global. doi:10.4018/978-1-4666-6260-5.ch007

Carels, R., Musher-Eizenman, D., Cacciapaglia, H., Pérez-Benítez, C., Christie, S., & O'Brien, W. (2004). Psychosocial functioning and physical symptoms in heart failure patients: A within-individual approach. *Journal of Psychosomatic Research, 56*(1), 95–101. doi:10.1016/S0022-3999(03)00041-2 PMID:14987970

Cassin, S. E., Sockalingam, S., Du, C., Wnuk, S., Hawa, R., & Parikh, S. V. (2016). A pilot randomized controlled trial of telephone-based cognitive behavioural therapy for preoperative bariatric surgery patients. *Behaviour Research and Therapy*, *80*, 17–22. doi:10.1016/j.brat.2016.03.001 PMID:26990279

Collins, E., Tranter, S., & Irvine, F. (2012). The physical health of the seriously mentally ill: An overview of the literature. *Journal of Psychiatric and Mental Health Nursing*, *19*(7), 638–646. doi:10.1111/j.1365-2850.2011.01831.x PMID:22070657

Cooper, G. J. (2010). Mental health management in New Zealand: The pathways model for client-based treatment. In W. Pease, M. Cooper, & R. Gururajan (Eds.), *Biomedical knowledge management: Infrastructures and processes for e-health systems* (pp. 253–266). Hershey, PA: IGI Global. doi:10.4018/978-1-60566-266-4.ch018

Cunningham, N. R., Jagpal, A., Tran, S. T., Kashikar-Zuck, S., Goldschneider, K. R., Coghill, R. C., & Lynch-Jordan, A. M. (2016). Anxiety adversely impacts response to cognitive behavioral therapy in children with chronic pain. *The Journal of Pediatrics*, *171*, 227–233. doi:10.1016/j.jpeds.2016.01.018 PMID:26879812

Dardas, L. A., & Simmons, L. A. (2015). The stigma of mental illness in Arab families: A concept analysis. *Journal of Psychiatric and Mental Health Nursing*, *22*(9), 668–679. doi:10.1111/jpm.12237 PMID:26118332

Deacon, B., Fawzy, T., Lickel, J., & Wolitzky-Taylor, K. (2011). Cognitive defusion versus cognitive restructuring in the treatment of negative self-referential thoughts: An investigation of process and outcome. *Journal of Cognitive Psychotherapy*, *25*(3), 218–232. doi:10.1891/0889-8391.25.3.218

DeNatale, L. M. (2013). Intersubjective experience of the infant and early childhood mental health consultant–program administrator consultee relationship. *Infant Mental Health Journal*, *34*(5), 470–482. doi:10.1002/imhj.21403

Dimidjian, S., & Davis, K. (2009). Newer variations of cognitive-behavioral therapy: Behavioral activation and mindfulness-based cognitive therapy. *Current Psychiatry Reports*, *11*(6), 453–458. doi:10.1007/s11920-009-0069-y PMID:19909667

Dowling, N., Thomas, N., Blair-West, S., Bousman, C., Yap, K., Smith, D. J., & Ng, C. H. (2016). Intensive residential treatment for obsessive-compulsive disorder: Outcomes and predictors of patient adherence to cognitive-behavioural therapy. *Journal of Obsessive-Compulsive and Related Disorders*, *9*, 82–89. doi:10.1016/j.jocrd.2016.04.006

Eapen, V., & Walter, A. (2016). Mind the gap: Developmental vulnerability and mental health. In R. Gopalan (Ed.), *Handbook of research on diagnosing, treating, and managing intellectual disabilities* (pp. 11–32). Hershey, PA: IGI Global. doi:10.4018/978-1-5225-0089-6.ch002

Espie, C. A., Barrie, L. M., & Forgan, G. S. (2012). Comparative investigation of the psychophysiologic and idiopathic insomnia disorder phenotypes: Psychologic characteristics, patients' perspectives, and implications for clinical management. *Sleep*, *35*(3), 385–393. PMID:22379245

Evans, E., Howlett, S., Kremser, T., Simpson, J., Kayess, R., & Trollor, J. (2012). Service development for intellectual disability mental health: A human rights approach. *Journal of Intellectual Disability Research*, *56*(11), 1098–1109. doi:10.1111/j.1365-2788.2012.01636.x PMID:23106753

Farrell, N. R., Deacon, B. J., Dixon, L. J., & Lickel, J. J. (2013). Theory-based training strategies for modifying practitioner concerns about exposure therapy. *Journal of Anxiety Disorders*, *27*(8), 781–787. doi:10.1016/j.janxdis.2013.09.003 PMID:24210013

Fleury, M. J., Bamvita, J. M., Farand, L., Aubé, D., Fournier, L., & Lesage, A. (2012). GP group profiles and involvement in mental health care. *Journal of Evaluation in Clinical Practice*, *18*(2), 396–403. doi:10.1111/j.1365-2753.2010.01597.x PMID:21114798

Foa, E. B., Liebowitz, M. R., Kozak, M. J., Davies, S., Campeas, R., Franklin, M. E., & Tu, X. (2005). Randomized, placebo-controlled trial of exposure and ritual prevention, clomipramine, and their combination in the treatment of obsessive-compulsive disorder. *The American Journal of Psychiatry*, *162*(1), 151–161. doi:10.1176/appi.ajp.162.1.151 PMID:15625214

Freedland, K. E., Carney, R. M., Rich, M. W., Steinmeyer, B. C., & Rubin, E. H. (2015). Cognitive behavior therapy for depression and self-care in heart failure patients: A randomized clinical trial. *JAMA Internal Medicine*, *175*(11), 1773–1782. doi:10.1001/jamainternmed.2015.5220 PMID:26414759

Georgakopoulos, P., Chatzidimitriou, M., & Tsolaki, M. (2015). A review of interventions with assistive technologies for patients with cognitive impairment. In P. Bamidis, I. Tarnanas, L. Hadjileontiadis, & M. Tsolaki (Eds.), *Handbook of research on innovations in the diagnosis and treatment of dementia* (pp. 118–129). Hershey, PA: IGI Global. doi:10.4018/978-1-4666-8234-4.ch006

Goldberg, D. P., Krueger, R. F., Andrews, G., & Hobbs, M. J. (2009). Emotional disorders: Cluster 4 of the proposed meta-structure for DSM-V and ICD-11. *Psychological Medicine*, *39*(12), 2043–2059. doi:10.1017/S0033291709990298 PMID:19796429

González-Prendes, A., & Resko, S. (2012). Cognitive-behavioral theory. In S. Ringel & J. Brandell (Eds.), *Trauma: Contemporary directions in theory, practice, and research* (pp. 14–40). Thousand Oaks, CA: Sage Publications. doi:10.4135/9781452230597.n2

Graham, D., Killoran, I., & Parekh, G. (2016). Supporting students' mental health and emotional well-being in inclusive classrooms. In M. Gordon (Ed.), *Challenges surrounding the education of children with chronic diseases* (pp. 86–116). Hershey, PA: IGI Global. doi:10.4018/978-1-4666-9452-1.ch005

Gulliksson, M., Burell, G., Vessby, B., Lundin, L., Toss, H., & Svärdsudd, K. (2011). Randomized controlled trial of cognitive behavioral therapy vs. standard treatment to prevent recurrent cardiovascular events in patients with coronary heart disease: Secondary prevention in Uppsala primary health care project (SUPRIM). *Archives of Internal Medicine*, *171*(2), 134–140. doi:10.1001/archinternmed.2010.510 PMID:21263103

Hadzic, M., & Dillon, D. S. (2010). Role of multi-agents system in creation of collaborative environments within mental health domain. In R. Paranjape & A. Sadanand (Eds.), *Multi-agent systems for healthcare simulation and modeling: Applications for system improvement* (pp. 196–214). Hershey, PA: IGI Global. doi:10.4018/978-1-60566-772-0.ch011

Hamdan-Mansour, A. M., Al-Gamal, E., Puskar, K., Yacoub, M., & Marini, A. (2011). Mental health nursing in Jordan: An investigation into experience, work stress and organizational support. *International Journal of Mental Health Nursing*, *20*(2), 86–94. doi:10.1111/j.1447-0349.2010.00716.x PMID:21371223

Happell, B., Byrne, L., Platania-Phung, C., Harris, S., Bradshaw, J., & Davies, J. (2014). Lived-experience participation in nurse education: Reducing stigma and enhancing popularity. *International Journal of Mental Health Nursing*, *23*(5), 427–434. doi:10.1111/inm.12077 PMID:24898260

Happell, B., & McAllister, M. (2014). Implementing a major stream in mental health nursing: Barriers to effectiveness. *International Journal of Mental Health Nursing*, *23*(5), 435–441. doi:10.1111/inm.12075 PMID:24890753

Happell, B., Palmer, C., & Tennent, R. (2010). Mental health nurse incentive program: Contributing to positive client outcomes. *International Journal of Mental Health Nursing*, *19*(5), 331–339. doi:10.1111/j.1447-0349.2010.00679.x PMID:20887607

Happell, B., & Platania-Phung, C. (2012). Mental health placements in a general health setting: No substitute for the real thing! *Journal of Clinical Nursing*, *21*(13/14), 2026–2033. doi:10.1111/j.1365-2702.2011.04016.x PMID:22564033

Happell, B., Platania-Phung, C., & Scott, D. (2011). Placing physical activity in mental health care: A leadership role for mental health nurses. *International Journal of Mental Health Nursing*, *20*(5), 310–318. doi:10.1111/j.1447-0349.2010.00732.x PMID:21896121

Happell, B., Platania-Phung, C., & Scott, D. (2013). Mental health nurse incentive program: Facilitating physical health care for people with mental illness? *International Journal of Mental Health Nursing*, *22*(5), 399–408. doi:10.1111/inm.12006 PMID:23279365

Happell, B., Scott, D., & Platania-Phung, C. (2013). Nurse views on the cardiometabolic health nurse as an approach to improving the physical health of people with serious mental illness in Australia. *International Journal of Mental Health Nursing*, *22*(5), 418–429. doi:10.1111/j.1447-0349.2012.00892.x PMID:23211091

Hardy, S., & Thomas, B. (2012). Mental and physical health comordibity: Political imperatives and practice implications. *International Journal of Mental Health Nursing*, *21*(3), 289–298. doi:10.1111/j.1447-0349.2012.00823.x PMID:22533336

Hashim, A. H., Kaur, M., Bahar, N., & Ismail, W. S. (2016). Mental health issues among family members of children with mental disability. In R. Gopalan (Ed.), *Handbook of research on diagnosing, treating, and managing intellectual disabilities* (pp. 54–81). Hershey, PA: IGI Global. doi:10.4018/978-1-5225-0089-6.ch004

Haug, T., Nordgreen, T., Ost, L. G., Tangen, T., Kvale, G., Hovland, O. J., & Havik, O. E. et al. (2016). Working alliance and competence as predictors of outcome in cognitive behavioral therapy for social anxiety and panic disorder in adults. *Behaviour Research and Therapy*, *77*, 40–51. doi:10.1016/j.brat.2015.12.004 PMID:26708332

Heller, S. S., Boothe, A., Keyes, A., Nagle, G., Sidell, M., & Rice, J. (2011). Implementation of a mental health consultation model and its impact on early childhood teachers' efficacy and competence. *Infant Mental Health Journal*, *32*(2), 143–164. doi:10.1002/imhj.20289

Ho, F. Y. Y., Chan, C. S., & Tang, K. N. S. (2016). Cognitive-behavioral therapy for sleep disturbances in treating posttraumatic stress disorder symptoms: A meta-analysis of randomized controlled trials. *Clinical Psychology Review*, *43*, 90–102. doi:10.1016/j.cpr.2015.09.005 PMID:26439674

Hoeve, M., Colins, O. F., Mulder, E. A., Loeber, R., Stams, G. J. J. M., & Vermeiren, R. R. J. M. (2015). The association between childhood maltreatment, mental health problems, and aggression in justice-involved boys. *Aggressive Behavior*, *41*(5), 488–501. doi:10.1002/ab.21586 PMID:25788428

Hsiao, C. Y., Lu, H. L., & Tsai, Y. F. (2015). Factors influencing mental health nurses' attitudes towards people with mental illness. *International Journal of Mental Health Nursing*, *24*(3), 272–280. doi:10.1111/inm.12129 PMID:25963120

Kasemsap, K. (2017a). Analyzing the role of health information technology in global health care. In N. Wickramasinghe (Ed.), *Handbook of research on healthcare administration and management* (pp. 287–307). Hershey, PA: IGI Global. doi:10.4018/978-1-5225-0920-2.ch017

Kasemsap, K. (2017b). The fundamentals of health literacy. In N. Wickramasinghe (Ed.), *Handbook of research on healthcare administration and management* (pp. 507–527). Hershey, PA: IGI Global. doi:10.4018/978-1-5225-0920-2.ch030

Kasemsap, K. (2017c). Promoting health literacy in global health care. In N. Wickramasinghe (Ed.), *Handbook of research on healthcare administration and management* (pp. 485–506). Hershey, PA: IGI Global. doi:10.4018/978-1-5225-0920-2.ch029

Kasemsap, K. (2017d). Promoting critical thinking in the modern learning environments. In R. Batko & A. Szopa (Eds.), *Strategic imperatives and core competencies in the era of robotics and artificial intelligence* (pp. 50–80). Hershey, PA: IGI Global. doi:10.4018/978-1-5225-1656-9.ch004

Kasemsap, K. (2017e). Advocating problem-based learning and creative problem-solving skills in global education. In C. Zhou (Ed.), *Handbook of research on creative problem-solving skill development in higher education* (pp. 351–377). Hershey, PA: IGI Global. doi:10.4018/978-1-5225-0643-0.ch016

Kasemsap, K. (2017f). Investigating the roles of neuroscience and knowledge management in higher education. In S. Mukerji & P. Tripathi (Eds.), *Handbook of research on administration, policy, and leadership in higher education* (pp. 112–140). Hershey, PA: IGI Global. doi:10.4018/978-1-5225-0672-0.ch006

Kasemsap, K. (2017g). Mastering cognitive neuroscience and social neuroscience perspectives in the information age. In M. Dos Santos (Ed.), *Applying neuroscience to business practice* (pp. 82–113). Hershey, PA: IGI Global. doi:10.4018/978-1-5225-1028-4.ch005

Kashikar-Zuck, S., Ting, T. V., Arnold, L. M., Bean, J., Powers, S. W., Graham, T. B., & Lovell, D. J. et al. (2012). Cognitive behavioral therapy for the treatment of juvenile fibromyalgia: A multisite, single-blind, randomized, controlled clinical trial. *Arthritis and Rheumatism*, *64*(1), 297–305. doi:10.1002/art.30644 PMID:22108765

Kauer, S., & Reid, S. (2015). Mobile tracking for mental health and wellbeing. In Z. Yan (Ed.), *Encyclopedia of mobile phone behavior* (pp. 860–870). Hershey, PA: IGI Global. doi:10.4018/978-1-4666-8239-9.ch071

Kidd, S., Kenny, A., & McKinstry, C. (2015). The meaning of recovery in a regional mental health service: An action research study. *Journal of Advanced Nursing*, *71*(1), 181–192. doi:10.1111/jan.12472 PMID:25040239

Knopp, J., Knowles, S., Bee, P., Lovell, K., & Bower, P. (2013). A systematic review of predictors and moderators of response to psychological therapies in OCD: Do we have enough empirical evidence to target treatment? *Clinical Psychology Review*, *33*(8), 1067–1081. doi:10.1016/j.cpr.2013.08.008 PMID:24077387

Krolikowski, A. M. (2013). The effectiveness of Internet-based mindfulness interventions for physical and mental illnesses: A narrative review. *International Journal of Cyber Behavior, Psychology and Learning*, *3*(4), 84–96. doi:10.4018/ijcbpl.2013100106

Kuyken, W., & Tsivrikos, D. (2009). Therapist competence, comorbidity and cognitive-behavioral therapy for depression. *Psychotherapy and Psychosomatics*, *78*(1), 42–48. doi:10.1159/000172619 PMID:19018156

Ledley, D. R., Marx, B. P., & Heimberg, R. G. (2011). *Making cognitive-behavioral therapy work: Clinical process for new practitioners*. New York, NY: The Guilford Press.

Levita, L., Duhne, P. G. S., Girling, C., & Waller, G. (2016). Facets of clinician's anxiety and the delivery of cognitive behavioral therapy. *Behaviour Research and Therapy*, *77*, 157–161. doi:10.1016/j.brat.2015.12.015 PMID:26764585

Lynch-Jordan, A. M., Sil, S., Peugh, J., Cunningham, N., Kashikar-Zuck, S., & Goldschneider, K. R. (2014). Differential changes in functional disability and pain intensity over the course of psychological treatment for children with chronic pain. *Pain*, *155*(10), 1955–1961. doi:10.1016/j.pain.2014.06.008 PMID:24954165

Marks, M., & Bowers, C. (2015). Technology and mental health. In M. Khosrow-Pour (Ed.), *Encyclopedia of information science and technology* (3rd ed., pp. 6455–6465). Hershey, PA: IGI Global. doi:10.4018/978-1-4666-5888-2.ch634

Martin, J., & McKay, E. (2014). Mental health, post-secondary education, and information communications technology. In *Assistive technologies: Concepts, methodologies, tools, and applications* (pp. 1209–1226). Hershey, PA: IGI Global. doi:10.4018/978-1-4666-4422-9.ch063

Matthews, M., Doherty, G., Coyle, D., & Sharry, J. (2008). Designing mobile applications to support mental health interventions. In J. Lumsden (Ed.), *Handbook of research on user interface design and evaluation for mobile technology* (pp. 635–656). Hershey, PA: IGI Global. doi:10.4018/978-1-59904-871-0.ch038

McCloughen, A., Foster, K., Huws-Thomas, M., & Delgado, C. (2012). Physical health and wellbeing of emerging and young adults with mental illness: An integrative review of international literature. *International Journal of Mental Health Nursing, 21*(3), 274–288. doi:10.1111/j.1447-0349.2011.00796.x PMID:22533335

McDaid, D., Knapp, M., & Raja, S. (2008). Barriers in the mind: Promoting an economic case for mental health in low- and middle-income countries. *World Psychiatry; Official Journal of the World Psychiatric Association (WPA), 7*(2), 79–86. doi:10.1002/j.2051-5545.2008.tb00160.x PMID:18560485

McKie, A., & Naysmith, S. (2014). Promoting critical perspectives in mental health nursing education. *Journal of Psychiatric and Mental Health Nursing, 21*(2), 128–137. doi:10.1111/jpm.12061 PMID:23552221

McKinlay, E., Garrett, S., McBain, L., Dowell, T., Collings, S., & Stanley, J. (2011). New Zealand general practice nurses' roles in mental health care. *International Nursing Review, 58*(2), 225–233. doi:10.1111/j.1466-7657.2010.00859.x PMID:21554297

Mendenhall, A. N., & Frauenholtz, S. (2015). Predictors of mental health literacy among parents of youth diagnosed with mood disorders. *Child & Family Social Work, 20*(3), 300–309. doi:10.1111/cfs.12078

Messer, S. B., & Wampold, B. E. (2002). Let's face facts: Common factors are more potent than specific therapy ingredients. *Clinical Psychology: Science and Practice, 9*(1), 21–25. doi:10.1093/clipsy.9.1.21

Morris, J., Belfer, M., Daniels, A., Flisher, A., Villé, L., Lora, A., & Saxena, S. (2011). Treated prevalence of and mental health services received by children and adolescents in 42 low-and-middle-income countries. *Journal of Child Psychology and Psychiatry, and Allied Disciplines, 52*(12), 1239–1246. doi:10.1111/j.1469-7610.2011.02409.x PMID:21554305

Moser, D., Dracup, K., Evangelista, L., Zambroski, C., Lennie, T., Chung, M., & Heo, S. et al. (2010). Comparison of prevalence of symptoms of depression, anxiety, and hostility in elderly patients with heart failure, myocardial infarction, and a coronary artery bypass graft. *Heart & Lung*, *39*(5), 378–385. doi:10.1016/j.hrtlng.2009.10.017 PMID:20561849

Namle, S., Ghapanchi, A. H., & Amrollahi, A. (2016). Information and communication technology for mental health: A systematic literature review. In M. Cruz-Cunha, I. Miranda, R. Martinho, & R. Rijo (Eds.), *Encyclopedia of e-health and telemedicine* (pp. 606–618). Hershey, PA: IGI Global. doi:10.4018/978-1-4666-9978-6.ch047

Newby, J. M., Twomey, C., Li, S. S. Y., & Andrews, G. (2016). Transdiagnostic computerised cognitive behavioural therapy for depression and anxiety: A systematic review and meta-analysis. *Journal of Affective Disorders*, *199*, 30–41. doi:10.1016/j.jad.2016.03.018 PMID:27060430

Newman, D., O'Reilly, P., Lee, S. H., & Kennedy, C. (2015). Mental health service users' experiences of mental health care: An integrative literature review. *Journal of Psychiatric and Mental Health Nursing*, *22*(3), 171–182. doi:10.1111/jpm.12202 PMID:25707898

O'Donnell, H., & Gormley, K. (2013). Service user involvement in nurse education: Perceptions of mental health nursing students. *Journal of Psychiatric and Mental Health Nursing*, *20*(3), 193–202. doi:10.1111/j.1365-2850.2012.01917.x PMID:22533371

Ohayon, M. M. (2002). Epidemiology of insomnia: What we know and what we still need to learn. *Sleep Medicine Reviews*, *6*(2), 97–111. doi:10.1053/smrv.2002.0186 PMID:12531146

Okajima, I., Komada, Y., & Inoue, Y. (2011). A meta-analysis on the treatment effectiveness of cognitive behavioral therapy for primary insomnia. *Sleep and Biological Rhythms*, *9*(1), 24–34. doi:10.1111/j.1479-8425.2010.00481.x

Palagini, L., Bruno, R. M., Gemignani, A., Baglioni, C., Ghiadoni, L., & Riemann, D. (2013). Sleep loss and hypertension: A systematic review. *Current Pharmaceutical Design*, *19*(13), 2409–2419. doi:10.2174/1381612811319130009 PMID:23173590

Patel, S. R., Malhotra, A., Gao, X., Hu, F. B., Neuman, M. I., & Fawzi, W. W. (2012). A prospective study of sleep duration and pneumonia risk in women. *Sleep*, *35*(1), 97–101. doi:10.5665/sleep.1594 PMID:22215923

Perils, M. L., & Smith, M. T. (2008). How can we make CBT-I and other BSM services widely available? *Journal of Clinical Sleep Medicine*, *4*(1), 11–13. PMID:18350955

Plaistow, J., Masson, K., Koch, D., Wilson, J., Stark, R. M., Jones, P. B., & Lennox, B. R. (2014). Young people's views of UK mental health services. *Early Intervention in Psychiatry*, *8*(1), 12–23. doi:10.1111/eip.12060 PMID:23773401

Prasad, B. V. (2017). *Chronic mental illness and the changing scope of intervention strategies, diagnosis, and treatment* (pp. 1–303). Hershey, PA: IGI Global. doi:10.4018/978-1-5225-0519-8

Robson, D., Haddad, M., Gray, R., & Gournay, K. (2013). Mental health nursing and physical health care: A cross-sectional study of nurses' attitudes, practice, and perceived training needs for the physical health care of people with severe mental illness. *International Journal of Mental Health Nursing*, *22*(5), 409–417. doi:10.1111/j.1447-0349.2012.00883.x PMID:23066812

Rosenberg, S., & McDermott, F. (2016). More than pills and beds: Contemporary challenges in social work practice and mental healthcare. In *Psychology and mental health: Concepts, methodologies, tools, and applications* (pp. 1111–1128). Hershey, PA: IGI Global. doi:10.4018/978-1-5225-0159-6.ch047

Samartzis, L., Dimopoulos, S., Tziongourou, M., & Nanas, S. (2013). Effect of psychosocial interventions on quality of life in patients with chronic heart failure: A meta-analysis of randomized controlled trials. *Journal of Cardiac Failure*, *19*(2), 125–134. doi:10.1016/j.cardfail.2012.12.004 PMID:23384638

Selene, G. C., Omar, C. I. F., & Silvia, A. P. (2016). Palliative care, impact of cognitive behavioral therapy to cancer patients. *Procedia: Social and Behavioral Sciences*, *217*, 1063–1070. doi:10.1016/j.sbspro.2016.02.110

Simpson, H. B., Foa, E. B., Liebowitz, M. R., Huppert, J. D., Cahill, S., Maher, M. J., & Campeas, R. (2013). Cognitive-behavioral therapy vs risperidone for augmenting serotonin reuptake inhibitors in obsessive-compulsive disorder: A randomized clinical trial. *JAMA Psychiatry*, *70*(11), 1190–1199. doi:10.1001/jamapsychiatry.2013.1932 PMID:24026523

Simpson, H. B., Foa, E. B., Liebowitz, M. R., Ledley, D. R., Huppert, J. D., Cahill, S., & Petkova, E. (2008). A randomized, controlled trial of cognitive-behavioral therapy for augmenting pharmacotherapy in obsessive-compulsive disorder. *The American Journal of Psychiatry*, *165*(5), 621–630. doi:10.1176/appi.ajp.2007.07091440 PMID:18316422

Smith, M. T., Perlis, M. L., Park, A., Smith, M. S., Pennington, J., Giles, D. E., & Buysse, D. J. (2002). Comparative meta-analysis of pharmacotherapy and behavior therapy for persistent insomnia. *The American Journal of Psychiatry*, *159*(1), 5–11. doi:10.1176/appi.ajp.159.1.5 PMID:11772681

Staner, L. (2010). Comorbidity of insomnia and depression. *Sleep Medicine Reviews*, *14*(1), 35–46. doi:10.1016/j.smrv.2009.09.003 PMID:19939713

Stanton, R., Reaburn, P., & Happell, B. (2015). Barriers to exercise prescription and participation in people with mental illness: The perspectives of nurses working in mental health. *Journal of Psychiatric and Mental Health Nursing*, *22*(6), 440–448. doi:10.1111/jpm.12205 PMID:25855247

Tully, P., Selkow, T., Bengel, J., & Rafanelli, C. (2014). A dynamic view of comorbid depression and generalized anxiety disorder symptom change in chronic heart failure: The discrete effects of cognitive behavioral therapy, exercise, and psychotropic medication. *Disability and Rehabilitation*, *1*, 1–8. PMID:24981015

Veale, D., Naismith, I., Miles, S., Gledhill, L. J., Stewart, G., & Hodsoll, J. (2016). Outcomes for residential or inpatient intensive treatment of obsessive-compulsive disorder: A systematic review and meta-analysis. *Journal of Obsessive-Compulsive and Related Disorders*, *8*, 38–49. doi:10.1016/j.jocrd.2015.11.005

Wahlbeck, K. (2015). Public mental health: The time is ripe for translation of evidence into practice. *World Psychiatry; Official Journal of the World Psychiatric Association (WPA)*, *14*(1), 36–42. doi:10.1002/wps.20178 PMID:25655149

Walker, S., & McAndrew, S. (2015). The same but different: Discussing the literature regarding mental health nurses' difficulty in meeting the physical health needs of service users, regardless of differing education programmes. *Journal of Psychiatric and Mental Health Nursing*, *22*(8), 640–646. doi:10.1111/jpm.12220 PMID:26337595

Wand, T. (2011). Real mental health promotion requires a reorientation of nursing education, practice and research. *Journal of Psychiatric and Mental Health Nursing*, *18*(2), 131–138. doi:10.1111/j.1365-2850.2010.01634.x PMID:21299725

Weist, M. D., Mellin, E. A., Chambers, K. L., Lever, N. A., Haber, D., & Blaber, C. (2012). Challenges to collaboration in school mental health and strategies for overcoming them. *The Journal of School Health*, *82*(2), 97–105. doi:10.1111/j.1746-1561.2011.00672.x PMID:22239135

Wilson, R. L., & Usher, K. (2015). Rural nurses: A convenient co-location strategy for the rural mental health care of young people. *Journal of Clinical Nursing*, *24*(17/18), 2638–2648. doi:10.1111/jocn.12882 PMID:26098196

Wynaden, D. (2010). There is no health without mental health: Are we educating Australian nurses to care for the health consumer of the 21st century? *International Journal of Mental Health Nursing*, *19*(3), 203–209. doi:10.1111/j.1447-0349.2010.00671.x PMID:20550644

Zachariae, R., Lyby, M. S., Ritterband, L. M., & O'Toole, M. S. (2016). Efficacy of Internet-delivered cognitive-behavioral therapy for insomnia: A systematic review and meta-analysis of randomized controlled trials. *Sleep Medicine Reviews, 30*, 1–10. doi:10.1016/j.smrv.2015.10.004 PMID:26615572

Ziller, E. C., Anderson, N. J., & Coburn, A. F. (2010). Access to rural mental health services: Service use and out-of-pocket costs. *The Journal of Rural Health, 26*(3), 214–224. doi:10.1111/j.1748-0361.2010.00291.x PMID:20633089

ADDITIONAL READING

Barrera, T. L., Mott, J. M., Hofstein, R. F., & Teng, E. J. (2013). A meta-analytic review of exposure in group cognitive behavioral therapy for posttraumatic stress disorder. *Clinical Psychology Review, 33*(1), 24–32. doi:10.1016/j.cpr.2012.09.005 PMID:23123568

Belleville, G., Guay, S., & Marchand, A. (2011). Persistence of sleep disturbances following cognitive-behavior therapy for posttraumatic stress disorder. *Journal of Psychosomatic Research, 70*(4), 318–327. doi:10.1016/j.jpsychores.2010.09.022 PMID:21414451

Bowers, H., Manion, I., Papadopoulos, D., & Gauvreau, E. (2013). Stigma in school-based mental health: Perceptions of young people and service providers. *Child and Adolescent Mental Health, 18*(3), 165–170. doi:10.1111/j.1475-3588.2012.00673.x

Chamberlain–Salaun, J., Mills, J., & Park, T. (2011). Mental health nurses employed in Australian general practice: Dimensions of time and space. *International Journal of Mental Health Nursing, 20*(2), 112–118. doi:10.1111/j.1447-0349.2010.00723.x PMID:21371226

Conners-Burrow, N., McKelvey, L., Sockwell, L., Ehrentraut, J. H., Adams, S., & Whiteside-Mansell, L. (2013). Beginning to "unpack" early childhood mental health consultation: Types of consultation services and their impact on teachers. *Infant Mental Health Journal, 34*(4), 280–289. doi:10.1002/imhj.21387

Cutcliffe, J., Stevenson, C., & Lakeman, R. (2013). Oxymoronic or synergistic: Deconstructing the psychiatric and/or mental health nurse. *International Journal of Mental Health Nursing, 22*(2), 125–134. doi:10.1111/j.1447-0349.2012.00850.x PMID:23066735

Espie, C. A., Kyle, S. D., Williams, C., Ong, J. C., Douglas, N. J., Hames, P., & Brown, J. S. L. (2012). A randomized, placebo-controlled trial of online cognitive behavioral therapy for chronic insomnia disorder delivered via an automated media-rich web application. *Sleep*, *35*(6), 769–781. doi:10.5665/sleep.1872 PMID:22654196

Fonagy, P., Luyten, P., & Strathearn, L. (2011). Borderline personality disorder, mentalization, and the neurobiology of attachment. *Infant Mental Health Journal*, *32*(1), 47–69. doi:10.1002/imhj.20283

Gee, A., & McGarty, C. (2013). Developing cooperative communities to reduce stigma about mental disorders. *Analyses of Social Issues and Public Policy (ASAP)*, *13*(1), 137–164. doi:10.1111/j.1530-2415.2012.01296.x

Germain, A. (2013). Sleep disturbances as the hallmark of PTSD: Where are we now? *The American Journal of Psychiatry*, *170*(4), 372–382. doi:10.1176/appi.ajp.2012.12040432 PMID:23223954

Goodyear, M., Hill, T. L., Allchin, B., McCormick, F., Hine, R., Cuff, R., & O'Hanlon, B. (2015). Standards of practice for the adult mental health workforce: Meeting the needs of families where a parent has a mental illness. *International Journal of Mental Health Nursing*, *24*(2), 169–180. doi:10.1111/inm.12120 PMID:25619407

Greenberg, J. L., Mothi, S. S., & Wilhelm, S. (2016). Cognitive-behavioral therapy for adolescent body dysmorphic disorder: A pilot study. *Behavior Therapy*, *47*(2), 213–224. doi:10.1016/j.beth.2015.10.009 PMID:26956653

Happell, B., McAllister, M., & Gaskin, C. J. (2015). Majors in mental health nursing: Issues of sustainability and commitment. *Perspectives in Psychiatric Care*, *51*(1), 28–35. doi:10.1111/ppc.12063 PMID:24606586

Harrison, C. A., Hauck, Y., & Hoffman, R. (2014). Choosing and remaining in mental health nursing: Perceptions of Western Australian nurses. *International Journal of Mental Health Nursing*, *23*(6), 561–569. doi:10.1111/inm.12094 PMID:25308149

Henderson, A. R., & Martyr, P. (2013). Too little, too late: Mental health nursing education in Western Australia, 1958–1994. *International Journal of Mental Health Nursing*, *22*(3), 221–230. doi:10.1111/j.1447-0349.2012.00861.x PMID:22809369

Kizito, O. (2015). Negative effects of home foreclosures on mental and physical health risks. *International Journal of Risk and Contingency Management*, *4*(2), 1–19. doi:10.4018/IJRCM.2015040101

Mehrotra, S., Tripathi, R., & Elias, J. K. (2013). Lay meanings of mental health in urban Indian college youth: Insights for mental health promotion. *Journal of Community & Applied Social Psychology*, *23*(4), 286–299. doi:10.1002/casp.2119

Miller, B. D., Blau, G. M., Christopher, O. T., & Jordan, P. E. (2012). Sustaining and expanding systems of care to provide mental health services for children, youth and families across America. *American Journal of Community Psychology*, *49*(3/4), 566–579. doi:10.1007/s10464-012-9517-7 PMID:22543719

Moxham, L., McCann, T., Usher, K., Farrell, G., & Crookes, P. (2011). Mental health nursing education in preregistration nursing curricula: A national report. *International Journal of Mental Health Nursing*, *20*(4), 232–236. doi:10.1111/j.1447-0349.2010.00735.x PMID:21385293

Parfitt, Y., & Ayers, S. (2014). Transition to parenthood and mental health in first-time partners. *Infant Mental Health Journal*, *35*(3), 263–273. doi:10.1002/imhj.21443 PMID:25798480

Potter, D. (2013). The social process behind inequalities in childrens mental health: Incorporating an illness career framework. *Social Compass*, *7*(9), 775–785. doi:10.1111/soc4.12061

Priddis, L. E., Matacz, R., & Weatherston, D. (2015). Building a workforce competency-based training program in infant/early childhood mental health. *Infant Mental Health Journal*, *36*(6), 623–631. doi:10.1002/imhj.21535 PMID:26514346

Semrau, M., Barley, E. A., Law, A., & Thornicroft, G. (2011). Lessons learned in developing community mental health care in Europe. *World Psychiatry; Official Journal of the World Psychiatric Association (WPA)*, *10*(3), 217–225. doi:10.1002/j.2051-5545.2011.tb00060.x PMID:21991282

Sloan, D. M., Feinstein, B. A., Gallagher, M. W., Beck, J. G., & Keane, T. M. (2013). Efficacy of group treatment for posttraumatic stress disorder symptoms: A meta-analysis. *Psychological Trauma: Theory, Research, Practice, and Policy*, *5*(2), 176–183. doi:10.1037/a0026291

Slominski, L., Sameroff, A., Rosenblum, K., & Kasser, T. (2011). Longitudinal pathways between maternal mental health in infancy and offspring romantic relationships in adulthood: A 30-year prospective study. *Social Development*, *20*(4), 762–782. doi:10.1111/j.1467-9507.2011.00610.x

Sturdy, S., Smith-Merry, J., & Freeman, R. (2012). Stakeholder consultation as social mobilization: Framing Scottish mental health policy. *Social Policy and Administration*, *46*(7), 823–844. doi:10.1111/j.1467-9515.2012.00848.x

Turner, H., Tatham, M., Lant, M., Mountford, V. A., & Waller, G. (2014). Clinicians' concerns about delivering cognitive-behavioural therapy for eating disorders. *Behaviour Research and Therapy*, *57*, 38–42. doi:10.1016/j.brat.2014.04.003 PMID:24793719

Ulmer, C. S., Edinger, J. D., & Calhoun, P. S. (2011). A multi-component cognitive-behavioral intervention for sleep disturbance in veterans with PTSD: A pilot study. *Journal of Clinical Sleep Medicine*, *7*(1), 57–68. PMID:21344046

van de Bovenkamp, H. M., & Trappenburg, M. J. (2012). Comparative review of family–professional communication: What mental health care can learn from oncology and nursing home care. *International Journal of Mental Health Nursing*, *21*(4), 366–385. doi:10.1111/j.1447-0349.2011.00798.x PMID:22510087

Waller, G., Stringer, H., & Meyer, C. (2012). What cognitive-behavioral techniques do therapists report using when delivering cognitive-behavioral therapy for the eating disorders? *Journal of Consulting and Clinical Psychology*, *80*(1), 171–175. doi:10.1037/a0026559 PMID:22141595

Wei, Y., Hayden, J. A., Kutcher, S., Zygmunt, A., & McGrath, P. (2013). The effectiveness of school mental health literacy programs to address knowledge, attitudes and help seeking among youth. *Early Intervention in Psychiatry*, *7*(2), 109–121. doi:10.1111/eip.12010 PMID:23343220

Wong, D. F. K., Zhuang, X. Y., Pan, J. Y., & He, X. S. (2014). A critical review of mental health and mental health-related policies in China: More actions required. *International Journal of Social Welfare*, *23*(2), 195–204. doi:10.1111/ijsw.12052

KEY TERMS AND DEFINITIONS

Anxiety: The uncomfortable feeling of worry about something that is happening or might happen in the future.

Behavior: The response of an individual or group to an action, environment, person, or stimulus.

Cognition: The utilization of conscious mental processes.

Cognitive Behavioral Therapy: The treatment for individuals suffering from mental illness that tries to change the way they think and behave.

Depression: The state of feeling very unhappy and without hope for the future.

Insomnia: The condition of being unable to sleep, over a period of time.

Mental Health: The condition of individuals' mind and whether or not they are suffering from any mental illness.

Mental Illness: The illness that affects the individuals' mind.

Therapy: The treatment that helps individuals feel better and grow stronger, especially after an illness.

Chapter 2
User Experiences and Perceptions of Internet Interventions for Depression

Filip Drozd
National Network for Infant Mental Health, Norway

Silje Marie Haga
National Network of Infant Mental Health, Norway

Caroline Emilie Andersen
University of Oslo, Norway

Kari Slinning
National Network for Infant Mental Health, Norway

Cato Alexander Bjørkli
University of Oslo, Norway

ABSTRACT

The purpose of this chapter is to review qualitative research on user experiences with internet interventions for depression and present original results from in-depth interviews from a preventive unguided intervention for postpartum depression. The first part reviews the literature on qualitative studies of client experiences and perceptions of internet interventions for depression. The next part describes original data from a study investigating participants' experiences using semi-structured interviews, following the modified SWOT-format (i.e., strengths, weakness, opportunities, and threats). In total, 10 pregnant and postpartum women aged 28 to 41 were interviewed. Insights from the current review and study are used as a point of departure for discussing future directions in research on internet interventions for depression. This chapter should be valuable for clinicians, researchers, and other health professionals interested in the applicability of internet interventions for their clients, design of future studies, and development of internet interventions.

DOI: 10.4018/978-1-5225-3241-5.ch002

INTRODUCTION

Depression is one of the leading causes of years lost due to disability and shortened life expectancy, affecting about 350 million people worldwide every year (Marcus, Yasamy, van Ommeren, Chisholm, & Saxena, 2012; World Health Organization, 2009). The estimated lifetime prevalence rate is about 20% with about 10% affected by depression each year (Mykletun, Knudsen, & Mathiesen, 2009). However, less than half (in some countries, fewer than 10%) have access to or seek professional help (World Health Organization, 2010). Internet interventions are suggested as a supplement to primary and secondary care to help overcome barriers to help-seeking associated with depression such as stigma, reluctance for emotional disclosure, undertreatment, and lack of trained providers and resources (Dennis & Chung-Lee, 2006; Goodman, 2009; Overland, Glozier, Krokstad, & Mykletun, 2007). Systematic reviews show that both unguided and therapist-supported internet interventions can be of benefit for people with depression (Cuijpers et al., 2011; Cuijpers, Donker, van Straten, Li, & Andersson, 2010). Such findings have contributed to the inclusion of guided internet-based cognitive behavior therapy (iCBT) in several national guidelines for treatment of mild-to-moderate depression (e.g., Australian Psychological Society, 2011; Norwegian Directorate of Health, 2009; The National Board of Health and Wellfare, 2010).

Despite promising studies of efficacy and the inclusion of iCBT in national guidelines, few studies have asked end-users to reflect on their experiences of internet interventions. Such reflections can provide a deeper and richer understanding of the uptake and use of internet interventions, the therapeutic processes, and generate hypotheses for future research. They can provide us with complementary knowledge to the many randomized trials and inform us about (1) why some users adhere to internet interventions and others do not, (2) how users change by using internet interventions (i.e., the therapeutic process), and (3) help to determine what internet interventions may be appropriate for whom. In addition, it would not be safe to assume that user experiences in face-to-face psychotherapy can be generalized to automated or computer-mediated protocols delivered over the internet. Therefore, this chapter starts by reviewing the literature on qualitative studies on user experiences and perceptions that can either facilitate or impede adherence to internet interventions, how internet interventions can instigate important therapeutic processes, and which interventions may be appropriate for whom. Finally, we present findings from a qualitative study on women's experiences from an unguided intervention designed to prevent postpartum depression.

LITERATURE REVIEW

A recent meta-synthesis of user experiences of computer-based interventions identified two overarching themes (Knowles et al., 2014); (1) First, interventions need to be more personalized and sensitive to the individual users' needs, so that users can identify with the program and relate the program content to themselves and their daily lives (e.g., use of role models, examples, and homework assignments). Second, the level of support and guidance, either by a professional or lay person, is experienced as contradictory. For some, support may help identify different clinical needs and relate program content to the user's situation, and recognize and acknowledge personal emotional and motivational difficulties. For others, support may be experienced negatively (e.g., perceptions of high demands or expectations from the therapist). The authors also concluded that these findings may not generalize to other user groups (e.g., ethnic minorities, elderly or pregnant women) and approaches other than cognitive behavior therapy (CBT). In addition, this synthesis included mixed qualitative studies on anxiety and depression, and 7 out of 8 included studies were desktop-based CBT interventions. Thus, it is necessary to examine experiences among other user groups, include different therapeutic approaches, and examine user experiences that are specifically related to internet interventions for depression.

Adherence

Accessibility, convenience, flexibility, and anonymity and privacy, are some of the major advantages of internet interventions for depression (e.g., completing the program at home and around family obligations, and reducing stigma), and important for uptake and adherence (Beattie, Shaw, Kaur, & Kessler, 2009; O'Mahen et al., 2015; Pugh, Hadjistavropoulos, Hampton, Bowen, & Williams, 2015). Those who persist with interventions for depression report intrinsic motivation such as valuing task completion, a sense of empowerment and control, and recognize the need for external motivators to aid the development of habits for program use (Donkin & Glozier, 2012; Wilhelmsen et al., 2013). They are proactive users of the programs and are able to identify with and relate the program content to their daily lives (Bendelin et al., 2011; Gerhards et al., 2011). Highly motivated users also take more time and words to describe their problems in the program and, hence, are better able to utilize the program and may expect greater improvements (Van Der Zanden et al., 2014). They attribute personal benefits to the program and usually go on to complete treatment as planned (Donkin & Glozier, 2012; Svartvatten, Segerlund, Dennhag, Andersson, & Carlbring, 2015). However, finding program content personally relevant is key for users to learn and acquire new knowledge and skills, but not all users succeed in translating program contents and adaptations to real life (e.g., Lillevoll et al., 2013).

According to a review that examined adherence to guided iCBT and individual face-to-face CBT, adherence to iCBT and CBT may be equal (van Ballegooijen et al., 2014), although the researchers did not take into account that in-person CBT usually consists of more sessions than guided iCBT (12–28 vs. 5–9 sessions). Thus, therapist-support may help balancing the need for privacy, independence, and active engagement, and the need for assistance, dependence, and help to restructure the newly acquired knowledge to user's problems, thereby ensuring adherence (Wilhelmsen et al., 2013). In a study by Lillevoll and colleagues (2013), users emphasized the importance of dialogue with a professional to ask questions, discuss issues with someone, receive trustworthy feedback, be supported and acknowledged. A lack of support or "check-ins" with a therapist (or lay person) may lead users to consider that how they engage with the program is irrelevant and decrease their motivation to use the program as prescribed or completing it (e.g., using filler-words such as "blah, blah, blah …" instead of completing a written assignment in a meaningful way; Donkin & Glozier, 2012; Gerhards et al., 2011). It reduces any obligations to log on to the program, feelings of commitment, and sense of accountability. At the same time, users have reported being stressed by high expectations and demands from the therapist (Bendelin et al., 2011). In addition, guided self-help may also generate concerns such as loss of anonymity, feeling of being more exposed, and becoming a more passive recipient of treatment. Overall, internet interventions may solve issues with accessibility, reduce stigma, provide users with a sense of control for taking action and seeking help, but it also introduces new issues. On the one hand, the free nature of unguided self-help programs may attract users and make them engage in help-seeking behaviors, but also cause users to place less value on completing it (i.e., that it was without costs, time restrictions, therapist guidance, etc.). On the other hand, a sense of obligation to others, can make some users more reluctant to seek internet interventions, but be important for those who engage and who, for example, have doubts about internet interventions or experience delayed perceptions of their usefulness.

The Change Process

There are concerns about users withholding and not disclosing personal and relevant information that may be important for a therapist, and users have reported that the mode of communication has limited their ability to meaningfully convey their feelings or the therapists' ability to fully understand their problem (Beattie et al., 2009). However, most users establish a good therapeutic relationship with their therapist rather quickly, which enables them to commit and be honest, and perhaps even more so by the idea of "anonymity" online (Andersson et al., 2012; Beattie et al., 2009). Since online communication with the therapist is mostly text-based, it also enables users to see and review their responses on the screen, reflect and let things sink in, and gives them time and opportunity to formulate their thoughts. These reflective processes are likely to occur with unguided interventions as well. However, the most interesting in the absence of therapist-support, is that users may anthropomorphize the system such as describing a fully automated intervention as a social agent they "didn't want to disappoint" (Farzanfar, Frishkopf, Friedman, & Ludena, 2007). Such findings are in line with the seminal work by Reeves and Nass (1996), Bickmore and Gruber (2010), and others who have demonstrated that it is possible to design systems that can build a sense of trust, rapport, and convey empathy, without therapist-support. However, fully automated responses and interventions may more easily come about as insensitive and be perceived more negatively (Gega, Smith, & Reynolds, 2013).

Case studies illustrate how therapists may work to instill hope, raise awareness, reinforce adherence, and build a therapeutic relationship, by offering support and an understanding of a user's needs, thoughts, and feelings. For example, Pugh, Hadjistavropoulos, and Fuchs (2014) described a program module focused on activity planning and, although the user was successful in scheduling and carrying out activities, how the therapist was able to address her needs and worries unrelated to activity planning, but to so-called "first experiences" with a newborn baby (e.g., the baby having her first cough or cold). At the present, no fully automated systems can follow the ebbs and flows, and adapt to the user's needs such as a human in this case. In another case study, Pugh, Hadjistavropoulos, Klein, and Austin (2014) demonstrated how a therapist assisted a depressed male, in reinforcing adherence and applying his newly acquired knowledge and skills. The user opened up regarding his difficulties with relaxation when feeling down. The therapist provided words of encouragement (e.g., "nice to hear that you tried the relaxation exercises despite feeling low"), normalized his feelings (e.g., "many find it difficult to practice relaxation techniques at first"), and assisted with considering an action plan for his down days (e.g., "It will be your go-to plan when you are feeling unmotivated. Do you have any ideas what this plan might look like?").

As a result of internet interventions, users may also start to question the validity of their own thoughts, avoid categorical thinking, reality-check their depressive ideas, and engage in more flexible thinking (e.g., exploring alternative interpretations; Lillevoll et al., 2013). Such changes may, in turn, instigate behavioral changes and break cycles of inactivity (e.g., starting to play with kids or going to a dinner party). It is also interesting how language use may be an indicator or marker of treatment progress. In one study, researchers found that improvements in depression was predicted by use of more discrepancy words during treatment (e.g., "should", "wish" or "hope"; Van Der Zanden et al., 2014). Discrepancy words may be a linguistic marker for future aspirations and not merely shortcomings in the past or present. In another study, Svartvatten and colleagues (2015) identified how the content in e-mail exchanges between therapists and users can serve as an indication of treatment progress. More specifically, they found that user statements related to "observing positive consequences" (e.g., "When I went for a walk when feeling down, I noticed how it put me in a better mood") and "alliance" (e.g., "Thank you for your ideas. I think this exercise might prove be useful to me") were positively related to changes in depressive symptoms. Thus, there are issues that may be more specific to internet interventions such as worries about being misunderstood or avoidance of difficult therapeutic tasks in the absence of anyone to "check in" on the user (Gega et al., 2013). However, it appears that the ingredients in the therapeutic processes such as alliance, regardless of whether the intervention is designed with or without therapist-support, are similar to traditional psychotherapy.

Adverse Effects

Barak and colleagues (2009, p. 5) define the purpose of internet interventions as "*... to create a positive change and/or improve/enhance knowledge, awareness, and understanding via the provision of sound health-related material and use of interactive web-based components*". Most will agree with the purpose to create a positive change, but it is also important not to forget that there may be negative changes as a consequence of using internet interventions. However, only one study has explicitly examined the side-effects of internet interventions (Rozental, Boettcher, Andersson, Schmidt, & Carlbring, 2015). As with face-to-face therapy, the researchers found that increased awareness and insight into the user's own problems occasionally lead to, at least, a temporary deterioration. Learning about their condition may cause users to pay more attention to negative events, feeling vulnerable, anxious or regretful, noticing new problems, facing problems that were previously avoided, or increase subjective health complaints (e.g., headaches or muscle tensions). Another side-effect was the exhausting program schedule (Rozental et al., 2015). Given that most internet interventions follow a regular schedule, some felt pressured by tight time schedules and lack of flexibility, particularly by having to complete many tasks during a short time interval, and eventually falling behind schedule and becoming frustrated. Life events, positive or negative, may also interfere with users' experiences and ability to adhere to internet interventions. In a study by O'Mahen and colleagues (2015), postpartum women reported that the demands of motherhood directly interfered with their ability to complete the program. This, in turn, increased their feelings of hopelessness which is characteristic of depression. Some women also felt overwhelmed by the program and found the flexibility and minimal support difficult to manage. In such a case, it is important that the failure to use and benefit from an internet intervention, does not add to the burden of being depressed and nourish feelings of hopelessness.

For Whom

Most studies have been concerned with experiences related to adherence and the change process as reviewed above. Based on this, it is clear that internet interventions may be appropriate for intrinsically motivated users (e.g., desire to learn more about themselves) and users who have perceptions of benefit (e.g., their general physician recommending a program that may be helpful). However, only one study has looked directly into who benefits from internet interventions for depression. Bendelin and colleagues (2011) identified three types of users; (a) readers, (b) strivers, and (c) doers. Readers were typically characterized as not able or willing to put their new insight into practice and working sporadically through the materials. The autonomy of working through the guided intervention proved to be an obstacle for adherence, and they wished for more help and support. Strivers worked with the program in a practical way and succeeded to integrate some of the program contents into everyday life. However, they also expressed ambivalence towards working on their own, had doubts about treatment effects, and were not able to fully profit from treatment. They wished for more contact with their therapist to overcome barriers during treatment, but, at the same time, felt stressed by the demands from the therapist. Doers applied the program to their daily experiences and real-life events, in structured and methodic manner. This systematic and practice-oriented approach seemed to help overcome many barriers, and was often described as the most valuable lessons. They also appreciated working on their own and the responsibility that came with the program. More research is, however, needed to investigate who these readers, strivers, and doers are, and whether these represent different groups of users for whom internet interventions may be appropriate (or not) and that can be reliably identified, or whether experiences can vary within users (Knowles et al., 2014).

MAIN PURPOSE OF THIS STUDY

The literature review shows that unguided and guided internet and computer-based interventions are experienced and perceived both positively and negatively in terms of adherence, the change process, and for whom such interventions may be appropriate. It also shows that more qualitative research is needed for preventive interventions and interventions using therapeutic approaches other than CBT, as most of the qualitative studies have been conducted on CBT programs for users with sub-clinical depression (e.g., Pugh et al., 2015; Svartvatten et al., 2015; Van Der Zanden et al., 2014; Wilhelmsen et al., 2013). The main objective for this study was, therefore, to gain insight into users' experiences of an internet intervention for perinatal depression by acquiring knowledge and an understanding of how the program is perceived among pregnant and postpartum women. The study was set up investigate positive and negative factors that could affect adherence to the program, and identify opportunities for further development and risks that need to be addressed. More generally, this study can contribute to the strategic planning and development of the current and future interventions.

METHODS

Study Design and Participants

This study used semi-structured interviews by following the strengths, weaknesses, opportunities, and threats (SWOT) format and surveying participant characteristics. Participants were recruited through a randomized controlled trial (RCT), after being randomly assigned to receive the internet intervention. All participants were enrolled for the study, the intervention, and invited for an interview, consecutively. Inclusion criteria for being invited for interview were either: (a) completing the intervention or (b) no program activity during the last 4 weeks or (c) lagging 3 or more sessions behind prescribed intervention schedule. The criteria for participation in the study was being 18 years or older, and being pregnant between gestation week 21 and 25. There were 10 participants partaking in the study, all females, who were either pregnant or had given birth at the time of the interview.

Measures

Demographic information such as age, due date, number of children, education, occupation and relationship status, and native country, was collected at baseline. In addition, participants completed the following measures:

The *Edinburgh Postnatal Depression Scale* (EPDS; Cox, Holden, & Sagovsky, 1987) which is a 10-item self-report scale that is used to assess depressive symptoms in the past 7 days among mothers, during pregnancy and after childbirth (e.g., "*I have been so unhappy that I have had difficulty sleeping*"). Items are scored on a scale from 0 to 3 and yield a total score from 0 to 30 with higher scores indicating more depressive symptomatology. A score of 10 or greater indicates a possible depression.

The *Satisfaction with Life Scale* (SWLS; Diener, Emmons, Larsen, & Griffin, 1985) is a 5-item self-report scale designed to assess people's overall cognitive judgment of their life. Participants rate items such as "*My life is in many ways close to my ideal*", on a scale from 1 ("*completely disagree*") to 7 ("*completely agree*"). Total scores range from 5 to 25 with higher scores indicating greater life satisfaction.

The *Positive and Negative Affect Schedule* (PANAS; Watson, Clark, & Tellegen, 1988) consists of two 10-item self-report scales that measure positive (e.g., "*alert*" and "*enthusiastic*") and negative (e.g., "*anger*" and "*nervousness*") dimensions of affect. Participants indicated to what extent they had felt this way during the past 7 days on a scale from 1 ("*Not at all*") to 5 ("*Very much*").

Interviews

In the present study, semi-structured interviews were conducted based on the open-ended Strengths, Weaknesses, Opportunities, and Threats (SWOT) format. The open-ended format encourages participants' free reflections on the use of the intervention, with minimal interruptions from the interviewer. It does, however, provide a certain structure to participant's reflections without specifying a particular type of answers (Lone et al., 2013). Each of the participants were asked the following four questions:

Please tell me about what you perceive as the advantages of and that seems to work well with Mamma Mia; we refer to this as the strengths of the program.

Please tell me about what you perceive as the disadvantages of and that does not seem to work well with Mamma Mia; we refer to this as the weaknesses of the program.

Please tell me about what you consider to be the possibilities of improving the quality of Mamma Mia; we refer to this as the opportunities of the program.

Please tell me about what you consider to be the obstacles to Mamma Mia; we refer to this as the threats to the program.

The first part of the interview consisted mainly of allowing participant to speak freely about the different SWOTs (i.e., open-ended part). This ensures that the interviewer influences the participant's answers or drives the conversation in a certain direction, only to a minimal degree. This open-ended structure generally results in a wider range of information retrieved. In the second part (i.e., explorative part), the interviewer used probing questions to obtain additional information and richer descriptions of the SWOTs identified in the open-ended part of the interview such as "Could you please provide an example of […]", "What do you mean by […]?", or "Do I understand you correctly when you say that [...]". Based on the answers given in part one, the interviewer systematically worked through the various SWOTs, as identified by the participant, to clarify specific issues. Two interviewers conducted the interviews separately. Interviews were conducted during the period of March to September in 2014. Five of the interviews were carried out at the Regional Center for Child and Adolescent Mental Health (RBUP), Eastern and Southern Norway, two at home visits, and three by telephone. The length of the interviews ranged between 30 minutes to 77 minutes (*mean* = 53.0 minutes). All interviews were recorded and transcribed electronically.

Mamma Mia

In this study, Mamma Mia was deployed as an unguided, universal intervention designed to (1) prevent the onset and development of perinatal depression and (2) enhance subjective well-being, among pregnant and postpartum women. The intervention consists of 44 sessions over a period of 11 ½ months, starting in pregnancy between gestational week 17 to 24, and lasts into the postpartum period, 6 months after childbirth. Mamma Mia is available on both PC/Mac, tablets, and mobile phones. The woman receives an e-mail with a unique hyperlink for every new session that becomes available. By clicking the hyperlink, she is directed to the unique program contents for that particular session. The core organizing principles for the delivery of the program and its contents is the tunneled design. This means that each session, which is designed to take 10 to 15 minutes, must be completed before proceeding to the next session. In a similar way, the program content is presented in a predetermined sequence on a page-by-page basis. There are 5 main components in the Mamma Mia program; (1) monitoring and identification of depressive symptoms by means of the EPDS, (2) help and support for managing depressive symptoms (e.g., ask for partner support), (3) mother's mental health and well-being (e.g., adopting a relaxing mindset), (4) partner relationship (e.g., expressing more positive emotions toward partner), and (5) the child and her development (e.g., demonstrating the infant's socio-emotional competence). These protective and risk factors have previously been identified as important with regard to the development of emotional distress in mothers and children during pregnancy and postpartum. For a comprehensive and systematic description of Mamma Mia, please access the intervention protocol (Drozd, Haga, Brendryen, & Slinning, 2015).

Data Analysis

Descriptives and frequencies were used to describe the sample characteristics. Interviews were transcribed verbatim, anonymized, and unitized into small, but meaningful statements, prior to the main qualitative analysis. A statement was defined as the smallest, meaningful analysis unit that expressed a logic, consistent, and separate point of view, and that can be a part of a sentence, several sentences or other fractions of communication (Hoff, Straumsheim, Bjørkli, & Bjørklund, 2009; Neuendorf, 2002). Data were then analyzed by the use of an inductive thematic analysis (Braun & Clarke, 2006), to identify women's experiences and perceptions of Mamma Mia. A thematic analysis is a flexible and inductive, data-driven approach, which is particularly compatible with the open-ended SWOT format. The analytic process was iterative, systematically going back to revise codes and themes in a non-linear fashion to improve analysis. In this regard, we employed participative inquiry, in which co-authors that did not take part of the thematic analysis, reviewed and commented on the coding along the way, ensuring reflection and refinement of the codes and coding process (Reason, 1994). Finally, residual statements that could not be coded onto any of the SWOTs were examined to determine whether these units contained any relevant information regarding women's experiences and perceptions of Mamma Mia.

RESULTS

Participants

All participating mothers were expecting one child and were aged from 28 to 41 with a mean age of 33.5 years. Seven women were first-time mothers, one had a child from before, and two women had two children prior to the current pregnancy. The women were highly educated, only one woman had a bachelor's degree, while three had a master's degree and six women had a degree requiring more than five years at a university or college. All of the participants were currently employed, either fulltime or part-time, or currently on maternity leave. Five of the women were married, while the remaining five women were living together with a partner. Seven women were native Norwegian and three were from Sweden, Denmark, and Iceland, respectively. By examining their depressive symptoms and subjective well-being, it was clear that these women had few symptoms of depression (*mean (M)* = 3.5; *standard deviation (SD)* = 2.7), were very much satisfied with their life (M = 22.9; SD = 1.6), and experienced more positive (M = 37.9; SD = 6.6) than negative emotions (M = 14.4; SD = 2.3).

SWOT Categories

Unitizing resulted in 790 statements with a mean of 79 (SD = 40) statements per participant. Three-hundred and forty (43.0%) statements were extracted from the open-ended part of the interview, 260 (32.9%) from exploration, and 190 (24.1%)

statements were unrelated to women's experiences with Mamma Mia (e.g., reflections on their pregnancy, partner or experiences from perinatal care). Consequently, 600 (75.9%) statements were identified and deemed relevant for analysis. Of these, 531 (88.5%) were coded onto one of the SWOT categories; 208 (34.7%) were coded as strengths, 114 (19.0%) as weaknesses, 170 (28.3%) as opportunities, and 39 (6.5%) as threats, not taking into account that some SWOTs may be counted several times. It is noted that 69 (11.5%) statements were coded as residuals (i.e., statements not captured by the SWOT dimensions). However, there were no emerging themes in the residual category that could add to the women's experiences with Mamma Mia. Thus, data from the residuals are not reported herein.

Key Themes

There were two emerging superordinate themes across each of the SWOT dimensions and that are related to; (1) the design of the program and (2) transition to motherhood. All women consistently emphasized both themes, but the fact that the themes were superordinate and spanned across the SWOTs, suggested that the program design and the way Mamma Mia supports women in their transition to becoming a mother, was a mixture of both positive and negative experiences.

Program Design

Strengths

First of all, women emphasized the accessibility of the program and using the internet as a channel for disseminating information, as one of its' major strengths. Being able to perform the program at home and at their own convenience was considered positive. The program contents and some of the exercises were seen as pleasant and rather easy to carry out, and conveyed in a light tone-of-voice. Especially, the combination of accessibility and pleasant exercises was highlighted.

For most of the time, I've been at home when I've done the exercises. That worked for me. If not, I wouldn't have bothered doing them. They are pleasant exercises. They help you find some peace [...] – Respondent 118

Mamma Mia came across as containing brief, yet quality assured information. It was often compared to other typical online sources of information many women often use during pregnancy and after giving birth. The participants favored Mamma Mia over other such websites and described it as more structured and trustworthy.

We receive so much input from all over, so the more information gathered ... it feels easy to deal with than that other mess. – Respondent 242

It was described as professional and highly credible, without being clinical. The credibility to the program was partly attributable to the fact that some women were recruited to the study at the hospital.

... it's good to have a service that is research-based and scientifically grounded, because if you look online ... on antenatal and postnatal mental health, it is easy to wind up on blogs where there are a lot of expressions of opinion... Those are not scientifically grounded, you get different answers, or you look for answers that you want, adapted to your situation. – Respondent 226

Weaknesses

The weaknesses related to the program design concerned the depth and relevance of information, and lack of flexibility. The content was, at times, perceived as obvious and lacking in depth, containing information easily retrieved from other sources such as magazines. The lack of depth was especially apparent among multiparous women, who emphasized that the program targeted young, first-time mothers, and was less suitable for multiparous women or women with pregnancy complications.

I feel like it appeals to first-time mothers who are in new relationships. And by young, I mean younger than twenty. I get a teenage-mom feeling, that they recently got together and wonder if they know each other. – Respondent 242

We had a different type of pregnancy than people generally have. There were no questions about that in the Mamma Mia program. Is the baby ill? Or do you know if you are getting a healthy baby? Our situation has been quiet different than those who get healthy babies. – Respondent 346

A lack of flexibility was reported, in general, as a weakness. Some women mentioned the lack of flexibility as not always finding an appropriate answer to the built-in EPDS in the program, or wanting to report the reason why they may, at times, have felt depressed, without being misunderstood or stigmatized.

[...] you had to answer for the last week if you felt overwhelmed. I thought to myself that I feel pretty tired, that's why things feel overwhelming, but in a manageable way. It's not like I'm about to slip into a depression kind of overwhelming. [...] I

get why the questions were as generic as they were, but I miss the opportunity to say why I answered as I did. – *Respondent 213*

This lack of flexibility was also mentioned in relation to subjects that women wanted to learn more about. Some sessions were considered too brief and superficial, with no links or suggestions as to where users could retrieve more information on the subject. This was clearly formulated by one woman who was annoyed by the "one-to-one problem-solution" formula.

There are too many times where only one approach is presented as a solution for a problem, without any alternative options. No possibility to ask for advice or be guided further if you tried something and it didn't work. – *Respondent 242*

Opportunities

Participants listed a number of opportunities for improvement, most of which were intended to deal with the weaknesses of the program (see above). However, they often made suggestions for new subjects regarding more practical care such as health behavior (e.g., indoor environment for babies), labor rights and workplace facilitation during pregnancy, and necessary safety-equipment. Further, the participants expressed a desire to manage the course of the program themselves, including choosing to go deeper into one subject of interest, or skip one. According to the women, this could also be resolved by adding links to other websites on various subjects, or connecting to a web portal with more information.

Threats

Threats were mostly concerned with the (automated) program schedule in the postpartum period. Due to a peak in depressive symptoms 4 to 6 weeks after birth, the frequency increases to three sessions per week for a period of 6 weeks. At the same time, the demands of motherhood, especially for new mothers, made it difficult to follow the program on a weekly basis postpartum. It felt a bit overwhelming and resulted in lagging behind schedule, which, in turn, was identified as a risk of discontinuing the program.

It's mostly the risk of not following through that I consider to be the biggest threat. Even though I have been healthy and had excess energy during my pregnancy, I thought it was a bit difficult. All of a sudden there were two or three sessions piled up. For instance, if I would struggle mentally, become apathetic, or had become depressed, then I would not have been able to do it. – *Respondent 167*

Transition to Motherhood

Strengths

Regarding the transition to motherhood, the program seemed comforting and preparing, being something the women looked forward to, and feeling like she was being taken care of and in good hands. Participants reported that the program was normalizing and non-judgmental, and has helped them look at things more positively in their everyday life.

...mental health is being talked about in a very nice and natural manner. I think that is great, that you can be prepared, knowing that many women go into a postpartum depression... – Respondent 167

It has also reminded me to be present, that's what the audio file [mindfulness exercise] highlights. So getting that reminder has helped me be more present when I walk to work, I notice the nice things around me, like birds and flowers. I am more attentive now. – Respondent 167

The psychoeducational information was also well received. They emphasized themes containing information about the baby as one of the strengths. The information createed awareness and self-reflection, and contained important reminders facilitating attachment and connecting with the baby.

I have a pretty hectic life, and when I sit down with the program, I fully focus on the pregnancy. This is pregnancy number three, so I barely remember what gestational week I'm in. It has just sort of run its course. So, that has been okay. I think it [the program] has made me pay more attention than I would normally. – Respondent 226

Weaknesses and Threats

Mamma Mia was perceived as not sufficiently taking into account the demands of motherhood (e.g., baby's irregular sleeping patterns, loss of energy, caretaking, etc.), which was both perceived as a weakness and a threat to the program. Women did not always have the time to complete the sessions as prescribed according to the program schedule, thus, falling behind and having more to do in the upcoming week. The relevance of information was thus affected by the tunneled design (i.e., having to complete one session before proceeding to the next). This resulted in perceiving the program as a nuisance or stressful. More importantly, by lagging behind, there was a risk of the information becoming irrelevant because it would no longer be aligned with, for example, gestational week during pregnancy or the baby's development after birth, eventually leading to discontinuation of the program.

Opportunities

Women suggested a parallel program dealing with problem-areas concerning difficulties relevant to multiparous women. Some participants also wished that the program facilitated more reflection, particularly self-reflection around subjects such as the partner relationship, transitioning into parenthood, and raising a child.

I think a well-designed program like this can lead to reflection or a conversation between partners. What do I really think, what do I really mean, how do I live my life? [...] Having these thoughts make me self-reflect. Or that my partner and me can clarify certain standpoints. I think a program like this should manage that. – Respondent 242

Including partner and significant others in what the mother is going through emotionally was also suggested, especially help to distinguish between postpartum blues and postpartum depression.

DISCUSSION

The purpose of this chapter was to review user experiences with internet and computer-based interventions for depression and add to this literature by presenting results from in-depth interviews of women's experiences from a preventive, unguided intervention for postpartum depression, and thereby identify factors that could potentially affect adherence and improve the quality of the program. There were two emerging, superordinate themes that spanned across the SWOTs; (1) program design and (2) transition to motherhood. Superordinate themes across SWOTs indicates that aspects of the program design and transition to motherhood were perceived both positively and negatively.

Women unanimously emphasized accessibility as a positive design characteristic. Designing accessible internet interventions addresses one of the important barriers for the prevention or treatment of perinatal depression, including lack of time and excess energy that many women experience during pregnancy (Goodman, 2009). The brief information in the program was valued, potentially contributing even further to the accessibility of Mamma Mia (i.e., being time-efficient). So far, the results from this study are aligned with the reviewed literature on user experiences with internet interventions for depression. However, despite that the content was considered trustworthy and generally likeable; several women emphasized its lack of depth as a weakness. This was particularly apparent among multiparous women, who claimed that parts of the content were irrelevant to their situation and contained things they already knew (e.g., from prior pregnancies), and that could possibly result in higher attrition among these women. Therapist-support could have been useful to help these women adapt program contents to their situation to some extent, but it is possible that multiparous women represent a different segment of the target population that are in need of different program content (e.g., sibling preparations or prior birth experiences).

The most consistent weakness of the program, however, was the intensity of the automated program schedule, in particular during the postpartum period. This was also considered a threat to adherence and relevance of the program, and unhelpful in the transition to motherhood. In the short term, this lead to irritation and stress, while in the longer term it contributed to a misalignment between the program content and the baby's actual age and development, thereby making the content personally irrelevant. Several women also explicitly and consistently expressed dissatisfaction with the tunneled sequence, which was characterized as inflexible. Tunneling, which does not allow skipping parts or going fast forward, could, in combination with the automated program schedule, contribute to sessions piling up and making it difficult use the program as prescribed.

Finally, Mamma Mia initiated cognitive processes such as increased awareness and reflection, and emotional processes such as comfort and normalization. They considered these processes to contribute to their well-being, attentiveness towards their pregnancy, and facilitating attachment to the baby. Furthermore, such cognitive and emotional processes could also prevent depressive symptoms and may potentially help women take early action when they start to feel more down (see e.g., Pugh, Hadjistavropoulos, Klein, et al., 2014).

SOLUTIONS AND RECOMMENDATIONS

The internet appears to be an important medium for the prevention of perinatal depression in terms of being accessible. The intention to use a program such as Mamma Mia, is dependent on its perceived unobtrusiveness and fit with users' daily lives (Drozd, Lehto, & Oinas-Kukkonen, 2012; O'Mahen et al., 2015). Once users start engaging with internet intervention, it should aim to instigate important cognitive and emotional processes that can promote maternal mental health and bonding with the baby by providing brief and concise contents. However, the brevity of information may lead to perceptions of program contents as lacking in depth or being superficial. There are several possible solutions to this problem;

First, is to include links to more information for those who are interested. Second, add dynamic content that goes more in-depth on certain subjects at a web portal or program home page. Third, add tailoring to adapt the contents to the individual user's needs and to make it more relevant (e.g., parity or prematurity). It is also important that interventions establish credibility early on. Credibility is important both for the uptake of interventions and their continued use (Jimison et al., 2008). In Mamma Mia, this is partly done by initially mentioning who has financed and developed the program (assuming that these are credible sources). It is unlikely that women would request more information in Mamma Mia, if they did not experience the program as credible. This may explain why women suggested more information on health behaviors such as physical activity and nutrition, practical information on workplace adaptations for pregnant women, safety equipment, and help to handle a changing body image.

Mamma Mia is a narrative-based program designed to build a relationship with the user and follow a certain program structure and chronology. This is the reason a tunneled design is used and, although it is known to have a negative effect on user's perception of efficiency (i.e., easy search and access to information in a program), tunneling leads to higher adherence (i.e., more time spent on website and pages visited) and increased knowledge gains (Crutzen, Cyr, & de Vries, 2012). This may, however, have unintended negative side effects in Mamma Mia and unguided interventions in general, especially in combination with an automated program schedule and a lengthy program (e.g., failure to adhere to the program may lead to increased hopelessness). As such, a module-based program with more separable components and/or some degree of (optional) support would seem beneficial for pregnant and postpartum women. In Norwegian perinatal care, midwives and public health nurses at well-baby clinics, and general physicians, are in position to provide such support. The anonymity and freedom of using internet self-help also seems to be a two-edged sword according to previous research. For some, this may motivate and lower the barrier to help-seeking, empower users, and provide a sense of mastery and control (e.g., Gerhards et al., 2011). For others, this may lead to a lack of commitment and lead to the discontinuation of the program unless some support is provided. Thus, Mamma Mia should be offered as both a guided and unguided option, depending on the woman's needs.

FUTURE RESEARCH DIRECTIONS

This study has two main limitations that are important to bear in mind while interpreting the results and directing future research. First, participant characteristics suggested that the women interviewed for this study were typically well-educated, employed, and living with partners. They also scored low on depressive symptoms and high on subjective well-being. After all, Mamma Mia is a program that is intended to be offered to all pregnant women. It is necessary to reach as many women as possible for preventing postpartum depression, including those who are doing well, because maternal mental health may change during pregnancy and postpartum (Wisner et al., 2013). The homogeneity of women in this study, however, does limit the generalizability of the results. Thus, a more diverse sample should be included in future studies by including women with lower socioeconomic status, single mothers, and women with a history of depressive disorders or current mild-to-moderate symptoms of depression (e.g., EPDS score ≥ 10).

This study adds to the literature by examining women's experiences with a program, which is based on principles other than CBT. However, a second limitation is the eclectic approach of Mamma Mia (see, Drozd et al., 2015). Mamma Mia is not limited to any one approach and utilizes principles from CBT, positive psychology, attachment-based methods, and several others. This adds a degree of uncertainty to the generalizability of the results to other internet interventions, particularly those based on a singular approach, although the findings in this study are recognizable from findings in other studies on women's experiences with iCBT (O'Mahen et al., 2015; Pugh, Hadjistavropoulos, & Fuchs, 2014). Therefore, on the one hand, future research should continue to examine user experiences with singular approaches to internet interventions other than CBT. On the other hand, more eclectic and module- or component-based approaches should be investigated. A meta-analysis of parent training programs has demonstrated that not all program components are equal (Wyatt Kaminski, Valle, Filene, & Boyle, 2008). Some are consistently associated with larger effects (e.g., parent-child interaction) and others with smaller effects (e.g., problem-solving). Consequently, future research should identify and test core program components that are consistently associated with larger effects and that can be combined in an eclectic approach (i.e., delivering evidence-based kernels), and potentially give a greater effect than any singular approach.

CONCLUSION

This chapter has reviewed the literature on user experiences with internet and computer-based interventions, and presented results from women's experiences with a universal, unguided intervention for the prevention of perinatal depression. The review showed that highly motivated users adhere to these programs and experience positive changes. The change process shares similarities with face-to-face therapy, but it is not entirely clear who may benefit from using internet interventions. Some of the results in the present study are aligned with the existing literature such as accessibility, but have also added implications for the future development of the design of unguided interventions for pregnant and postpartum women. These should offer more flexibility and support, which is particularly important to avoid adverse effects of using Mamma Mia in a hectic period in life and better support women in their transition to motherhood. Nevertheless, women found the program to be accessible and requested more content that could be attributable to the credibility of the program. Mamma Mia also offered comfort, self-reflection, and maternal bonding with the baby, and seemed to provide a viable platform for the prevention of perinatal depression.

ACKNOWLEDGMENT

Mamma Mia was developed by Changetech in collaboration with the Regional Centre for Child and Adolescent Mental Health (RBUP) for the Norwegian Women's Public Health Association (N.K.S.). This research was funded by the Norwegian Women's Public Health Association (project no.: H3/2013) and the Research Council of Norway (project no.: 213737).

REFERENCES

Andersson, G., Paxling, B., Wiwe, M., Vernmark, K., Felix, C. B., Lundborg, L., & Carlbring, P. et al. (2012). Therapeutic alliance in guided internet-delivered cognitive behavioural treatment of depression, generalized anxiety disorder and social anxiety disorder. *Behaviour Research and Therapy*, *50*(9), 544–550. doi:10.1016/j.brat.2012.05.003 PMID:22728647

Australian Psychological Society. (2011). *Guidelines for providing psychological services and products using the internet and telecommunications technologies*. Melbourne, Australia: Australian Psychological Society.

Barak, A., Klein, B., & Proudfoot, J. G. (2009). Defining Internet-supported therapeutic interventions. *Annals of Behavioral Medicine*, *38*(1), 4–17. doi:10.1007/s12160-009-9130-7 PMID:19787305

Beattie, A., Shaw, A., Kaur, S., & Kessler, D. (2009). Primary-care patients expectations and experiences of online cognitive behavioural therapy for depression: A qualitative study. *Health Expectations*, *12*(1), 45–59. doi:10.1111/j.1369-7625.2008.00531.x PMID:19250152

Bendelin, N., Hesser, H., Dahl, J., Carlbring, P., Nelson, K. Z., & Andersson, G. (2011). Experiences of guided Internet-based cognitive-behavioural treatment for depression: A qualitative study. *BMC Psychiatry*, *11*(1), 107. doi:10.1186/1471-244X-11-107 PMID:21718523

Bickmore, T. W., & Gruber, A. (2010). Relational agents in clinical psychiatry. *Harvard Review of Psychiatry*, *18*(2), 119–130. doi:10.3109/10673221003707538 PMID:20235777

Braun, V., & Clarke, V. (2006). Using thematic analysis in psychology. *Qualitative Research in Psychology*, *3*(2), 77–101. doi:10.1191/1478088706qp063oa

Cox, J. L., Holden, J. M., & Sagovsky, R. (1987). Detection of postnatal depression. Development of the 10-item Edinburgh Postnatal Depression Scale. *The British Journal of Psychiatry*, *150*(6), 782–786. doi:10.1192/bjp.150.6.782 PMID:3651732

Crutzen, R., Cyr, D., & de Vries, N. K. (2012). The role of user control in adherence to and knowledge gained from a website: Randomized comparison between a tunneled version and a freedom-of-choice version. *Journal of Medical Internet Research*, *14*(2), e45. doi:10.2196/jmir.1922 PMID:22532074

Cuijpers, P., Donker, T., Johansson, R., Mohr, D. C., van Straten, A., & Andersson, G. (2011). Self-guided psychological treatment for depressive symptoms: A meta-analysis. *PLoS ONE*, *6*(6), e21274. doi:10.1371/journal.pone.0021274 PMID:21712998

Cuijpers, P., Donker, T., van Straten, A., Li, J., & Andersson, G. (2010). Is guided self-help as effective as face-to-face psychotherapy for depression and anxiety disorders? A systematic review and meta-analysis of comparative outcome studies. *Psychological Medicine*, *40*(12), 1943–1957. doi:10.1017/S0033291710000772 PMID:20406528

Dennis, C. L., & Chung-Lee, L. (2006). Postpartum depression help-seeking barriers and maternal treatment preferences: A qualitative systematic review. *Birth*, *33*(4), 323–331. doi:10.1111/j.1523-536X.2006.00130.x PMID:17150072

Diener, E., Emmons, R. A., Larsen, R. J., & Griffin, S. (1985). The satisfaction with life scale. *Journal of Personality Assessment*, *49*(1), 71–75. doi:10.1207/s15327752jpa4901_13 PMID:16367493

Donkin, L., & Glozier, N. (2012). Motivators and motivations to persist with online psychological interventions: A qualitative study of treatment completers. *Journal of Medical Internet Research*, *14*(3), e91. doi:10.2196/jmir.2100 PMID:22743581

Drozd, F., Haga, S. M., Brendryen, H., & Slinning, K. (2015). An Internet-based intervention (Mamma Mia) for postpartum depression: Mapping the development from theory to practice. *JMIR Research Protocols*, *4*(4), e120. doi:10.2196/resprot.4858 PMID:26476481

Drozd, F., Lehto, T., & Oinas-Kukkonen, H. (2012). Exploring perceived persuasiveness of a behavior change support system: A structural model. In M. Bång & E. Ragnmalm (Eds.), *The 7th Conference on Persuasive Technology* (pp. 157–168). Linköping, Sweden: Springer-Verlag. doi:10.1007/978-3-642-31037-9_14

Farzanfar, R., Frishkopf, S., Friedman, R., & Ludena, K. (2007). Evaluating an automated mental health care system: Making meaning of human-computer interaction. *Computers in Human Behavior*, *23*(3), 1167–1182. doi:10.1016/j.chb.2004.11.015

Gega, L., Smith, J., & Reynolds, S. (2013). Cognitive behaviour therapy (CBT) for depression by computer vs. therapist: Patient experiences and therapeutic processes. *Psychotherapy Research*, *23*(2), 218–231. doi:10.1080/10503307.2013.766941 PMID:23390994

Gerhards, S. A. H., Abma, T. A., Arntz, A., de Graaf, L. E., Evers, S. M. A. A., Huibers, M. J. H., & Widdershoven, G. A. M. (2011). Improving adherence and effectiveness of computerised cognitive behavioural therapy without support for depression: A qualitative study on patient experiences. *Journal of Affective Disorders*, *129*(1-3), 117–125. doi:10.1016/j.jad.2010.09.012 PMID:20889214

Goodman, J. H. (2009). Womens attitudes, preferences, and perceived barriers to treatment for perinatal depression. *Birth*, *36*(March), 60–69. doi:10.1111/j.1523-536X.2008.00296.x PMID:19278385

Hoff, T., Straumsheim, P., Bjørkli, C. A., & Bjørklund, R. A. (2009). An external validation of two psychosocial work environment surveys - A SWOT approach. *Scandinavian Journal of Organization Psychology*, *1*(1), 12–19.

Jimison, H. B., Gorman, P., Woods, S., Nygren, P., Walker, M., Norris, S., & Hersh, W. (2008). *Barriers and drivers of health information technology use for the elderly, chronically ill, and underserved*. Rockville, MD: Agency for Healthcare Research and Quality.

Knowles, S. E., Toms, G., Sanders, C., Bee, P., Lovell, K., Rennick-Egglestone, S., & Bower, P. et al. (2014). Qualitative meta-synthesis of user experience of computerised therapy for depression and anxiety. *PLoS ONE*, *9*(1), e84323. doi:10.1371/journal.pone.0084323 PMID:24465404

Lillevoll, K. R., Wilhelmsen, M., Kolstrup, N., Høifødt, R. S., Waterloo, K., Eisemann, M., & Risør, M. B. (2013). Patients experiences of helpfulness in guided internet-based treatment for depression: Qualitative study of integrated therapeutic dimensions. *Journal of Medical Internet Research, 15*(6), e126. doi:10.2196/jmir.2531 PMID:23786763

Lone, J. A., Bjørklund, R. A., Østerud, K. B., Anderssen, L. A., Hoff, T., & Bjørkli, C. A. (2014). Assessing knowledge-intensive work environment: General versus situation-specific instruments. *European Journal of Work and Organizational Psychology, 23*(3), 469–482. doi:10.1080/1359432X.2012.750449

Marcus, M., Yasamy, M. T., van Ommeren, M., Chisholm, D., & Saxena, S. (2012). *Depression: A global public health concern*. Geneva, Switzerland: World Health Organization.

Mykletun, A., Knudsen, A. K., & Mathiesen, K. S. (2009). *Psykiske lidelser i Norge: Et folkehelseperspektiv* [Mental disorders in Norway: A public health perspective]. Oslo, Norway: Norwegian Institute of Public Health.

Neuendorf, K. A. (2002). *The content analysis guidebook*. Thousand Oaks, CA: Sage Publications Inc.

Norwegian Directorate of Health. (2009). *Nasjonale retningslinjer for diagnostisering og behandling av voksne med depresjon i primær- og spesialisthelsetjenesten* [National guidelines for diagnosis and treatment of adults with depression in primary and secondary care]. Oslo, Norway: Norwegian Directorate of Health.

O'Mahen, H. A., Grieve, H., Jones, J., McGinley, J., Woodford, J., & Wilkinson, E. L. (2015). Womens experiences of factors affecting treatment engagement and adherence in internet delivered behavioural activation for postnatal depression. *Internet Interventions, 2*(1), 84–90. doi:10.1016/j.invent.2014.11.003

Overland, S., Glozier, N., Krokstad, S., & Mykletun, A. (2007). Undertreatment before the award of a disability pension for mental illness: The HUNT Study. *Psychiatric Services, 58*(11), 1479–1482. doi:10.1176/ps.2007.58.11.1479 PMID:17978260

Pugh, N. E., Hadjistavropoulos, H. D., & Fuchs, C. M. (2014). Internet therapy for postpartum depression: A case illustration of emailed therapeutic assistance. *Archives of Women's Mental Health, 17*(4), 327–337. doi:10.1007/s00737-014-0439-2 PMID:24965602

Pugh, N. E., Hadjistavropoulos, H. D., Hampton, A. J. D., Bowen, A., & Williams, J. (2015). Client experiences of guided internet cognitive behavior therapy for postpartum depression: A qualitative study. *Archives of Women's Mental Health, 18*(2), 209–219. doi:10.1007/s00737-014-0449-0 PMID:25109484

Pugh, N. E., Hadjistavropoulos, H. D., Klein, B., & Austin, D. W. (2014). A case study illustrating therapist-assisted internet cognitive behavior therapy for depression. *Cognitive and Behavioral Practice, 21*(1), 64–77. doi:10.1016/j.cbpra.2013.08.002

Reason, P. (1994). Co-operative inquiry, participatory action research, and action inquiry: Three approaches to participative inquiry. In N. K. Denzin & Y. S. Lincoln (Eds.), *Handbook of qualitative research* (pp. 324–339). Thousand Oaks, CA: Sage.

Reeves, B., & Nass, C. (1996). *The media equation: How people treat computers, television and new media like real people and places*. Stanford, CA: Cambridge University Press.

Rozental, A., Boettcher, J., Andersson, G., Schmidt, B., & Carlbring, P. (2015). Negative effects of internet interventions: A qualitative content analysis of patients experiences with treatments delivered online. *Cognitive Behaviour Therapy, 44*(3), 223–236. doi:10.1080/16506073.2015.1008033 PMID:25705924

Svartvatten, N., Segerlund, M., Dennhag, I., Andersson, G., & Carlbring, P. (2015). A content analysis of client e-mails in guided internet-based cognitive behavior therapy for depression. *Internet Interventions, 2*(2), 121–127. doi:10.1016/j.invent.2015.02.004

The National Board of Health and Wellfare. (2010). *Nationella riktlinjer för vård vid depression och ångestsyndrom 2010 - stöd för styrning och ledning* [National guidelines for care in cases of depression and anxiety disorders]. Stockholm, Sweden: The National Board of Health and Wellfare.

van Ballegooijen, W., Cuijpers, P., Van Straten, A., Karyotaki, E., Andersson, G., Smit, J. H., & Riper, H. (2014). Adherence to internet-based and face-to-face cognitive behavioural therapy for depression: A meta-analysis. *PLoS ONE, 9*(7), e100674. doi:10.1371/journal.pone.0100674 PMID:25029507

Van Der Zanden, R., Curie, K., Van Londen, M., Kramer, J., Steen, G., & Cuijpers, P. (2014). Web-based depression treatment: Associations of clients word use with adherence and outcome. *Journal of Affective Disorders, 160*, 10–13. doi:10.1016/j.jad.2014.01.005 PMID:24709016

Watson, D., Clark, L. A., & Tellegen, A. (1988). Development and validation of brief measures of positive and negative affect: The PANAS Scales. *Journal of Personality and Social Psychology, 54*(6), 1063–1070. doi:10.1037/0022-3514.54.6.1063 PMID:3397865

Wilhelmsen, M., Lillevoll, K. R., Risør, M. B., Høifødt, R. S., Johansen, M.-L., Waterloo, K., & Kolstrup, N. et al. (2013). Motivation to persist with internet-based cognitive behavioural treatment using blended care: A qualitative study. *BMC Psychiatry, 13*(1), 296. doi:10.1186/1471-244X-13-296 PMID:24199672

Wisner, K. L., Sit, D. K. Y., Mcshea, M. C., Rizzo, D. M., Zoretich, R. A., Hughes, C. L., & Hanusa, B. H. et al. (2013). Onset timing, thoughts of self-harm, and diagnoses in postpartum women with screen-positive depression findings. *Journal of American Medical Association Psychiatry, 70*(5), 490–498. doi:10.1001/jamapsychiatry.2013.87.Onset

World Health Organization. (2009). *Global health risks: Mortality and burden of disease attributable to selected major risks*. Geneva, Switzerland: World Health Organization; doi:10.2471/BLT.09.070565

World Health Organization. (2010). Depression. Retrieved February 19, 2016, from http://www.who.int/mental_health/management/depression/en/

Wyatt Kaminski, J., Valle, L. A., Filene, J. H., & Boyle, C. L. (2008). A meta-analytic review of components associated with parent training program effectiveness. *Journal of Abnormal Child Psychology, 36*(4), 567–589. doi:10.1007/s10802-007-9201-9 PMID:18205039

KEY TERMS AND DEFINITIONS

Internet-Based Cognitive Behavioral Therapy (iCBT): The most commonly used psychotherapeutic approach for treating mental health problems on the internet based on the same principles as in-person cognitive behavior therapy.

Mamma Mia: An unguided internet intervention designed to prevent pre- and postnatal depression and promote subjective well-being among pregnant and postpartum women.

Perinatal Depression: Onset or elevated symptoms of depression during pregnancy and the first 6 months following childbirth.

Strengths, Weaknesses, Opportunities, and Threats (SWOT): A systematic method and tool for assessment of internal and external environments to support strategic planning and decision-making, and development of products, organizations, and services.

Subjective Well-Being: Refers to people's experience of the quality of their lives and encompasses cognitive evaluations of life and emotional reactions.

Tunneled Design: A directive information architecture that guides users step-by-step through a predetermined sequence of web pages and/or sessions in order to improve the chances of achieving a goal.

Unguided Intervention: A fully automated and self-guided internet intervention without any therapist-support or human involvement.

Chapter 3
Treating Sleep Disorders with an ACT-Based Behavior Change Support System

Sitwat Usman Langrial
Sur University College, Oman

Päivi Lappalainen
University of Jyväskylä, Finland

Harri Oinas-Kukkonen
University of Oulu, Finland

Raimo Lappalainen
University of Jyväskylä, Finland

ABSTRACT

Suitable duration and appropriate quality of sleep are essential for mental and cognitive wellbeing. Sleep disorders, whether mild or severe, have proven to have adverse effects on general wellbeing. One's quality of life could be disturbed as a consequence of various mental conditions, sleep disorders being one of them. Researchers have started paying attention to designing, implementing and evaluating eHealth interventions to address sleep disorders. In this chapter, we highlight findings from a field study that was conducted to evaluate effect of software features on a Web-based intervention for sleep disorders. Tyyne is a Web-based eHealth intervention that will be repeatedly mentioned as Behavior Change Support Systsm (BCSS). Tynne offered weekly modules that were drawn from Acceptance and Commitment Therapy (ACT). From an Information system's perspective, the modules were identified and applied as a persuasive software feature that is promoted by the Persuasive Systems Design Model (PSD Model). The duration of the Web-based intervention was 6 weeks.

DOI: 10.4018/978-1-5225-3241-5.ch003

Upon completion of the intervention, about one third (37.2%) of the participants reported that they could better manage their sleep problems. We argue that a relatively low percentage is still highly encouraging, as treatment of sleep-related disorders is a complicated and understudied area. Manifestly, longitudinal studies would help determine the effect of ACT-incorporated Web-based interventions. However, the chapter underscores the effect of persuasive software features incorporated with ACT-based components as a step towards managing sleep disorders.

1. INTRODUCTION

Suitable duration and decent quality of sleep are crucial for mental and cognitive wellbeing. Sleep disorders, whether mild or severe, have proven adverse effects on general wellbeing. One's quality of life could be poor as a consequence of various mental conditions, sleep disorders being one of them. Sleeplessness both in terms of quality and/or quantity, leads to serious health issues such as cognitive functioning (Frenda & Fenn, 2016), mood disorder (Kahn-Greene et al. 2007), depression (Hemmeter et al. 2010), obesity (Patel & Hu, 2008), metabolic disorders and diabetes (Knutson & Van Cauter, 2008). There could be various reasons for people's unhealthy lifestyles. Because of their detrimental effect on one's mental and general health, sleep disorders are a research area (Langrial et al. 2014; Alhola & Polo-Kantola, 2007). Literature provides reassuring indications that sleep disorders are negatively correlated with an individual's health and mental wellbeing irrespective of age, gender and social status. According to van Straten and Cuijpers (2009), sleep related disorders, including insomnia, are common among individuals. Sleep deprivation and insomnia have several negative consequences for individuals; for example, fatigue, mood instabilities, psychological stress and addictive disorders (van Straten &Cuijpers, 2009; Gillin, 1998). Sleep disorders are regularly associated with poor life quality, reduced work productivity, fear, despair, and alcoholism (Walsh, 2004). Further, lack of sleep could adversely affect neurocognitive functioning, as stated earlier. The growing number of the population suffering from sleep disorders is indicative that it has now become a widespread issue (Morin et al. 2006). More than 20% of the adult population alone suffers from sleep disorders (Goel et al. 2009). The effects of sleep disorders on general well-being are frightening (Faubel et al. 2009).

It is a promising sign to note that sleep disorders have received increasing attention because of their negative psychological consequences (Espie et al. 2012; Vincent & Lewycky, 2009; Ström et al. 2004; Moul et al. 2004). Existing literature has a rich body of studies that focus on healthy diet and regular exercise, and that good sleep quality is vital for health (Choe et al. 2011). EHealth interventions that promote nourishing diet (Purpura et al. 2011) and energetic lifestyles (Albanina et al.

2009) have been well studied. Surprisingly, sleep disorders have gained researchers' attention in more recent times. Mental health conditions, including sleep disorders, pose on-going challenges for researchers from the field of Information Systems, Behavior Change Interventions and Clinical Psychology. Developing and evaluating effective eHealth interventions for sleep disorders calls for creativity leading to novel solutions.

Behavioral Psychology that incorporates Persuasive Software Features has opened up new opportunities to develop novel Cognitive Behavioral Interventions for people with mental health conditions. Promising effects of such interventions have been repeatedly reported, especially when information systems (interventions) are incorporated with Cognitive Behavioral Therapies (Kuonanoja et al. 2015; Andersson & Cuijpers, 2009; Amstadter et al. 2009; Kiropoulus et al. 2008; Ybarra & Eaton, 2005).

Several research studies have been conducted in Medicine and Behavioral Psychology. Findings from such studies underline the potential of CBT-based eHealth interventions in better managing sleep-related disorder. For example, Vincent and Lewycky (2009) evaluated the effect of an online intervention for insomnia. The intervention included pyschoeducation and cognitive therapy. Vincent and Lewycky (2009) highlight statistically significant improvements in subjects' sleep quality. Earlier, Ritterband et al. (2009) examined effects of CBT-based intervention for people suffering from insomnia. The intervention was based on face-to-face therapy. Ritterband et al. (2009) conclude that the treatment / intervention was effective and people developed positive sleep routines.

A number of factors are known that prevent people with mental disorders from using traditional (face-to-face) treatments. Some of the identified factors include lack of motivation, hesitation to share personal experiences, poor health care facilities, relatively higher treatment costs, privacy concerns and social stigma (Aromaa et al. 2011; Thom & Campbell, 1997).

There is a recent trend among the Human-Computer Interaction (HCI) researchers relating with studying and investigating eHealth technologies aimed at behaviour change (Consolvo et al. 2009). In order to overcome the above-mentioned barriers, several information systems (interventions) have been designed. Researchers have identified promising outcomes from several studies where online cognitive therapies are delivered using persuasive design software (Kuonanoja et al. 2015). Among the studied domains, are, to name a few, smoking cessation, obesity, diabetes, anxiety, stress and depression (e.g. Hamari et al. 2014). Persuasive Information Systems are interactive technologies that are developed with a special focus on helping people change their attitudes and/or behaviours (Fogg, 2002). Another requisite for persuasive information systems is that they do not employ coercion or deception as proposed by (Oinas-Kukkonen & Harjumaa, 2009).

Realizing the growing and persistent challenge of sleep disorders among general population, presented intervention was designed and examined using a Web-based Behavior Change Support System (Oinas-Kukkonen, 2010, 2013). A Behavior Change Support System can be considered as an extension of Persuasive Information Systems (Langrial, 2012). The main objective of the intervention was to examine and identify likely impact of reminders on task adherence and Acceptance and Commitment-based online rehearsal on the ability to manage sleep behaviors respectively. Online or more specifically, virtual rehearsal is advocated as a persuasive software feature that can help people practice and consequently learn new behaviors (Langrial et al. 2014). As stated earlier, very little research has been conducted on virtual rehearsal (Kelders et al. 2012), especially in the research fields of HCI and eHealth for mental wellbeing.

Psychologists have been emphasizing on the need for developing effective solutions for mental conditions such as sleep disorders. Lim and Dinges (2008) have been persistent in arguing that there is an urgent need to help people manage sleep disorders. Unexpectedly, a limited amount of published literature is available that examines probable explanations and solutions for sleep disorders. For example, Manber et al. (2008) conducted a study to examine the impact of Cognitive Behavioral Therapy on sleeplessness. They suggest that symptom-focused cognitive Behavioral Therapy has promising effects for people suffering for sleeplessness, as well as depression. Langrial et al. (2012) worked on a BCSS for sleep deprivation. They carried out a pilot study and evaluated a web-based BCSS using software features from the Persuasive Systems Design model (Oinas-Kukkonen &Harjumaa, 2009). The pilot study was conducted to identify whether virtual rehearsal could be used to help people learn new behaviors related with sleep deprivation.

This chapter presents outcomes of a six-week field study. A Web-based eHealth intervention (BCSS) was designed and implemented to support participants learning and practicing new skills to better manage sleep problems. The chapter is structured to report participants' pre- intervention expectations, post- intervention remarks and finally identified differences in pre- and post- intervention psychological measures.

2. BACKGROUND

Oh et al. (2005) define eHealth as delivering of healthcare solutions using technological platforms such as information systems. The potential advantages of eHealth interventions have been highlighted in terms of reach, ease of access, accessibility, cost effectiveness, and novel sustainable solutions (Murray, 2012). Ritterband and Tate (200) further endorse eHealth interventions for healthcare by highlighting Web-based healthcare interventions as scalable and efficient. It does not come as a surprise that Health Psychology-related research has been utilizing the Internet as a delivery medium frequently (Kraft &Yardley, 2009).

Current studies reveal success of CBT-based eHealth interventions delivered through the Internet (Andersson and Cuijpers, 2009). Seligman et al. (2011) support the effectiveness of CBT-based eHealth interventions for mental health by proposing that such interventions have indicated noteworthy medical and statistical results. Similarly, Sivertsen et al. (2006) have performed studies on sleeplessness. They propose that CBT-based eHealth interventions are superior when compared with Zoplicone treatment. Cognitive Behavior literature offers adequate support pertaining to the use of CBT-based eHealth interventions.

Yet few studies have reported the use of *acceptance* and *value-based* eHealth interventions that employ (Lappalainen et al. 2015) Acceptance and Commitment Therapy (ACT) (e.g. Gaudiano & Herbert, 2006; Forman et al. 2007). ACT is known to increase psychological flexibility because it is positively correlated with improved mental health (Lappalainen et al. 2015; Hayes et al. 2005). Thoughtful works have been performed to develop and assess eHealth for mental well-being with a specific focus on task adherence (Makai et al. 2014), user satisfaction (Kim & Chang, 2007) and overall psychological outcomes. Adequate sleep is positively correlated with improved health; however, issues related with sleep disorders remain an understudied area. Although reasonable research has been conducted to address the issue in Medical Informatics and Clinical Psychology, still there is manifest lack of investigation about sleep disorders in the fields of Information Systems (Langrial et al. 2012).

It is an encouraging observation that people have shown keen interest and willingness to try out different forms of treatments before deciding to contact healthcare professionals (Morin et al. 2005). Such observations underline noteworthy premises and open opportunities for researchers to overcome identified research gaps. More importantly, it is proposed that people with sleep disorders do not necessarily seek medical treatments. They are eager to try alternative options (Langrial et al. 2012).

HCI researchers have stressed on designing eHealth interventions that can bring envisioned change in users' behaviors. Identifying the scope for treating sleep disorders through Information Technology, Choe et al. (2011) propose that technological innovations could be used to improve poor sleep habits. They further argue that designing eHealth interventions for sleep disorders is a challenging task and therefore it is essential to have a thorough understanding of factors including culture, privacy and individual sleep habits. Their work highpoints the importance of improving sleep disorders through eHealth interventions, and at the same time indicates that there are design prospects for developing such interventions. While Choe et al. (2011) offer an appealing framework for developing eHealth interventions for sleep disorders, we suggest that their framework does not provide explicit guidelines. Consolvo et al. (2009) emphasize on utilizing behavior change theories when designing eHealth interventions. Their design strategies are valuable; however, to the best of our knowledge, evaluating the effect of definite persuasive software features has been fairly disregarded. This particular gap is evident when it comes to persuasive software features such as virtual rehearsal. Rehearsal or learning through practice (Thorpe et al. 1987) has largely been expended in CBT-related studies. Psychological specialists have recognized intellectual improvements through performance-based process. Importance of rehearsal as a behavior change method has further been testified by (Thorpe et al. 1987) who uphold that rehearsal is a beneficial method for refining self-efficacy.

There is some evidence that supports practicality of rehearsal for learning new behaviors. Jaafar and Nur (2009) studied virtual rehearsal for educating children with an aim to ease dental anxiety. However, the implemented software was more related with simulation, which is different from virtual rehearsal (Oinas-Kukkonen &Harjumaa, 2009). Similarly, Fogg (2002) promotes virtual rehearsal as a means to provide a setting where people can exercise and learn new behaviors. Rehearsal has also been studied in other settings, for example computer training (Davis &Yi, 2004). They highlight Social Cognitive Theory (SCT) by Bandura (1986). SCT proposes that learning process is primarily "an information processing activity in which information about the structure of behavior and about environmental events is transformed into symbolic representations that serve as cognitive guides for the construction of complex modes of behavior" (Bandura, 1986, p.51). Niemi et al. (2003) have worked on Web-based learning environments. They grounded their work on Self-regulation, Self-determination and Self-efficacy as core psychological procedures that in their opinion can lead to empowering users (Fetterman, 2001). Niemi et al. (2003) state that for learning new skills, rehearsal, critical thinking, and connecting previous and new information are the keys. In their work, Nakanishi et al. (2005) suggest that virtual training simplifies learning process. They conclude that it is comparatively hard to learn new behaviors through reading and simulation, thus supporting the potential of virtual rehearsal as an appropriate method.

We opted to examine selected persuasive software features and their probable effect on the efficiency of a Web-based eHealth intervention (BCSS) for sleep disorder. As stated by Oinas-Kukkonen and Harjumaa (2009), interactive Information Systems are expected to provide immediate feedback and simplify task completion. In other words, we categorize Web-based eHealth interventions as BCSSs that are persuasive in nature, integrated with persuasive software features including, but not limited to, reminders and virtual rehearsal. According to Oinas-Kukkonen (2012), a BCSS is defined as "an information system designed to form, alter or reinforce attitudes, behaviors or an act of complying without using deception, coercion or inducements". Building on Fogg's (2002) seminal work, Oinas-Kukkonen and Harjumaa (2009) proposed a theoretical framework otherwise known as the Persuasive Systems Design model. The model is about methodically designing and evaluating persuasive information systems, in this case the eHealth intervention. Usually, a persuasive system would remind users to perform target behaviors when they are engaged in the interaction. Reminders can improve eHealth interventions (BCSSs) to facilitate task completion (Oinas-Kukkonen &Harjumaa, 2009). Reminders can be of varying designs; for instance, they could be combined as subtle messages (Fry &Neff, 2009) and can be delivered through different media with varying frequencies. Reminders have regularly been used in persuasive systems for improving general and mental health. Different techniques have been examined to advance the efficiency of reminders with, for example, personalized content. One of the persistent challenges for eHealth interventions is low adherence (task completion/compliance) and learning new skills to manage mental health (Mohr et al. 2010). For the presented study, we formulated the following research questions:

RQ1: How do participants perceive persuasive reminders to help them complete virtual rehearsal tasks?

RQ2: How do participants perceive usefulness of virtual rehearsal in helping them overcome sleep difficulties?

3. METHODOLOGGY

3.1 Recruitment

The study was conducted between October 2013 and November 2013. Participants were recruited through newspaper advertisements. It was explained in the advertisements that we were looking for those individuals who felt that they were suffering from sleep disorders. The eligibility criteria were: 1) Access to Internet/ email, 2) that participants would not take lengthy breaks during the intervention, 3) access to telephone, 4) not being a part of a therapy or study in parallel, 5) Finnish as mother language and 6) age 18 years or older.

In response to the advertisements, a total of 122 individuals (76 via email and 46 via phone) contacted the university clinic and were screened over phone on the 7th and 8th of October 2013. In addition, those who contacted the university clinic through email were screened on the 17th and 19th of October, 2013. Of the 122 individuals who were initially selected for the study, 14 were excluded because they did not fulfil the eligibility criteria. Further, 22 participants were not included in the study because the number of interested participants was too high and we had rather limited resources to carry out the study in a professional manner. Therefore, the final number of participants was 86 (N=86). Later, measurement packages explaining the objective of the study and informed consent forms were sent out to eligible participants. As the study included actual patients of sleep disorder, ethical approval was formally obtained from the Ethical Committee at the University of Jyväskylä, Finland.

3.2 Participants' Randomization

Randomization was performed using the tool (https://www.random.org/lists/) on the 9th of October 2013. Participants were randomized into two groups: (1) Intervention group (n = 43) that received the measurements, had access to the intervention (BCSS), received bi-weekly email-based reminders and had access to weekly rehearsal modules, and (2) Wait-list control group (n = 43). For ethical reasons, the wait-list control group received the same program (but reminders were not sent) and URL as an access point to the Web-based intervention (BCSS) was sent out when the intervention group had completed the program. The study commenced on the 21st of October and concluded on the 25th of November 2013. This chapter presents results from the intervention group only. A total of 12 (27.9%) males and 31 (72.1%) females aged between 24 to 73 years comprised the sample (Mean = 55.74, Std. Deviation = 10.99) A majority of participants (58.5%) had obtained higher education either and college or university level.

3.3 The eHealth Intervention (BCSS Tynne)

A research group from the Department of Information Processing Science, University of Oulu, Finland devised and implemented the BCSS (*Tynne*). It was a perplexing task and took several iterations and testing stages before being finalised. A research team from the Department of Psychology, University of Jyväskylä, Finland developed the content for the eHealth intervention (BCSS *Tynne*), especially the content of ACT-based virtual rehearsal modules. ACT-based rehearsal modules were incorporated with novel techniques for managing sleep disorders. Virtual rehearsal as a software feature was used with an aim to improve mindfulness, acceptance skills, psychological flexibility and commitment towards value-based actions among participants by applying a variety of metaphors, experiential exercises (both audio and video) for mindfulness and Behavioral activation (Hayes et al. 2005). Table 1 presents a brief overview of the ACT themes used for the rehearsal content.

Table 1. Acceptance and commitment therapy themes and content

Week	Theme	Content
1	Values and value-based actions	Knowing what matters the most for an individual in his/her life and acting in accordance
2	The present moment	Living in the present moment (mindfulness)
3	Cognitive defusion	Understanding that an individual's thoughts could be different
4	The observer stance	Learning to view one's thoughts and feelings from an observer's stance
5	Acceptance	Accepting one's feelings, and thoughts and admitting that one cannot change things
6	Summary	Rehearsing ACT exercises from the previous weeks.

3.4 The Persuasive Systems Design Model

The research field of Persuasive Technology was introduced by Fogg (2002). Generally speaking, persuasive technologies are designed to bring a positive change in people's behaviors. Building upon Fogg's seminal work (Fogg, 2002), Oinas-Kukkonen and Harjumaa (2009) redefined the research area by adding that persuasive systems help people change their behaviors without the use of coercion or deception. Further, use of a persuasive information system has to be on a voluntary basis (Karppinen & Oinas-Kukkonen, 2013). Oinas-Kukkonen and Harjumaa proposed a theoretical framework else known as the Persuasive Systems Design Model that enables systematic evaluation of the persuasion context (the intent, the event and the persuasion strategy). The model provides a range of persuasive software features and functionalities for developing persuasive eHealth interventions (BCSSs). The four distinct categories outlined in the PSD model are primary task, user-system dialogue, credibility and social support features. Researchers have employed the PSD model in different contexts, for example, Lehto and Oinas-Kukkonen (2011), Räisanen et al. (2010), Stibe et al. (2013), Drozd et al. (2012), Wiafe et al. (2012) and Yetim (2011). The PSD model has also been applied in the area of ubiquitous applications that are developed for general well-being (Langrial et al. 2012), personal wearable devices for physical training (Harjumaa et al. 2009), and information systems that promote healthy behavior (Purpura et al. 2011). Kelders et al. (2012) support the use of the PSD model for Web-based interventions. The model does not promote integration of all the proposed software features to develop an effective intervention meaning thereby the persuasiveness of a given eHealth intervention for behavior change is by no means guaranteed in terms of the quantity of incorporated persuasive software features. On the contrary, it is the features of selected software that could lead to an effective intervention or BCSS.

3.5 Use of Virtual Rehearsal and Reminders

The study was planned in a way that the participants were advised to complete and practice one ACT-based virtual rehearsal module before moving on to the next step in the following week. This was intended for two reasons: 1) to provide adequate time for participants to practice and 2) to bring in the element of incremental behavior change process, which is promoted by the PSD model (Oinas-Kukkonen & Harjumaa, 2009). The main objective of sending Email-based reminders was to inspire the participants to interact with the intervention without being obtrusive. Each week three Email-based (automated) reminders were sent out to the participants with an aim to initiate interaction between participants and the intervention (BCSS). The first reminder was to praise the participants for successful completion of the allocated task. For example, the first reminder was sent upon completing rehearsals for week 1, the second reminder was sent to motivate users to continue practicing skills that they had learned, and the third reminder was sent to advise that participants could access the next rehearsal module and start practicing new skills.

3.6 Data Collection About Participants' Experiences

System effectiveness and users' overall experience with the intervention (BCSS) were assessed using Likert-scale (Likert, 1932) questionnaires at the beginning and end of the intervention. For data collection, we developed pre- and post-study questionnaires. The questionnaires consisted of two parts. The first part included demographic-related questions formulated to gather information about the participants, their computing skills and experience related with Internet use. The second part in the pre- study questionnaire comprised of questions about participants' anticipations and perceived usefulness of the intervention (BCSS). The post- study questionnaire was developed to gather information about real experiences of the participants after having used the intervention (BCSS). Special emphasis was laid on system usefulness, ease of use; impact of reminders on task completion, effect of virtual rehearsal on sleep management skills, and participants' observations about the efficiency of virtual rehearsal. We used seven-point rating scales for all items (1 = Strongly disagree; 7 = Strongly agree) (Likert, 1932). Finally, participants were interviewed in a post- study satisfaction (exit) survey to get a better picture of their experiences with the intervention.

3.7 Measures for Well-Being

We used Beck Depressive Inventory–II (BDI-II) (Beck et al. 1961) and Epworth Sleepiness Scale (ESS) (Johns, 1991) for measuring psychological outcomes. Beck

Depressive Inventory II includes of 21 questions about depressive symptoms and their severity. The scale ranges from 0 – 63 (where 0 – 13 no or few depressive symptoms, 14 -19 indicate mild depression, 20 – 28 indicate moderate depression and 29 – 63 indicate severe depression). BDI-II has been acknowledged to have reliability and validity in both among clinical and non-clinical populations. Epworth Sleepiness Scale (ESS) is a self-administrated eight-item questionnaire (Johns, 1992). It establishes the level of sleepiness during daytime (Johns, 1991). An ESS score that is greater than 16 indicates a high level of daytime sleepiness. The ESS has proven to be reliable and internally consistent tool (Johns, 1992).

DATA EVALUATION

We applied the PSD model to evaluate the effectiveness of the intervention. The model outlines 28 distinct persuasive software features; however for the purpose of this study, only reminders and virtual rehearsal were chosen as key software features. The goal of the study was to examine the effect of reminders on task completion and / or compliance. The major task for the participants was to learn new behaviors through practice for better managing sleep disorders through ACT-based virtual rehearsal modules. Particular emphasis was placed upon the said software features to understand how a combination of the two could be further utilized to develop operative and effective eHealth interventions (BCSSs) for sleep disorders. In addition, we aimed to investigate participants' anticipations from the intervention in terms of system usefulness, ease of use, expected enjoyment, whether participants perceived virtual rehearsal useful software feature, their willingness to use the system, and whether participants considered reminders to be effective. Using structured questionnaires, we opted for collecting qualitative date.

Participants completed pre- and post- study questionnaires representing their replies both in terms of anticipations and real experiences respectively. Finally, participants were given an option to give additional remarks about the intervention. For the purpose of the analyses and to answer aforementioned questions, we followed a qualitative research methodology. We used elements of the Grounded Theory (Strauss & Corbin, 1998). It allows using previously defined themes and, at the same time provides an opportunity to collect emerging themes as stated by Fereday and Muir-Ccochrane (2008). Further, we evaluated frequency distribution between pre- and post- measurements using Chi-square test.

FINDINGS

Table 2 exemplify participants' responses for both pre- and post- study questionnaires. The table exhibits pre- and post- intervention responses in percentage (Agreed; Unsure or Disagreed), pre- and post- intervention mean sores and standard deviation (SD), and t-test revealing statistical differences between pre- and post- mean values.

3.8 Psychological Measures

Symptoms of sleeplessness were assessed at the beginning and the end of the study. For measuring psychological symptoms, Beck Depression Inventory–II (BDI-II) (Beck et al. 1961) and Epworth Sleepiness Scale (ESS) (Johns, 1991) were used as primary measures. BDI-II (Beck et al. 1961) was used as a primary measure because depression is a common reason for sleeplessness and other sleep disorders (Hall et al. 2000). ESS (Johns, 1991) provides valid measurements of sleep propensity in adults. Outcomes from the analysis for pre- and post- BDI-II measurements revealed statistically significant decreases in the intervention group where mean values dropped from 12.20 to 8.15 ($t = 5.54$, $df = 38$, $p < 0.01$). Similarly, promising results were observed when ESS was analysed. Outcomes from the pre- and post- study for ESS showed notable decrease in mean values from 6.98 to 5.63 (t 0 2.59, $df = 37$, $p < 0.05$). Mean values for the psychological measurements provide evidence that support overall effectiveness of the intervention. Figure 1 exhibits scores for Mean and Standard Deviation for Intervention group.

Figure 1. Mean scores and standard deviations for psychological measures

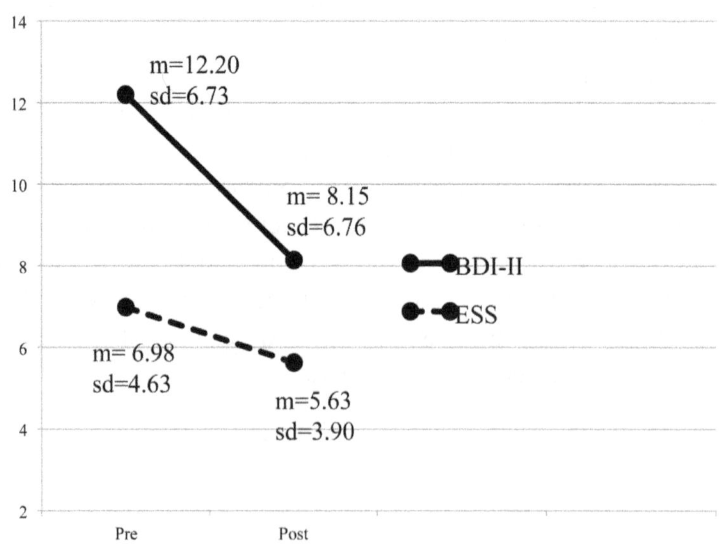

Table 2. Pre- and post- study responses depicting statistical outcomes

Question/Theme	Pre % (n)	Post % (n)	χ^2 3.7.1.1.1.1.1.1.2	Pre: Mean (sd)	Post: Mean (sd)
The intervention(BCSS) will improve my sleep habits/helped me improve my sleep habits				2.91 (.29)	2.54 (.67)
Agreed	90.7% (39)	60.5% (26)	χ^2=9.83; df = 2 p < 0.01		
Unsure or Disagreed	9.3% (4)	34.9% (15)			
The intervention (BCSS) will be/was easy to interact with				2.77 (.48)	2.95 (.26)
Agreed	79.1% (36)	90.7% (39)	χ^2 = 2.85; df = 2 p = 0.09		
Unsure or Disagreed	20.9% (7)	4.7% (2)			
Web-based interventions(BCSSs) for sleep disorders is a good idea				2.88 (.50)	2.83 (.38)
Agreed	93.0% (40)	79.1% (34)	χ^2 = 4.22; df = 2 p = 0.12		
Unsure or Disagreed	7.0% (3)	16.3% (7)			
Learning new skills through Web-based interventions (BCSSs) is a good idea				2.93 (.258)	2.98 (.156)
Agreed	93.0% (40)	93.0% (40)	χ^2 =0.93; df = 1 p = 0.33		
Unsure or Disagreed	7.0% (3)	2.3% (1)			
Reminders will help people complete Web-based interventions				2.95 (.213)	2.68 (.610)
Agreed	95.3% (41)	72.1% (31)	χ^2 =7.12; df = 2 p = 0.03		
Unsure or Disagreed	4.7% (2)	23.3% (10)			
After using the intervention (BCSS), I will be/am able to manage my sleep problems better				2.88 (.324)	2.32 (.610)
Agreed	88.4% (38)	37.2% (16)	χ^2 = 22.63; df = 2 p = < 0.01		
Unsure or Disagreed	11.6% (5)	58.2% (25)			

3.9 Participants' Open Comments

Of the 43 participants, 41 volunteered to complete post- study questionnaires. Several observations were noticed and themes were identified. Keeping in mind the identified themes, below are some of the exemplary comments:

3.9.1 Need for Extended Interaction

A little more interaction (prolonged period of study) would have been better (desirable) otherwise it was a good experience. (Female; 45 years)

I had high expectations but I did not have enough time for the system (to interact with the system). (Female; 45 years)

The program (intervention) did not help me. The study period should have been longer. (Male; 53 years)

The period of the study (intervention) was too short". (Male; 58 years)

3.9.2 Reminders are Beneficial

The system met my expectations. Reminders worked fine. Adding SMS-based reminders would have been better. (Male; 53 years)

The system was good! I found reminders and rehearsal to be beneficial. (Female; 62 years)

I expected a little more from the system. The rehearsals were good and so were the reminders (they were much needed). (Female; 62 years)

3.9.3 Virtual Rehearsal is a Suitable Method

I got to know myself (better) and now I have new (better) viewpoints (about my life). (Female; 65 years)

I am highly grateful! I am (feel calm) about my waking up during night time and (now) I (manage) to sleep gain. (Female; 65 years)

I had no problems using the intervention (BCSS). It was (indeed) a positive experience. The program (intervention) was well built (designed) both technically and content wise. There was enough information given the short study (intervention) period. My sleep did not improve. The process of improvement was just starting (to happen). I learned new views (techniques) to think about my life. (Female; 67 years)

There was a lot of new information. The program provided broad (comprehensive) approaches towards sleep problems, it was engaging. Although, my sleep problems are the same I will continue to rehearse. (Male; 67 years)

The system (BCSS) was easy to use. Rehearsals were reasonable (logical). It was an interesting experience. I (would) highly recommend using the (same) system. Now, I can sleep easily and (also) breathe better. (Female; 50 years)

I cannot compare this (experience) to anything else. The memories are pleasant. I would like to take part in something similar (intervention) in future. (Female; 63 years)

The system met my expectations. It was a positive experience. Working out the exercises (rehearsing) has improved my situation. (Female; 57 years)

The system was good. It did not resolve my insomnia but I still feel it (the BCSS) was useful. (Female; 47 years)

Very surprising and exciting experience. I committed (myself) to the program (intervention) and learnt new skills. The best results are thoughtfulness that I have achieved in six weeks. (Female; 56 years)

The system taught me to listen, breathe and meditate well. It helped me accept that there are bad times. Thank you. (Female; 56 years)

My expectations were met and exceeded. Quality of sleep has increased remarkably. Length of sleep is bit better. Not so much of awakening during night. Best of all, I have almost quit using sleeping pills. (Female; 50 years)

3.10 General Remarks

I did not have any expectations (that my sleep problems will be solved). (Female; 60 years)

I expected a more from the system (intervention). However, my own laziness (has) influenced my (learning) progress. (Male; 51 years)

The system met my expectations. I had problems because of my Internet connection. (Female; 64 years)

I am still practising (rehearsing). Let us see what happens. (Female; 56 years)

The program (intervention) was positive (good). I just did not have much time. It was worth a try. (Male; 59 years)

4. DISCUSSION

The central objective of the study was to evaluate (1) how do participants perceive reminders support them completing weekly tasks and, (ii) how do they perceive likely effect of virtual rehearsal in overcoming sleep disorder. According to Oinas-Kukkonen and Harjumaa (2009). effective dialogue support features should be integrated to keep the users motivated in continuing to interact with the system / intervention and supporting them to reach their goals. It has been stated that features supporting users' primary task are necessary for persuasion (Oinas-Kukkonen and Harjumaa 2009). Additionally, primary task support features aim to improve users' self-efficacy by reducing rational burden and perplexity (Webster & Ahuja 2006). This study demonstrates how the PSD model can be utilized in developing and evaluating an eHealth intervention (BCSS).

It is apparent that the participants had high hopes from the intervention; however upon completion of the intervention, the post- study survey responses indicate a relatively different picture. We had two research questions for this study. RQ1 was aimed to examine how and to what extent reminders helped users in task completion/ compliance. Post- study results suggest that reminders were perceived as helpful. This is especially evident in participants' open comments, where majority of the participants (72.1%) commended reminders as an appropriate technique for task completion/compliance in both pre- and post- study questionnaires. RQ2 was developed to examine the extent to which virtual rehearsal could help participants learn new behaviours. An overwhelming majority of participants (93.1%) favoured virtual rehearsal as an effective feature for learning new behaviours. In addition, participants' open comments provide evidence that support usefulness of virtual rehearsal. Several participants expressed their desire for an extended period of the intervention.

A prominent limitation of presented work is that the time duration of the intervention was relatively short. Chronic mental conditions such as sleep disorder require a prolonged interaction between users and the intervention (BCSS). However, our work opens new opportunities for e-Health researchers to further investigate selected software features that could improve effectiveness of interventions that are designed for sleep disorders.

5. CONCLUSION

This chapter highlights findings from evaluation of a Web-based eHealth intervention (BCSS) for sleep disorders. The software features were drawn from the PSD model, however; the main focus was to examine the potential effect of reminders and virtual rehearsal. Majority of the participants agreed that the intervention was helpful. Nearly all the participants agreed that learning new skills through Web-based interventions was a good idea. Although most of the participants agreed at the beginning of the intervention that reminders might help them in task completion, the number decreased significantly upon completion of the intervention. A high majority of the participants expected that upon completion of the intervention, they would be able to manage their sleep problems better. However, it was observed that several participants' expectations were not met.

Nevertheless, 16 participants agreed that they could better manage their sleep problems, 22 participants were unsure and 3 participants disagreed upon completion of the intervention. One major reason for this outcome is relatively short time period of the intervention. Although the intervention lasted for a period of six weeks only, still the findings are encouraging because the entire intervention was carried without face-to-face therapy and a significant number of participants evaluated the intervention positively.

We believe that our work is a good starting point to develop and evaluate novel eHealth interventions that are designed with intent to help people suffering from mental conditions such as sleep disorders. Our work has several implications for eHealth, HCI and IS researchers especially those who wish to analyse the effect of reminders on task completion and virtual rehearsal such interventions.

6. ACKNOWLEDGMENT

The study was a part of the OASIS research group of Martti Ahisaari Institute, University of Oulu, Finland. The SalWe Research Program supported it for Mind and Body (Tekes – The Finnish Funding Agency for Technology & Innovation grant 1104/10). The contribution made by the research group at the Department of Psychology, University of Jyväskylä cannot be overlooked. The authors thank the entire team for the effort and contribution in completing the study.

REFERENCES

Albaina, I. M., Visser, T., van der Mast, C. A., & Vastenburg, M. H. (2009, April). Flowie: A persuasive virtual coach to motivate elderly individuals to walk. *Proceedings of the 3rd International Conference on Pervasive Computing Technologies for Healthcare Pervasive Health '09* (pp. 1-7). IEEE. doi:10.4108/ICST.PERVASIVEHEALTH2009.5949

Alhola, P., & Polo-Kantola, P. (2007). Sleep deprivation: Impact on cognitive performance. *Neuropsychiatric Disease and Treatment*, *3*(5), 553. PMID:19300585

Amstadter, A. B., Broman-Fulks, J., Zinzow, H., Ruggiero, K. J., & Cercone, J. (2009). Internet-based interventions for traumatic stress-related mental health problems: A review and suggestion for future research. *Clinical Psychology Review*, *29*(5), 410–420. doi:10.1016/j.cpr.2009.04.001 PMID:19403215

Andersson, G., & Cuijpers, P. (2009, December). Internet-based and other computerized psychological treatments for adult depression: A Meta-analysis. *Cognitive Behaviour Therapy*, *38*(4), 196–205. doi:10.1080/16506070903318960 PMID:20183695

Andersson, G., & Cuijpers, P. (2009). Internet-based and other computerized psychological treatments for adult depression: A meta-analysis. *Cognitive Behaviour Therapy*, *38*(4), 196–205. doi:10.1080/16506070903318960 PMID:20183695

Aromaa, E., Tolvanen, A., Tuulari, J., & Wahlbeck, K. (2011). Personal stigma and use of mental health services among people with depression in a general population in Finland. *BMC Psychiatry*, *11*(1), 52. doi:10.1186/1471-244X-11-52 PMID:21453504

Bandura, A. (1986). *Social foundations of thought and action* (pp. 5–107). Englewood Cliffs, NJ: Prentice Hall.

Beck, A. T., Ward, C., & Mendelson, M. (1961). Beck depression inventory (BDI). *Archives of General Psychiatry*, *4*(6), 561–571. doi:10.1001/archpsyc.1961.01710120031004 PMID:13688369

Briñol, P., & Petty, R. E. (2009). Persuasion: Insights from the self-validation hypothesis. *Advances in Experimental Social Psychology*, *41*, 69–118.

Choe, E. K., Consolvo, S., Watson, N. F., & Kientz, J. A. (2011, May). Opportunities for computing technologies to support healthy sleep behaviors. *Proceedings of the SIGCHI Conference on Human Factors in Computing Systems* (pp. 3053-3062). ACM. doi:10.1145/1978942.1979395

Consolvo, S., McDonald, D. W., & Landay, J. A. (2009, April). Theory-driven design strategies for technologies that support behavior change in everyday life. *Proceedings of the SIGCHI Conference on Human Factors in Computing Systems* (pp. 405-414). ACM. doi:10.1145/1518701.1518766

Davis, F. D., & Yi, M. Y. (2004). Improving Computer Skill Training: Behavior Modeling, Symbolic Mental Rehearsal, and the Role of Knowledge Structures. *The Journal of Applied Psychology*, *89*(3), 509–523. doi:10.1037/0021-9010.89.3.509 PMID:15161409

Dey, A. K. (2001). Understanding and using Context. *Pers. Ubiquit. Comput.* 5, 1, 4–7.

Drozd, F., Lehto, T., & Oinas-Kukkonen, H. (2012). Exploring perceived persuasiveness of a behavior change support system: a structural model. In Persuasive Technology. Design for Health and Safety (pp. 157-168). Springer Berlin Heidelberg. doi:10.1007/978-3-642-31037-9_14

Espie, C. A., Kyle, S. D., Williams, C., Ong, J. C., Douglas, N. J., Hames, P., & Brown, J. S. (2012). A randomized, placebo-controlled trial of online cognitive behavioral therapy for chronic insomnia disorder delivered via an automated media-rich web application. *Sleep*, *35*(6), 769–781. doi:10.5665/sleep.1872 PMID:22654196

Faubel, R., Lopez-Garcia, E., Guallar-Castillón, P., Balboa-Castillo, T., Gutiérrez-Fisac, J. L., Banegas, J. R., & Rodríguez-Artalejo, F. (2009). Sleep duration and health-related quality of life among older adults: A population-based cohort in Spain. *Sleep*, *32*(8), 1059. PMID:19725257

Fereday, J., & Muir-Cochrane, E. (2008). Demonstrating rigor using thematic analysis: A hybrid approach of inductive and deductive coding and theme development. *International Journal of Qualitative Methods*, *5*(1), 80–92.

Fetterman, D. M. (2001). Foundations of empowerment evaluation. *Sage (Atlanta, Ga.).*

Fogg, B. J. (2002). Persuasive technology: Using computers to change what we think and do. *Ubiquity*, *2002*(December), 5. doi:10.1145/764008.763957

Fogg, B. J. (2009, April 26 - 29). A behaviour model for persuasive design. In *Proceedings of the 4th International Conference on Persuasive Technology Persuasive '09*, Claremont, CA.. ACM, New York, NY. doi:10.1145/1541948.1541999

Forman, E. M., Herbert, J. D., Moitra, E., Yeomans, P. D., & Geller, P. A. (2007). A randomized controlled effectiveness trial of acceptance and commitment therapy and cognitive therapy for anxiety and depression. *Behavior Modification, 31*(6), 772–799. doi:10.1177/0145445507302202 PMID:17932235

Frenda, S. J., & Fenn, K. M. (2016). Sleep Less, Think Worse: The Effect of Sleep Deprivation on Working Memory. *Journal of Applied Research in Memory and Cognition, 5*(4), 463–469. doi:10.1016/j.jarmac.2016.10.001

Fry, J. P., & Neff, R. A. (2009, April-June). Periodic Prompts and Reminders in Health Promotion and Health Behavior Interventions: Systematic Review. *Journal of Medical Internet Research, 11*(2), e16. doi:10.2196/jmir.1138 PMID:19632970

Gaudiano, B. A., & Herbert, J. D. (2006). Acute treatment of inpatients with psychotic symptoms using Acceptance and Commitment Therapy: Pilot results. *Behaviour Research and Therapy, 44*(3), 415–437. doi:10.1016/j.brat.2005.02.007 PMID:15893293

Gefen, D., & Straub, D. (2000). The relative importance of perceived ease of use in IS adoption: A study of e-commerce adoption. *Journal of the Association for Information Systems, 1*(1). Retrieved from http://aisel.aisnet.org/jais/vol1/iss1/8

Gillin, J. C. (1998). Are sleep disturbances risk factors for anxiety, depressive and addictive disorders? *Acta Psychiatrica Scandinavica, 98*(s393), 39–43. doi:10.1111/j.1600-0447.1998.tb05965.x PMID:9777046

Goel, N., Rao, H., Durmer, J. S., & Dinges, D. F. (2009, September). Neurocognitive consequences of sleep deprivation. []. NIH Public Access.]. *Seminars in Neurology, 29*(4), 320–339. doi:10.1055/s-0029-1237117 PMID:19742409

Hall, M., Buysse, D. J., Nowell, P. D., Nofzinger, E. A., Houck, P., Reynolds, C. F. III, & Kupfer, D. J. (2000). Symptoms of stress and depression as correlates of sleep in primary insomnia. *Psychosomatic Medicine, 62*(2), 227–230. doi:10.1097/00006842-200003000-00014 PMID:10772402

Hamari, J., Koivisto, J., & Pakkanen, T. (2014, May). Do persuasive technologies persuade?-a review of empirical studies. *Proceedings of the International Conference on Persuasive Technology* (pp. 118-136). Springer International Publishing. doi:10.1007/978-3-319-07127-5_11

Harri, O.-K. (2013, August). A foundation for the study of behavior change support systems. *Personal and Ubiquitous Computing*, *17*(6), 1223–1235. doi:10.1007/s00779-012-0591-5

Hassenzahl, M., & Tractinsky, N. (2006). User experience – a research agenda. *Behaviour & Information Technology*, *25*(2), 91–97. doi:10.1080/01449290500330331

Hayes, S. C., Luoma, J. B., Bond, F. W., Masuda, A., & Lilles, J. (2005). Acceptance and Commitment Therapy: Model, Processes and Outcomes. *Behaviour Research and Therapy*, *44*(1), 1–25. doi:10.1016/j.brat.2005.06.006 PMID:16300724

Hemmeter, U. M., Hemmeter-Spernal, J., & Krieg, J. C. (2010). Sleep deprivation in depression. *Expert Review of Neurotherapeutics*, *10*(7), 1101–1115. doi:10.1586/ern.10.83 PMID:20586691

Jaafar, W. A., & Nur, S. (2009). Applying Virtual Rehearsal Principle in Developing a Persuasive Multimedia Learning Environment (PMLE). In Visual Informatics: Bridging Research and Practice (pp. 427-435). Springer Berlin Heidelberg.

Johns, M. W. (1991). A new method for measuring daytime sleepiness: The Epworth sleepiness scale. *Sleep*, *14*(6), 540–545. doi:10.1093/sleep/14.6.540 PMID:1798888

Johns, M. W. (1992). Reliability and factor analysis of the Epworth Sleepiness Scale. *Sleep*, *15*(4), 376–381. PMID:1519015

Kahn-Greene, E. T., Killgore, D. B., Kamimori, G. H., Balkin, T. J., & Killgore, W. D. (2007). The effects of sleep deprivation on symptoms of psychopathology in healthy adults. *Sleep Medicine*, *8*(3), 215–221. doi:10.1016/j.sleep.2006.08.007 PMID:17368979

Karppinen, P., & Oinas-Kukkonen, H. (2013, April). Three approaches to ethical considerations in the design of behavior change support systems. *Proceedings of the International Conference on Persuasive Technology* (pp. 87-98). Springer Berlin Heidelberg. doi:10.1007/978-3-642-37157-8_12

Kelders, S. M., Kok, R. N., Ossebaard, H. C., & Van Gemert-Pijnen, J. E. (2012). Persuasive system design does matter: A systematic review of adherence to web-based interventions. *Journal of Medical Internet Research*, *14*(6), e152. doi:10.2196/jmir.2104 PMID:23151820

Kim, D., & Chang, H. (2007). Key functional characteristics in designing and operating health information websites for user satisfaction: An application of the extended technology acceptance model. *International Journal of Medical Informatics*, *76*(11), 790–800. doi:10.1016/j.ijmedinf.2006.09.001 PMID:17049917

Kiropoulos, L. A., Klein, B., Austin, D. W., Gilson, K., Pier, C., Mitchell, J., & Ciechomski, L. (2008). Is internet-based CBT for panic disorder and agoraphobia as effective as face-to-face CBT? *Journal of Anxiety Disorders*, *22*(8), 1273–1284. doi:10.1016/j.janxdis.2008.01.008 PMID:18289829

Knutson, K. L., Spiegel, K., Penev, P., & Van Cauter, E. (2007). The metabolic consequences of sleep deprivation. *Sleep Medicine Reviews*, *11*(3), 163–178. doi:10.1016/j.smrv.2007.01.002 PMID:17442599

Knutson, K. L., & Van Cauter, E. (2008). Associations between sleep loss and increased risk of obesity and diabetes. *Annals of the New York Academy of Sciences*, *1129*(1), 287–304. doi:10.1196/annals.1417.033 PMID:18591489

Kraft, P., & Yardley, L. (2009). Current issues and new directions in Psychology and Health: What is the future of digital interventions for health behaviour change?.

Kuonanoja, L., Langrial, S., Lappalainen, R., Lappalainen, P., & Oinas-Kukkonen, H. (2015). Treating depression with a behavior change support system without face-to-face therapy. *AIS Transactions on Human-Computer Interaction*, *7*(3), 192–210.

Langrial, S. (2012). From digital interventions to behavior change support systems: Understanding persuasive systems' development and evaluation process. *Proceedings of IRIS*, *2012*, 1–16.

Langrial, S., Oinas-Kukkonen, H., Lappalainen, P., & Lappalainen, R. (2014). *Influence of Persuasive reminders and Virtual Rehearsal on Information Systems for Sleep Deprivation* (p. 228). PACIS.

Langrial, S., Oinas-Kukkonen, H., & Wang, S. (2012). Design of a Web-Based Information System for Sleep Deprivation–A Trial Study. In *Exploring the Abyss of Inequalities* (pp. 41–51). Springer Berlin Heidelberg. doi:10.1007/978-3-642-32850-3_4

Lappalainen, P., Langrial, S., Oinas-Kukkonen, H., Tolvanen, A., & Lappalainen, R. (2015). Web-based acceptance and commitment therapy for depressive symptoms with minimal support: A randomized controlled trial. *Behavior Modification*, *39*(6), 805–834. doi:10.1177/0145445515598142 PMID:26253644

Lee, E.-J. (2009). I like you, but I wont listen to you: Effects of rationality on affective and Behavioral responses to computers that flatter. *International Journal of Human-Computer Studies*, *67*(8), 628–663. doi:10.1016/j.ijhcs.2009.03.003

Lehto, T., & Oinas-Kukkonen, H. (2011). Persuasive features in web-based alcohol and smoking interventions: A systematic review of the literature. *Journal of Medical Internet Research, 13*(3), e46. doi:10.2196/jmir.1559 PMID:21795238

Likert, R. (1932). A technique for the measurement of attitudes. *Archives de Psychologie*.

Lim, J., & Dinges, D. F. (2008). Sleep deprivation and vigilant attention. *Annals of the New York Academy of Sciences, 1129*(1), 305–322. doi:10.1196/annals.1417.002 PMID:18591490

Lockton, D., Harrison, D., & Stanton, N. (2008, June 4-6). Design with intent: Persuasive technology in a wider context. *Proceedings of the 3rd International Conference on Persuasive Technology Persuasive '08*, Oulu, Finland, LNCS (*Vol. 5033*, pp. 274-278). Springer-Verlag, Berlin, Heidelberg. doi:10.1007/978-3-540-68504-3_30

Makai, P., Perry, M., Robben, S. H., Schers, H. J., Heinen, M. M., Rikkert, M. G. O., & Melis, R. F. (2014). Evaluation of an eHealth intervention in chronic care for frail older people: Why adherence is the first target. *Journal of Medical Internet Research, 16*(6), e156. doi:10.2196/jmir.3057 PMID:24966146

Manber, R., Edinger, J. D., Gress, J. L., San Pedro-Salcedo, M. G., Kuo, T. F., & Kalista, T. (2008). Cognitive behavioral therapy for insomnia enhances depression outcome in patients with comorbid major depressive disorder and insomnia. *sleep, 31*(4), 489.

Mohr, D. C., Duffecy, J., Jin, L., Ludman, E. J., Lewis, A., Begale, M., & McCarthy, M. Jr. (2010). Multimodal e-mental health treatment for depression: A feasibility trial. *Journal of Medical Internet Research, 12*(5), e48. doi:10.2196/jmir.1370 PMID:21169164

Morin, C. M., Beaulieu-Bonneau, S., LeBlanc, S., & Savard, M. (2005). Self-help Treatment for Insomnia: A Randomized Controlled Trial. *Sleep*, 28. PMID:16295218

Morin, C. M., LeBlanc, M., Daley, M., Gregoire, J. P., & Merette, C. (2006). Epidemiology of insomnia: Prevalence, self-help treatments, consultations, and determinants of help-seeking behaviors. *Sleep Medicine, 7*(2), 123–130. doi:10.1016/j.sleep.2005.08.008 PMID:16459140

Moul, D. E., Hall, M., Pilkonis, P. A., & Buysse, D. J. (2004). Self-report measures of insomnia in adults: Rationales, choices, and needs. *Sleep Medicine Reviews, 8*(3), 177–198. doi:10.1016/S1087-0792(03)00060-1 PMID:15144961

Murray, E. (2012). Web-based interventions for behavior change and self-management: potential, pitfalls, and progress. *Medicine 2.0, 1*(2), e3.

Nakanishi, H., Shimizu, S., & Isbister, K. (2005). Sensitizing social agents for virtual training. *Applied Artificial Intelligence, 19*(3-4), 341–361. doi:10.1080/08839510590910192

Niemi, H., Nevgi, A., & Virtanen, P. I. (2003). Towards self-regulation in web-based learning. *Journal of Educational Media, 28*(1), 49–71. doi:10.1080/1358165032000156437

Oinas-Kukkonen, H. (2010, June 7-10). Behaviour change support systems: A research model and agenda. In *Proceedings of the 5th International Conference on Persuasive Technology,* Copenhagen, Denmark, LNCS (Vol. 6137, pp. 4-14). Springer-Verlag, Berlin, Heidelberg. doi:10.1007/978-3-642-13226-1_3

Oinas-Kukkonen, H., & Harjumaa, M. (2008, June 4-6). A Systematic Framework for Designing and Evaluating Persuasive Systems. *Proceedings of the 3rd International Conference on Persuasive Technology Persuasive '08*, Oulu, Finland, LNCS (*Vol. 5033*, pp. 164-176). Springer-Verlag, Berlin, Heidelberg. doi:10.1007/978-3-540-68504-3_15

Oinas-Kukkonen, H., & Harjumaa, M. (2009). Persuasive systems design: Key issues, process model, and system features. *Comm. Assoc. Inform. Sys.,* 24(1). Retrieved from http://aisel.aisnet.org/cais/vol24/iss1/28

Patel, S. R., & Hu, F. B. (2008). Sleep deprivation and obesity. *Obesity epidemiology*, 320.

Portnoy, D. B., Scott-Sheldon, L. A. J., Johnson, B. T., & Carey, M. P. (2010). Computer delivered interventions for health promotion and Behavioral risk reduction: A meta-analysis of 75 randomized controlled trials. *Preventive Medicine*, *47*(1), 3–16. doi:10.1016/j.ypmed.2008.02.014 PMID:18403003

Purpura, S., Schwanda, V., Williams, K., Stubler, W., & Sengers, P. (2011, May). Fit4life: the design of a persuasive technology promoting healthy behavior and ideal weight. *Proceedings of the SIGCHI Conference on Human Factors in Computing Systems* (pp. 423-432). ACM. doi:10.1145/1978942.1979003

Räisänen, T., Lehto, T., & Oinas-Kukkonen, H. (2010). Practical findings from applying the PSD model for evaluating software design specifications. In *Persuasive Technology* (pp. 185–192). Springer Berlin Heidelberg. doi:10.1007/978-3-642-13226-1_19

Ritterband, L. M., & Tate, D. F. (2009). The science of internet interventions.

Ritterband, L. M., Thorndike, F. P., Gonder-Frederick, L. A., Magee, J. C., Bailey, E. T., Saylor, D. K., & Morin, C. M. (2009). Efficacy of an Internet-based behavioral intervention for adults with insomnia. *Archives of General Psychiatry*, *66*(7), 692. doi:10.1001/archgenpsychiatry.2009.66 PMID:19581560

Seligman, L. D., & Ollendick, T. H. (2011). Cognitive behavioral therapy for anxiety disorders in youth. *Child and Adolescent Psychiatric Clinics of North America*, *20*(2), 217–238. doi:10.1016/j.chc.2011.01.003 PMID:21440852

Sivertsen, B., Omvik, S., Pallesen, S., Bjorvatn, B., Havik, O. E., Kvale, G., & Nordhus, I. H. et al. (2006). Cognitive behavioral therapy vs zopiclone for treatment of chronic primary insomnia in older adults. *Journal of the American Medical Association*, *295*(24), 2851–2858. doi:10.1001/jama.295.24.2851 PMID:16804151

Stibe, A., & Oinas-Kukkonen, H. (2012, October). Exploring the Effects of Social Influence on User Behavior Targeted to Feedback Sharing. In B. White (Ed.), *Proceedings of the IADIS WWW/Internet Conference (ICWI), Madrid, Spain.*

Stibe, A., Oinas-Kukkonen, H., & Lehto, T. (2013, January). Exploring Social Influence on Customer Engagement: A Pilot Study on the Effects of Social Learning, Social Comparison, and Normative Influence. *Proceedings of the 2013 46th Hawaii International Conference on System Sciences (HICSS)* (pp. 2735-2744). IEEE.

Straus, A., & Corbin, J. (1998). Basics of qualitative research: Techniques and procedures for developing grounded theory (2nd ed.).

Ström, L., Pettersson, R., & Andersson, G. (2004). Internet-based treatment for insomnia: a controlled evaluation. *Journal of consulting and clinical psychology, 72*(1), 113.

Thom, D. H., & Campbell, B. (1997). Patient-physician trust: An exploratory study. *The Journal of Family Practice*, *44*(2), 169–177. PMID:9040520

Thorpe, G. L., Hecker, J. E., Cavallaro, L. A., & Kulberg, G. E. (1987). Insight Versus Rehearsal in Cognitive-Behavior Therapy: A Crossover Study with Sixteen Phobics. *Behavioural Psychotherapy*, *15*(4), 319–336.

Tørning, K., & Oinas-Kukkonen, H. (2009, April). Persuasive system design: state of the art and future directions. *Proceedings of the 4th International Conference on Persuasive Technology* (p. 30). ACM. doi:10.1145/1541948.1541989 van Straten, A., & Cuijpers, P. (2009). Self-help therapy for insomnia: A meta-analysis. *Sleep Medicine Reviews*, *13*(1), 61–71. doi:10.1016/j.smrv.2008.04.006 PMID:18952469

Vincent, N., & Lewycky, S. (2009). Logging on for better sleep: RCT of the effectiveness of online treatment for insomnia. *Sleep*, *32*(6), 807–815. PMID:19544758

Walsh, J. K. (2004). Clinical and socioeconomic correlates of insomnia. *The Journal of Clinical Psychiatry*, *65*(8), 13–19. PMID:15153063

Webb, T. L., Joseph, J., Yardley, L., & Michie, S. (2010). Using the internet to promote health behavior change: A systematic review and meta-analysis of the impact of theoretical basis, use of behavior change techniques, and mode of delivery on efficacy. *Journal of Medical Internet Research*, *12*(1), e4. doi:10.2196/jmir.1376 PMID:20164043

Webster, J., & Ahuja, J. S. (2006). Enhancing the design of web navigation systems: The influence of user disorientation on engagement and performance. *Management Information Systems Quarterly*, *30*(3), 661–678.

Wiafe, I., Nakata, K., Moran, S., & Gulliver, S. (2011). Considering user attitude and behaviour in persuasive systems design: The 3D-RAB MODEL. Proceedings of ECIS '11. Retrieved from http://aisel.aisnet.org/ecis2011/186

Ybarra, M. L., & Eaton, W. W. (2005). Internet-based mental health interventions. *Mental Health Services Research*, *7*(2), 75–87. doi:10.1007/s11020-005-3779-8 PMID:15974154

Yetim, F. (2011). A set of critical heuristics for value sensitive designers and users of persuasive systems.

Chapter 4
From Science to Practice:
Implementation and Clinical Guidelines for an Internet Intervention for Postpartum Depression

Filip Drozd
National Network for Infant Mental Health, Norway

Silje Marie Haga
National Network of Infant Mental Health, Norway

Kari Slinning
National Network for Infant Mental Health, Norway

ABSTRACT

This chapter provides a practical hands-on blueprint needed to design and plan the implementation of internet interventions, addressing all the important aspects of the implementation process. The guidelines are based on the active implementation framework by Fixsen and colleagues (2005) and provide readers with a case example of an internet intervention in Norwegian primary care. They describe the "how-to" of implementation from presenting the background of the intervention, the theory behind implementation, actual implementation planning, evaluation, and clinical work. This serves to give stakeholders a common framework for understanding the requirements for implementing an intervention in practice, the activities and resources needed, and may guide an organization through the implementation process. The case example also shows that implementation and clinical guidelines are mutually affected by each other, and should be developed and viewed together.

DOI: 10.4018/978-1-5225-3241-5.ch004

INTRODUCTION

Internet interventions have shown positive effects for preventing and treating mental health problems (Andersson, Cuijpers, Carlbring, Riper, & Hedman, 2014). However, when interventions are imported, replicated or scaled up, it is critical not only to understand whether an intervention works, but also how to translate and integrate the intervention effectively into practice. Effective interventions that are implemented with low quality are not going to benefit users and provide safer and better healthcare services (Blase & Fixsen, 2013; Proctor & Rosen, 2007), and may even have unintended negative consequences (Barnoski & Aos, 2004). Thus, it is of utmost importance that the implementation of internet interventions is considered and studied to the same extent as their efficacy and effectiveness. However, to date, no studies of internet interventions have any hard data about their implementation. A recent review of internet interventions for depression demonstrated the absence of research and information about their implementation, in particular on aspects of leadership and organization (Drozd, et al., 2016). None of the identified studies examined the relationship between the implementation quality and intervention outcomes, and few studies were even considered to investigate the effects of specific implementation strategies. There are some articles describing "lessons learned" in the development and delivery of internet-based cognitive behavior therapy (e.g., Hadjistavropoulos et al., 2011), case studies (e.g., Christensen & Griffiths, 2007), and methodological papers (e.g., Andrews & Williams, 2015). However, few provide any direct input for implementation. Consequently, the implementation of internet interventions must be better documented and studied to accelerate their uptake in practice.

MAIN FOCUS OF THIS CHAPTER

The purpose of this chapter is to provide a practical, hands-on blueprint for the implementation of internet interventions presented by a case for the prevention of perinatal depression in well-baby clinics. This can contribute to a systematic and comprehensive description and reporting of the implementation of internet interventions, which, in turn, may contribute to speed the translation of research findings into routine practice. The guidelines are based on the Active Implementation Framework (AIF) by Fixsen and colleagues (2005) and The Norwegian Center for Child Behavioral Development's implementation of comprehensive programs in Norway (Gomez, Grønlie, Kristiansen, & Richardsen, 2014). In addition, the guidelines are based on the National Network for Infant Mental Health's extensive knowledge and experiences of implementing nationwide programs over the past decade, including the internet intervention used as a case herein. These guidelines serve to provide stakeholders with a common framework and understanding of what is required to offer an intervention in an organization, and guide the organization in the implementation process.

IMPLEMENTATION GUIDELINES

The guidelines are structured and organized in four sections. Section 1 briefly presents the historical background for the intervention, its research and development, and describes the intervention, its target group, and the context for implementation. Section 2 presents the theory behind the guidelines to provide stakeholders with a common understanding of the different concepts of implementation. Section 3 translates the theory into practice, illustrated with examples from a plan for the implementation of an internet intervention for perinatal depression in well-baby clinics. Finally, section 4 includes the clinical guidelines for the use of the intervention with pregnant women. The clinical and implementation guidelines affect each other mutually and must be viewed together. Implementation, for example, affects the timing of guided support and guided support, in turn, influences the contents of training and coaching.

SECTION 1: BACKGROUND ON THE INTERVENTION AND NEW PRACTICE

Between 10 to 15% of women experience depressive symptoms during pregnancy and following childbirth (Banti et al., 2011; Gavin et al., 2005). In Norway, this equals to 6 000 to 9 000 mothers *and* their children and partners per year. The postpartum period has usually been considered the risk period for developing depression, but recent research shows that the onset of depression during pregnancy occurs almost as frequently as after childbirth (Wisner et al., 2013). In addition, about 1 in 4 women experience the onset of a depression predating their pregnancy. Therefore, it is important to intervene early in pregnancy to prevent the onset and/or development of depressive symptoms and promote maternal mental health. Also, because depression during pregnancy, often remains undetected and many women thus do not receive adequate help and support (Flynn et al., 2006). This is a serious concern because most of these women continue to struggle with their depression after birth, in contrast to those who receive effective treatment (see e.g., Yazici et al., 2015). This has societal consequences as well, with estimated social costs of mental illness for each annual cohort of births of approximately £1.2 billion (Bauer, Parsonage, Knapp, Iemmi, & Adelaja, 2014). These were some of the considerations behind the Norwegian

Women's Public Health Association's (N.K.S.) decision to finance the development of an internet-based early intervention, developed by Changetech in collaboration with the National Network for Infant Mental Health (NNIMH). N.K.S. is a non-profit, voluntary organization that in 1914 established what became the precursor to the modern, Norwegian well-baby clinic. Naturally, one of the early stated goals was to examine whether the intervention could be implemented in well-baby clinics. In addition, an increasing amount of research has shown that providing some degree of support with internet interventions generally results in larger effects (Johansson & Andersson, 2012). Women who used the program, often also requested personal contact and follow-up, even those who have undergone a good pregnancy and postnatal period (Drozd, Andersen, Haga, Slinning, & Bjørkli, 2017).

Mamma Mia

Mamma Mia was originally developed as an unguided, self-help program available for PC/Mac, mobile phones, and tablets. The goal of the program is to (1) prevent the onset or development of depression and (2) enhance subjective well-being during pregnancy and the postpartum period. It follows the pregnant woman and her child from registration during gestational week 17–24 and up to 6 months after birth, and contains a total of 44 sessions over a period of approximately 11 ½ months. For each session, the woman receives a reminder e-mail with a unique link to the program and may log in via the program website. The main program components include (1) identification and monitoring of depressive symptoms, (2) help and support for depressive symptoms, (3) maternal mental health and quality of life, (4) couple relationship and (5) the child and the child's development, which are described in greater detail elsewhere (Drozd, Haga, Brendryen, & Slinning, 2015; for a demonstration, see: Changetech, 2015).

Initial research has examined the feasibility of the program (Haga, Drozd, Brendryen, & Slinning, 2013) and assured its quality through interviews with pregnant and postpartum women (Drozd, Andersen, Haga, Slinning, & Bjørkli, 2017). The unguided program is currently being tested in a randomized trial (Drozd, 2013), but has since been developed further as a guided intervention by means of the clinical and implementation guidelines presented in this chapter, for use at well-baby clinics. The National guidelines for prenatal care (Norwegian Directorate of Health, 2005), postnatal care (Norwegian Directorate of Health, 2013), and guidelines to regulations (Norwegian Directorate of Health, 2004; The Ministry of Health and Care Services, 2003), have been important in the design of the clinical and implementation guidelines, to ensure program fit with the well-baby clinics and their tasks and responsibilities. The overall goal with the well-baby clinic is to promote physical and mental health and prevent injuries and disease, and ensure a continuity of care for its users (Norwegian Directorate of Health, 2004). This has consequences for the implementation of Mamma where it is necessary that midwives and public health nurses (PHNs) engage in multidisciplinary work to ensure the delivery Mamma Mia for continuous care since the program starts in pregnancy and continues up to the baby is 6 months.

Guidelines for Prenatal Care

According to guidelines for prenatal care, it is recommended that the midwife should provide the expecting mother with an opportunity for an open dialogue and discussion based on the woman's wants and needs (Norwegian Directorate of Health, 2005). However, many pregnant women find it difficult to disclose their feelings which may be reinforced by health professionals' occasional reluctance to respond to her emotional needs (Dennis & Chung-Lee, 2006). As such, Mamma Mia may provide both the midwife and woman an opening for a dialogue about mental health during pregnancy, and provide a certain structure to this dialogue based on the key topics presented in the program. Furthermore, it is recommended that midwives identify women in need of extended care, and supplement verbal information by offering written materials and courses (Norwegian Directorate of Health, 2005, p. 30). In this regard, Mamma Mia can be a useful tool for the midwife whom can offer the program both as a preparatory course and as part of extended care. First, the program prepares the woman of becoming a parent and promotes the development of an emotional bond between the mother and baby. Second, the program requires her to report on symptoms of depression at six different times and may be particularly suitable for women with previous mild-to-moderate depressions. More specifically, this should occur during the third consultation, which occurs in gestational week 24 and coincides with recommended program startup. Furthermore, by the fifth and sixth consultation in gestational week 32 and 36 the midwife should, according to the guidelines, (a) prepare the woman on breastfeeding and (b) provide information with an opportunity to discuss her concerns. As mentioned, [Anonymized] may provide the midwife and woman with an opening to discuss mental health, and includes information about breastfeeding and other feeding options.

Guidelines for Postnatal Care

According to guidelines to regulations of the well-baby clinics' program for health promotion and prevention in primary care 0–5 years (Norwegian Directorate of Health, 2004), it is recommended that the first home-visit from the PHN to new parents occurs about 2 weeks after birth, and consists of parental guidance and somatic health exams. Mamma Mia is a contribution and supplement to this end for the PHN and new mothers. In fact, the program covers 6 (54.5%) out of 11 checklist items, as described under parental guidance at the first home-visit. More specifically, Mamma Mia can cover (a) topics that the parents want to discuss, (b) the child's well-being, (c) breastfeeding and alternative feeding options, (d) parent-child interaction, (e) maternal mental health, and (f) parental role, family situation, and social support network. In addition, Mamma Mia can supplement the PHN's somatic exams and parents when it comes to learning about the child's behavior, temperament, and contact initiatives. Furthermore, according to guidelines for postnatal care (Norwegian Directorate of Health, 2013), it is recommended one home-visit by a midwife after discharge from hospital care. For women at risk, which are offered additional home visits from a midwife during the first week after birth, the midwife and PHN may coordinate the implementation and clinical use of the program. At the next consultation with the PHN, about 4–6 weeks after birth, Mamma Mia may supplement 4 (57.1%) out of 7 checklist items listed under parental guidance; (a) breastfeeding, (b) maternal mental health, (c) parent-child interaction, and (d) sleep, and somatic items related to the baby's development and ability for social contact. Overall, Mamma Mia appears to fit well with national guidelines for well-baby clinics as described above, and can be a useful tool and catalyst for dialogues about maternal and infant mental health, both for the health professional and the mother.

SECTION 2: IMPLEMENTATION THEORY

Both the intervention *and* its implementation must be effective in order to create positive effects for the intervention's intended target population. Therefore, there are certain requirements for organizations that want to implement and use interventions such as Mamma Mia, which is important that all involved parties understand. Understanding the concepts and theories of implementation helps to draw attention to the factors that are important for implementation, and to ensure that Mamma Mia and other interventions become integrated in routine practice. Implementation is defined as "a planned and purposeful process with a specified set of activities designed to put into practice an activity or program of known dimensions" (Fixsen, Naoom, Blase, Friedman, & Wallace, 2005, p. 5). Those activities are identified as the core components that need be addressed for successful implementation. These core components are described as "… the most essential and indispensable components of an implementation practice or program" (Fixsen, Naoom, Blase, Friedman, & Wallace, 2005, p. 24), and include (1) recruitment, (2) training, (3) coaching, (4) performance assessment, (5) decision-support, (6) administrative support, (7) system intervention, and (8) leadership. These are considered universal, and apply to all implementation efforts, and compensatory such that weaknesses in one of the components may be overcome by the strengths in other components (e.g., high-quality supervision and performance assessments may compensate for poor training). Thus, it is not the applied number of components that determines the quality of implementation (i.e., the more, the better), but rather the quality of how these are carried out.

At first, there needs to be a selection of personnel that can deliver the intervention to the population and in the organization. This includes practitioners, leaders, administrative personnel, and other staff members, that either are affected by or can contribute directly to its implementation. Thereafter, practitioners and other staff members will need to acquire new knowledge and skills, which require some form of training and coaching. Knowledge and skills can be introduced in training, but are mostly learned through experience and practice on the job with the support from a coach. Coaching can expand on the learned knowledge and skills; provide emotional support, and assessments and feedback (e.g., how to improve on their practice). However, performance assessments should also include evaluations at multiple levels in the organization and include all aspects of the implementation. Thus, it is essential to establish decision-support systems to assess key aspects of the overall performance to support decision-making, assure the implementation of the intervention and benefits for the target population. In support of the implementation, it may be necessary to make changes to internal, administrative routines and procedures to reduce barriers and facilitate the use of the intervention in the organization (e.g., practitioner workload, job descriptions, or changes in IT-configurations). However, all organizations exist in relation to wider systems and may have to change external policies, secure funding, inform the target population and other stakeholders, collaborate with external agencies, and monitor the environment for system-related changes that can affect the organization and implementation (e.g., updated national guidelines or new local funding scheme). A supportive leadership is thus needed to navigate through the implementation, not only through their formal position of power, but also because leaders can prioritize, provide direction, and maintain stability while the organization is undergoing change during implementation.

SECTION 3: IMPLEMENTATION OF THE INTERVENTION

Since there is little research with direct input for implementation of internet interventions (Drozd, et al., 2016), it is difficult to recommend specific implementation strategies. It is up to each organization to develop and specify a plan based on local conditions, needs, and priorities. The AIF framework does, however, help to structure and guide planning to meet the needs of the local organization without fundamentally changing the intervention or its implementation (Fixsen, et al., 2005; Gomez, et al., 2014), although the specific strategies for the core implementation components may vary between organizations. The examples from Mamma Mia presented in this section are italicized and gray-scaled, and may be adapted or replaced for other interventions.

Background for the Implementation

Before actual implementation, the organization should conduct a needs assessment and readiness evaluation. A needs assessment recognizes, describes, and analyzes a problem to determine whether there is an actual need for an intervention (e.g., prevalence or unmet needs in a population), while readiness evaluates whether the organization is prepared for the demands of an intervention and can successfully deliver this as part of their service. In essence, this includes identifying potential barriers and facilitators of implementation (see "Assessment" below for examples and suggested readings). Once a readiness assessment is completed, indicating that the conditions for implementation are right, the decision to proceed with an intervention should be explicitly described together with a timeframe for the plan:

- *Plan for implementation of Mamma Mia at [location or site]*
- *Valid for the period from [date] to [date]*

On [date], the well-baby clinic will start pre-service training in Mamma Mia at the National Network for Infant Mental Health (NNIMH). The decision to invest in Mamma Mia is based on the well-baby clinic's strategically important position for early prevention among pregnant women and their families at the lowest level of intervention in the municipality. About 50% of pregnant women go to their midwife at the clinic, while almost 100% of women go with their newborns to the public health nurse. The well-baby clinic focuses on Mamma Mia as a priority for promoting maternal mental health and provide practitioners with new, modern tools in their clinical work. Mamma Mia appears to fit with the values and philosophy of the clinic and stakeholders' interests.

Next, official plans and documents for the organization that are relevant for the implementation of the intervention should be identified. This may include different types of strategy plans, action plans, business plans, reports, financial plans, and other documents. It is advisable to include and incorporate new interventions in new, existing, or revised plans to secure their sustainability such as in this example:

Plans that are relevant for Mamma Mia include:

- *Strategic plan for prevention among children, adolescents, and families 2017-2020, goal 2.1: The municipality prioritizes primary prevention*
- *Action plan for mental health 2015-2020, no. 1.1: Municipal early intervention*
- *Competency plan for the well-baby clinic 2015-2020, no. 3.2: training in mental health for all midwives and PHNs according to action plan*

Organization

The implementation must then be organized such that there is a group of people who have the formal and overall responsibility for planning and executing the work that needs to be done.

Steering Committee

It is desirable to identify and involve leaders and other key staff members in a steering committee that has the overall responsibility for the implementation, with the authority to make decisions, and devise strategies for implementation. This includes opinion leaders that can influence on the adoption of the intervention and leaders who can declare the priority of the intervention and mandate change. The steering committee should have at least one representative from the workgroup.

Mandate

The steering committee will plan and direct the implementation process and have the authority to make decisions in the implementation of the intervention. The committee's tasks and responsibilities include:

- Develop an implementation plan for Mamma Mia
- Review the implementation plan on a regular basis to ensure progress and/or make necessary changes to the plan
- Ensure organizational commitment so that leaders and staff members support the use of Mamma Mia and its practitioners

Table 1. List of all members of the steering committee

Position	Name	Service	Role
Clinical lead			Head of the committee
Midwife			Committee member
PHN			Committee member

- Allocate sufficient time and resources to the implementation of Mamma Mia
- Incorporate Mamma Mia in the well-baby clinic's and/or municipality's plans and policy documents
- Keep an open dialogue and preserve the information flow between stakeholders (e.g., staff members, external agencies, politicians, and target population)

Workgroup

The workgroup are running the day-to-day operations of the intervention and are responsible for executing the implementation plan decided upon in the steering committee. The workgroup usually consists of staff members who have received training in the intervention, and key personnel in the implementation. The tasks and the persons involved in the workgroup may vary over time and can involve personnel for a limited time to solve specific tasks. The workgroup can also include partners external to the organization and should list all of its members and their assigned implementation roles.

Mandate

The workgroup will carry out the implementation in practice and are responsible for executing the decisions made by the steering committee. The workgroup's tasks and responsibilities include:

- Establish a steering committee.
- Establish and maintain contact with the National Network for Infant Mental Health (NNIMH; i.e., unit responsible for training and implementation support).
- Write, initiate, and activate the implementation plan.
- Disseminate information about Mamma Mia to relevant stakeholders, including the target group.
- Arrange regular meetings with the steering committee, workgroup, and other stakeholders.

Table 2. List of all members of the workgroup and their assigned roles in the implementation

Position	Name	Service	Role
Midwife		Well-baby clinic	Clinical lead on Mamma Mia
PHN		Well-baby clinic	Implementation lead on Mamma Mia
Midwife		Local hospital	Lead in external agency

- Establish the collection and summary of clinical performance data over time and pass it on to the steering committee, practitioners, and relevant stakeholders.
- Monitor and report adverse effects to the NNIMH.

Initiating and Operating the Intervention

Unless an intervention is part of a comprehensive national or public program or funding scheme, staff who have received training will oftentimes need to recruit personnel, form partnerships, provide necessary educational sessions for leaders, co-workers, and other stakeholders, among many other things, to implement new knowledge or interventions in the organization.

Recruitment

Recruiting leaders and co-workers may be necessary for the provision of the intervention in practice. This may also include administrative staff that can manage booking processes or offer technical support (e.g., referring a woman to a Mamma Mia practitioner or providing women with the link to the program homepage, but not psychological support). For example, in Mamma Mia, it is required that the midwives and PHNs at the clinic collaborate since the program starts during pregnancy and continues up to six months after birth. It is also recommended that general physicians or psychologists working at the clinic are included, if extended or more intensive care is needed. A plan with procedures and criteria for selecting and recruiting personnel are described such as here:

Recruitment Manager: [Name of a designated person responsible for recruitment].

For the recruitment of new practitioners, the following criteria are emphasized:

- A bachelor's degree in health and social sciences such as medicine, psychology or nursing, preferably with post-graduation in midwifery or public health nursing

Table 3. Plan and describe recruitment activities

Date	Activity	Responsible
	Recruit the clinical lead at the clinic to the steering committee	Clinical lead on Mamma Mia
	Devise a contingency plan for turnover and leaves of absence	Implementation lead

- Motivation, commitment, and interest in primary prevention, mental health, internet interventions, and/or maternal and child well-being
- Previous experience from professional developmental work

Training

To enable administrative staff, partners, newly hired staff, and other personnel, to contribute to the implementation, it is important that trained personnel plan and provide necessary information, training, and guidance, in the organization. This may include the use of powerpoint presentations, reading research articles, reviewing the program contents, and practicing the clinical guidelines.

Trainer: [Name of a designated person].

Referral Routines and Case Coordination

It is expected that organizations use existing routines for referrals for higher levels of intervention (e.g., intensive medical care). However, internal routines may have to be established such that it becomes easy for, for example, pregnant women requesting the program to sign up when the inclusion criteria are satisfied, and receive guided support when needed. However, since program registration in Mamma Mia must occur within gestational week 25, efficient case management is required for a coordinated delivery of service.

Coordinator: [Name of a designated person].

Table 4. Plan and describe training activities

Date	Time	Location	Target Population	Training Activity	Responsible
			All leaders and staff members at the well-baby clinic	Provide information about Mamma Mia and the plan for implementation at the clinic	Workgroup leader
			Newly hired staff members	Read research articles on Mamma Mia	New staff members
			Newly hired staff members	Run a demonstration of Mamma Mia	Clinical lead
			Administrative staff and web editor	How to manage inquiries about Mamma Mia from pregnant women, journalists, and others	Implementation lead

- Inform pregnant women about Mamma Mia before gestational week 17
- Offer pregnant women enrollment for Mamma Mia between gestational week 17 and 24
- Registered women are offered support and guidance by a Mamma Mia practitioner, according to the clinical guidelines
- Inquiries from women concerning Mamma Mia should be directed to the coordinator, which quickly coordinates the cases among practitioners
- Design a referral form for midwives, PHNs, and external agencies who are not Mamma Mia practitioners
- Use existing or establish new referral routines for women who need alternative or more intensive care (e.g., medical treatment or psychologist)
- Create and maintain a proper practice of transferring women from midwives to PHNs (including record keeping, archiving, and confidentiality)

Documentation and Reporting

All staff members must adhere to national or local guidelines for documentation in the organization including record keeping, archiving, and confidentiality, and any intervention-specific requirements. In Mamma Mia, all practitioners must enroll pregnant women by using a unique link for their clinic that they are provided during pre-service training. The clinic receives performance data on the *implementation* during training, but clinics are expected to establish routines for collecting and summarizing *clinical* performance data to monitor, evaluate, modify practitioner behavior, and provide feedback to administrators and leaders.

Maintenance and Quality Assurance

A program will usually require a set of minimum requirements for the practice of an intervention, which are necessary to maintain and assure the quality of competence and expertise. Thus, any routines for maintenance and quality assurance must be described and planned:

Quality Assurance Manager: [Name of a designated person].

- Complete 2-days pre-service training organized by the NNIMH
- Participate in monthly (group) supervision between pre-service and final training
- Attend the final 2-day training, share experiences from practice, and participate in course evaluation

- Revise the implementation plan after final training and have the implementation plan approved by the NNIMH
- Review implementation progress on a regular basis
- Regularly evaluate the implementation plan and use of Mamma Mia in practice
- Continuously use Mamma Mia in clinical work
- Participate in meetings with the case coordinator

Information Strategy

Developing a plan to ensure that the right people receive the right information at the right time, may support decision-making, facilitate better communication, avoid conflicts and resistance, and contribute to the dissemination of the intervention.

Information Manager: [Name of a designated person].

Table 5. Describe past and future information activities

Date	Time	Location	Target Group	Information Activity	Responsible
			All leaders and staff members of the well-baby clinic	Present Mamma Mia and the implementation plan	Workgroup leader
			Employees at the local hospital working with pregnant women	Presentation of Mamma Mia on a staff meeting	Clinical lead
			Local population, politicians, and pregnant women	Write and publish an article on the clinic's website	Implementation lead
			Local population, politicians, and pregnant women	Send a press release to the local newspaper	Clinical lead
			Pregnant women	Print and hand out brochures in the waiting room at the clinic	Practitioner1
			Mamma Mia practitioners and relevant leaders	Send a newsletter twice a year and to inform about the status of the work and objectives	Clinical lead

Implementation

Timeline

Many implementation efforts can quickly become complicated and require many steps. A timeline will be necessary to provide a "snapshot" of the activities and progress, and in getting the plan completed in reasonable time. The timeline should account for all major activities, as proposed for the implementation of Mamma Mia, and consider all the core components in the plan, including clinical work. Activities may be added or removed as needed.

Implementation Goals

It is important to set realistic goals based on the activities and timeline in the plan, and the number of clients expected to utilize the service, during the valid period of the plan, to guide the implementation.

Estimated total number of pregnant women at the clinic per year: _____ women
Estimated number of women offered Mamma Mia per year: _____ women
Estimated number of women registered for Mamma Mia per year: _____ women

Assessment

Resources

To allocate and secure sufficient time and resources to the implementation, it is helpful to record resource use. This may be especially important for practitioners to balance their time between clinical work and implementation practice. It will be beneficial if the person, who will be least involved in clinical work initially, to take the lead role for the implementation, although this may change over time. At well-baby clinics, this will most often be a PHN since women first visit the midwife:

In [the clinic] there are [number] practitioners. Each practitioner has participated in training, supervision, and other implementation activities (e.g., internal education of co-workers and/or external partners or prepared record keeping practices). This work has accounted for about [estimated percentage] of the employees' position(s). On this basis, the steering committee has come to the following resource allocation for this period:

Table 6. Describe and plan the implementation activities for the designated period

Date	Item	Implementation Activity	Responsible
	Steering committee	Appoint a steering committee	Workgroup
	Workgroup	Appoint a workgroup	
	Readiness assessment	Identify barriers and facilitators for implementation	Workgroup
	Recruitment	Identify and recruit collaborative partners	Recruitment manager
	Training	Describe and plan necessary educational activities	Trainer
	Referrals	Describe and plan referral procedures and case coordination	Coordinator
	Documentation	Prepare the link for registration of women at the clinic, link to the program homepage, and email address to technical support	Quality assurance manager
	Documentation	Prepare routines for record keeping and transfer of cases from midwives to PHNs	Quality assurance manager
	Quality assurance	Describe and plan minimum requirements for maintenance of Mamma Mia	Quality assurance manager
	Quality assurance	Make appointments for supervision with the NNIMH	Quality assurance manager
	Information strategy	Develop and execute the information plan	Information manager
	Implementation	Finalize the implementation plan	Workgroup
	Clinical guidelines	Start to inform women about Mamma Mia	Midwife
	Clinical guidelines	Start to enroll women for Mamma Mia	Midwife
	Clinical guidelines	Provide guided support to women in the program	Midwife & PHN
	Evaluation	Review and approval of the implementation plan by the head of clinic	Evaluator
	Evaluation	Review and approval of the implementation plan by the NNIMH	Evaluator
	Resources	Conduct an assessment of resources to implement Mamma Mia	Evaluator
	Costs	Conduct a cost assessment	Evaluator
	Evaluation	Evaluate the entire implementation of Mamma Mia by the end of the plan period	Steering committee

- Practitioner 1, midwife, 2–3 minutes per consultation to inform women about Mamma Mia prior to gestational week 17. Thereafter, 5 minutes to recruitment of women between week 17 to 24 and 10 minutes per consultation to follow-up in week 32-36, primarily clinical work

- Practitioner 2, PHN, 10 minutes to provide guided support at the first home-visit after birth and 6-week consultation, mainly clinical work. She will also assist with implementation, primarily training and information activities
- Practitioner 3, psychologist, workgroup leader with the overall responsibility for the implementation. S/he will spend 10% of his/her position on implementation activities as described in this plan
- The workgroup has allocated one bi-weekly meeting to coordinate cases and work on the implementation

Costs

During implementation, there may be aspects of the implementation, intervention or organization itself that lead to (un-)foreseen costs. Therefore, it is necessary to keep a record of all expenses, because it is important to allocate and secure sufficient financial resources to sustain the intervention. After training, there are no direct costs related to the NNIMH. New information and materials related to Mamma Mia and its implementation will be sent to clinics unless these are proprietary, copyrighted, or entail costs for the NNIMH. In such cases, materials can be purchased by the clinic from the publisher. The clinic must cover all expenses related to the implementation and operation of Mamma Mia (e.g., print materials, locations, catering, etc.)

Barriers and Facilitators for Implementation

There are number of factors that may affect the implementation of an intervention in practice. Regularly assessing barriers and facilitators before, during, and after the installment of an intervention, can help the organization to get an overview and specify areas in need of work. There are several instruments that can be used or adapted for internet interventions (see e.g., Cabana et al., 1999; Gravel, Légaré, & Graham, 2006; Murray, May, & Mair, 2010; Shea, Jacobs, Esserman, Bruce, & Weiner, 2014). Regardless of the choice of instruments, these should be used to reveal barriers and their potential solutions, and help the organization learn to change their approach early and prevent later problems.

Evaluator: [Name of a designated person].

The staff at the well-baby clinic experienced their work as demanding because of the different site locations. The clinic was to be re-organized to co-locate all employees in one location. The clinic management was supportive of Mamma Mia, but the implementation of the program was no priority at this point. The steering committee thus decided to 'go slow', stretch the timeline for the implementation to allow for the re-organization, and conduct small clinical tests with a few women to provide feedback to the management. The goal was to maintain clinical skills and expertise and convince the management to make Mamma Mia a priority after the re-organization.

Evaluation

Implementation plans will often need adjustments and should be assessed regularly in the steering committee. However, the overall implementation must also be evaluated before the period for the implementation plan expires:

By the end of the period for this plan [expiration date], the implementation is evaluated by the members of the workgroup. The workgroup must consider the overall implementation, including all core components in the implementation plan and feedback from users of Mamma Mia. The workgroup presents their evaluation for the steering committee who should give a clear recommendation for the future work and operation of Mamma Mia.

SECTION 4: CLINICAL GUIDELINES

Step 1: Preparation

When: Before registration of women for Mamma Mia
Who: Midwife
Purpose: Facilitate recruitment, registration, and guided support
Task: Save the link to Mamma Mia easily accessible for registration of women, preferably as a shortcut on the desktop or bookmark in the internet browser. Ask IT-department for support, if needed.

Step 2: Orientation

When: Gestational week 8–12
Who: Midwife
Purpose: Inform about Mamma Mia

- Internet-based program accessed through your e-mail
- Starts in GW 17–24 and continues until your baby is 6 months
- Each session takes about 10 minutes
- Support from midwife and PHN
- Prevent perinatal depression and promote well-being
- Learn about your baby and form an early emotional bond

- Learn about yourself, your thoughts, and feelings
- Learn about strengthening your relationship and support each other, before becoming parents

Task: Print and hand out information brochure about Mamma Mia to pregnant women

Step 3: Registration

When: Gestational week 17–24
Who: Midwife
Purpose and Task: Recruitment and enrollment of pregnant women for Mamma Mia

The following exclusion criteria may apply if women report:

1. No or limited access to the internet (i.e., < 3 days per week)
2. Problematic internet use (e.g., excessive online gambling, shopping, or internet addiction)
3. Acute crisis (e.g., separation, substance abuse, or domestic violence)
4. Being a single mother

These criteria were developed because it is unlikely that women in these situations will be able to use and benefit from Mamma Mia. However, the midwife should always use clinical judgment to determine if some of the criteria are present and which suggest that the woman may experience adverse effects of using Mamma Mia (e.g., problematic internet use). Here, we present some examples of a few, simple questions the midwife can ask to explore the exclusion criteria.

Internet Use

We have an internet-based program – Mamma Mia – which is designed to prevent perinatal depression, promote maternal mental health, and support you on your way to becoming a mother. Is it okay if I ask you a some questions to see if Mamma Mia may be appropriate for you?

If given permission, continue with the following questions:

Do you have access to the internet via a computer, smartphone or tablet?

How often are you online each week?

If a woman reports being online or having access to the internet at least 3 times per week, she may be able to use and benefit from Mamma Mia. You may also probe what information she is typically searching for:

Online Health Information

Do you search for pregnancy-related information, information about the child and child development, couple relationship, or similar?

The midwife is listening for information about:

- Maternal mental health (e.g., stress, worries, sadness, etc.)
- Partner relationship (e.g., partner involvement, expectations, support, etc.)
- Child and child development (e.g., growth, breastfeeding, sleep, etc.)
- Attachment (e.g., how establish an emotional bond to your baby)
- Parent-child interaction (e.g., how to comfort your baby)
- Parenting skills (e.g., stress and emotion regulation)

Women who do not search for this kind of information are not to be excluded. This information is only to help the midwife to target those women who are most likely to benefit from using Mamma Mia.

Problematic Internet Use

For most, the internet is a useful tool. However, for some, the internet is a two-edged sword. They spend too much time or money online; have a constant urge to check their e-mail, engage in downward comparisons to other parents on Facebook, or get stressed by being available all the time. How is that for you?

Adopt an open and non-judgmental attitude, and acknowledge that the internet has many positive aspects, but that it is important to rule out negative consequences of internet use such as:

- Addictive problems (e.g., gambling, shopping, overuse of social media)
- Downward social comparisons (e.g., not being "good enough" compared to other parents)
- Financial, psychological, social, school or work-related problems (e.g., debt, avoidance, productivity loss)
- Loneliness and isolation

- Beliefs that one's own physical and mental health is poor or worse off than others
- Safety-seeking behaviors (e.g., excessive symptom-checking online)

Problematic internet use such as described above, is characterized by being repeated over time, compulsive, and affecting the woman's daily functioning.

Single Mothers

Today, it is not possible to opt out of the partner component in Mamma Mia, which may be emotionally distressing for some women (e.g., remind them about a recent break-up or unwanted pregnancy). No women have yet reported any serious adverse effects from this but it may cause mild irritation or make them feel sad. It is, therefore, important to ask the following:

Are you currently in a partner relationship?

If the woman reports being single, it is the midwife's responsibility to inform her that Mamma Mia has a partner component:

Since you and your partner recently broke up, I should say that Mamma Mia has a partner component, which you cannot skip. Women in your situation have either quickly browsed through this part of the program or tried to use what they learn in their relationship to significant others such as grandparents or close friends. How do you think that would be for you?

Acute Crisis

In the case of an acute crisis such as marital separation, divorce, substance abuse, or domestic violence, use the organization's existing referral procedures. Negative life events such as incarceration, death of a close family member, personal injury, illness or health problems (incl. pregnancy complications), are also contraindications to the use of Mamma Mia, primarily because the woman is unlikely to use or benefit from the program.

Refusal

Women who meet one or more criteria, must receive specific feedback why Mamma Mia is considered unsuitable for her:

Based on what we have talked about, Mamma Mia does not seem to be right for you. The reason is that ... What do you think?

If she still wants to use the program, she should be offered guided support like all other women. Women for whom the program does not appear to be appropriate, may be exactly those who need support and extended care from the clinic.

Registration

Each clinic is provided with their unique link and should provide women access to the internet for registration via computers, tablets or other mobile devices, at the clinic. The midwife may also assist to register the woman, if needed. If the woman does not want guided support, she can still use Mamma Mia as an unguided program. Women who sign-up for Mamma Mia via the Norwegian Women's Public Health Association, may also be provided guided support like women who sign-up via the clinic.

Step 4: First Dialogue

Who: Midwife
Purpose: Open up for emotional disclosure, discuss topics from Mamma Mia, and encourage future use

Open-Ended Part

During the first part of this dialogue, it is important to be open-minded and listen actively. This entails to listen to what is being said, understand what is important for the woman, and recognize the many meanings and nuances in communication. Listen with an even, receptive attention, without further exploration or interpretation. What is said during this first part is referred to as *events*, which form the basis for exploration later in the dialogue.

In the second trimester, you registered for Mamma Mia.

Tell me about your experiences and perceptions of Mamma Mia so far?

If necessary, ask 3–4 probing questions to obtain their experiences and ask for specific descriptions and examples. Probing questions without interpretation are intended to create spontaneous and open reflections on her experiences, without interruptions from health personnel. In this way, the dialogue is not limited by the health professional's assumptions or pre-conceptions, and does not require any pre-determined or specific answers.

Examples of probing questions include:

What else?

Tell me more about the [positive/negative] aspects of Mamma Mia that you experienced.

What have been some of the (dis-)advantages of Mamma Mia for you?"

What have you learned by using Mamma Mia so far?

What has been difficult or challenging to understand in Mamma Mia so far?

Tell me about some of your other experiences?

Can you give an example?

Women's perceptions of benefits may be reinforced by being given an opportunity to put the observed positive consequences into words. Women who do not find it beneficial, may help to identify any adverse consequences of using Mamma Mia or need help to translate and integrate the lessons learned in real life. Importantly, the midwife should thus be sensitive to these specific issues:

Lack of Practice or Integration

A persistent lack of use of Mamma Mia, the program contents, or homework assignments, may be due to a lack of understanding of the program components or difficulties translating these to everyday life. In the former case, health professionals should socialize the woman in the program such as explaining its preventive perspective or strengthening the couple relationship. In the latter case, health professionals should support women applying the program contents to her daily experiences and real-life events, in a systematic and structured manner. This practice-oriented approach is likely to help overcome many barriers and make the program contents more personally relevant.

Misuse of Tasks and Exercises

Some women may use the tasks and exercises from the program incorrectly. For example, using attention training to avoid negative thoughts or repeatedly perform mindfulness exercises that are anxiety-provoking. Using exercises and techniques as an avoidance strategy, distraction, or attempt to control emotional distress, may interfere with emotional processing and contribute to maintain negative thoughts or feelings. In such cases, it would be useful to explain how incorrect use of tasks and exercises may be counterproductive and help correct their use (e.g., practicing the attention training technique on the bus to work, rather than every time she experiences negative thoughts).

Exploration

Upon closing the open part, it is important to join the dialogue. This involves asking clarifying or exploratory questions, reflecting, and interpreting what is being said. The transition to the exploration phase should be done seamlessly, for example, by reconnecting into the last experience that is mentioned. Alternatively, health professionals may meta-communicate and explain how they will start from the beginning to review and explore some of her experiences.

The dialogue follows an inner logic and structure that is familiar for many health professionals, and often used in clinical work (e.g., Brudal, 2014). An important purpose of this second part is to raise awareness and draw attention to emotional issues and to help the woman make sense of her experiences during the perinatal period. Issues may be triggered by using Mamma Mia (i.e., behavior) and can help the woman to identify her concerns (i.e., events), feelings (i.e., affect), thoughts (i.e., cognitions), and how this may be understood, integrated, and managed, through sense-making with a health professional (see Figure 1). In this regard, the following questions may be useful:

"What did you feel when …?" *[Affect consciousness]*
"What do you think about … now?" *[Reflection]*
"What I understand you are telling me, is that …" *[Coherence and meaning-making]*

Step 5: Second Dialogue

When: 2–3 weeks after childbirth, at home-visit
Who: Public health nurse (or midwife)
Purpose: Assist the woman to resume Mamma Mia and encourage continued use. Open up for emotional disclosure, discuss topics from the program.

The second dialogue is based on the same internal logic and structure as the first dialogue. The timing of this dialogue is a window of opportunity to build a mutual relationship and understanding of the new mother's emotional concerns and

Figure 1. The triangular ABC-model for guided support in Mamma Mia

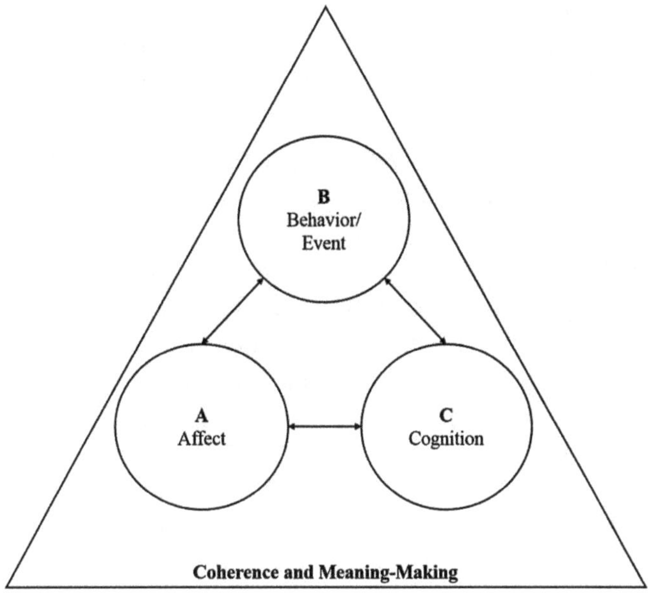

preoccupations, particularly in cases where the woman has been transferred from the midwife to the PHN.

I talked with your midwife and understand that you are using Mamma Mia.

I am curious to hear what you think about it and whether you have started using it after childbirth

Use the probing and explorative questions explained in the first dialogue above to elicit and integrate her experiences to a coherent and meaningful narrative. Importantly, Mamma Mia is not the main concern at this point in the mother's and baby's lives, and may quickly become forgotten, even though she has the intention of using the program. Therefore, a key objective during this dialogue is to remind her about the program, explore if she wants to continue, and assist her to resume the program, if needed.

There are essentially three ways the woman may resume the program:

1. Check if she has received any recent e-mails from Mamma Mia
2. Log in via the program homepage
3. Send a text message with a code to a designated phone number

The woman is encouraged to continue her use of Mamma Mia whenever possible. However, if she expresses any concerns, uncertainties or ambivalence towards the use of Mamma Mia, it is the PHN's task to help her clarify the ambivalence. The following principle is based on the work by Bagozzi, Bergami, and Leone (2003) that developed a framework for eliciting the idiographic, hierarchical representation of people's motives, and to uncover context-specific motives, their interconnections, and go beyond the surface-level. First, a woman is asked to list her personal reasons for starting Mamma Mia. After listing her reasons, she is asked to return to her first reason given and to justify why her *first reason* was important to her. Next, she is asked to explain why her *justification* is important to her. This can continue to one or more additional levels of self-interpretation, but typically third-level explanations are sufficient. Finally, the above procedure may be repeated for each of the original reasons given. Here is an example taken from a nurse eliciting a woman's motivation for using Mamma Mia:

PUBLIC HEALTH NURSE (PHN): *It sounds that you are not sure whether you have the time to use the program. Is that right?*

WOMAN: *Uhm-hm.*

PHN: *If I may ask, what was the reason you decided to use Mamma Mia in the first place?*

WOMAN: *Well, when I first heard about it, I thought it was a good initiative to prevent postpartum depression. It was positive that the well-baby clinic offered this ... What seemed like a fun, modern online program for a problem many women seem to experience, but few talk about.*

PHN: *Why is the prevention of postpartum depression important for you?*

WOMAN: *To be honest, I had a depressive episode in my early twenties. Although that was many years ago, I still remember it. That was tough. And I really, really do not want to experience it again, especially not now that I have become a mother.*

PHN: *Why is that so important for you now as a mother?*

WOMAN: *I'm afraid that I might ruin my relationship with my baby if I get depressed. I mean ... a baby has to have a lot of attention and care ... A mother that looks at her, talks to her, plays with her ... She cannot just feed off, of a mother that can barely get out of bed in the morning and cries all the time.*

PHN: *So, you are currently doing great ... but have these concerns, which you describe, changed in any way since you started Mamma Mia?*

WOMAN: *(Shakes her head) No, not really.*

PHN: *Okay. It sounds that you are still concerned about experiencing a new episode of depression and how that may affect your baby, which is the reason you started Mamma Mia. With this in mind ... Would you be willing to continue with the program?*
WOMAN: *Yeah, I suppose I should give it a try.*

Examples of questions to elicit and clarify ambivalence and motivations may include:

"What made you start with Mamma Mia" *[Motivation]*
"Why is [..] important to you? Has this changed?" *[Core motivation]*
"What do you think about continue using Mamma Mia?" *[Reflection]*
"Is it okay if I tell just a bit about what is ahead of you in the program?" *[Ask for permission]*

Other similar approaches to clarifying ambivalence and motivation may be used instead of, or in conjunction, with the approach proposed herein, such as motivational interviewing (Miller & Rollnick, 2002) or solution-focused approaches (de Shazer & Dolan, 2007). However, regardless of approach, clarification of ambivalence occurs in a friendly and respectful way. The health professional may be curious and explore her wish to discontinue the program, but should ultimately support the woman in clarifying her ambivalence and help her reach a decision that is best for her.

Step 6: Third Dialogue

When: Approximately 6 weeks postpartum
Purpose: Open up for emotional disclosure, discuss topics from Mamma Mia, and encourage future use.

Symptoms of depression usually reaches a peak at about 6 weeks postpartum, which is when the final dialogue should take place. For details on how to respond to each of the steps in this script, please see the preceding dialogues above, which follow the same internal logic and structure.

It has been a while since you started Mamma Mia and you have been using the program for quite some time now. Please tell me about your experiences and perceptions of Mamma Mia?

Be open-minded and actively listen. If necessary, ask 3–4 probing questions, to obtain their experiences and ask for specific descriptions and examples. In particular, listen for:

- Lack of practice or integration
- Misuse of tasks and exercises

After the open part of the dialogue, use the triangular ABC-model in your exploration of her experiences and perceptions as described in Figure 1 above. Among women who have not adhered to the program as prescribed, it may also be helpful to assure the quality of the program by asking:

What is the reason that you have not used Mamma Mia?

For women in need of more long-term follow-up, supportive counseling, intensive care or treatment, the well-baby clinic must use their pre-existing and established referral routines.

ACKNOWLEDGMENT

Mamma Mia was developed by Changetech in collaboration with the National Network for Infant Mental Health for The Norwegian Women's Public Health Association (N.K.S.). This research was funded by N.K.S. (project no. H3/2013) and the Research Council of Norway (project no. 213737).

REFERENCES

Andersson, G., Cuijpers, P., Carlbring, P., Riper, H., & Hedman, E. (2014). Guided Internet-based vs. face-to-face cognitive behavior therapy for psychiatric and somatic disorders: A systematic review and meta-analysis. *World Psychiatry; Official Journal of the World Psychiatric Association (WPA)*, *13*(3), 288–295. doi:10.1002/wps.20151 PMID:25273302

Andrews, G., & Williams, A. D. (2015). Up-scaling clinician assisted internet cognitive behavioural therapy (iCBT) for depression: A model for dissemination into primary care. *Clinical Psychology Review*, *41*, 40–48. doi:10.1016/j.cpr.2014.05.006 PMID:25043445

Bagozzi, R. P., Bergami, M., & Leone, L. (2003). Hierarchical representation of motives in goal setting. *The Journal of Applied Psychology*, *88*(5), 915–943. doi:10.1037/0021-9010.88.5.915 PMID:14516253

Banti, S., Mauri, M., Oppo, A., Borri, C., Rambelli, C., Ramacciotti, D., & Cassano, G. B. et al. (2011). From the third month of pregnancy to 1 year postpartum. Prevalence, incidence, recurrence, and new onset of depression. Results from the Perinatal Depression-Research & Screening Unit study. *Comprehensive Psychiatry*, *52*(4), 343–351. doi:10.1016/j.comppsych.2010.08.003 PMID:21683171

Barnoski, T., & Aos, S. (2004). *Outcome evaluation of Washington State's research-based programs for juvenile offenders*. Washington, DC: Washington State Institute for Public Policy.

Bauer, A., Parsonage, M., Knapp, M., Iemmi, V., & Adelaja, B. (2014). *The costs of perinatal mental health problems*. London, UK: London School of Economics & Centre for Mental Health.

Blase, K. A., & Fixsen, D. L. (2013). *Core intervention components: Identifying and operationalizing what makes programs work*. Washington, DC: US Department of Health and Human Services.

Brudal, L. H. (2014). *Empatisk kommunikasjon: Et verktøy for menneskemøter* [Empathic communication: The missing link]. Oslo: Gyldendal Akademisk.

Cabana, M. D., Rand, C. S., Powe, N. R., Wu, A. W., Wilson, M. H., Abboud, P.-A. C., & Rubin, H. R. (1999). Why dont physicians follow clinical practice guidelines? A framework for improvement. *Journal of the American Medical Association*, *282*(15), 1458–1465. doi:10.1001/jama.282.15.1458 PMID:10535437

Christensen, H., & Griffiths, K. (2007). Reaching standards for dissemination: A case study. *Studies in Health Technology and Informatics*, *129*(Pt 1), 459–463. PMID:17911759

de Shazer, S., & Dolan, Y. (2007). *More than miracles: The state of the art of solution-focused brief therapy*. New York, NY: Routledge.

Dennis, C. L., & Chung-Lee, L. (2006). Postpartum depression help-seeking barriers and maternal treatment preferences: A qualitative systematic review. *Birth (Berkeley, Calif.)*, *33*(4), 323–331. doi:10.1111/j.1523-536X.2006.00130.x PMID:17150072

Drozd, F. (2013). A web-based program for depressive symptoms and life satisfaction during pregnancy and after childbirth. Retrieved June 24, 2015, from http://www.webcitation.org/6ZWKG3j4P

Drozd, F., Andersen, C. A., Haga, S. M., Slinning, K., & Bjørkli, C. A. (2017). User experiences and perceptions of internet interventions for depression. In S. U. Langrial & A. Sharieh (Eds.), *Web-based behavioral therapies for mental disorders* (pp. 27–52). Hershey, PA: IGI Global.

Drozd, F., Haga, S. M., Brendryen, H., & Slinning, K. (2015). An Internet-based intervention (Mamma Mia) for postpartum depression: Mapping the development from theory to practice. *JMIR Research Protocols*, *4*(4). doi:10.2196/resprot.4858

Drozd, F., Vaskinn, L., Bergsund, H. B., Haga, S. M., Slinning, K., & Bjørkli, C. A. (2016). The implementation of internet interventions for depression: A scoping review. *Journal of Medical Internet Research*, *18*(9), e236. doi:10.2196/jmir.5670 PMID:27608548

Fixsen, D. L., Naoom, S. F., Blase, K. A., Friedman, R. M., & Wallace, F. (2005). *Implementation research: A synthesis of the literature*. Tampa, FL: National Implementation Research Network, University of Florida.

Flynn, H. A., Blow, F. C., & Marcus, S. M. (2006). Rates and predictors of depression treatment among pregnant women in hospital-affiliated obstetrics practices. *General Hospital Psychiatry*, *28*(4), 289–295. doi:10.1016/j.genhosppsych.2006.04.002 PMID:16814627

Gavin, N., Gaynes, B. N., Lohr, K., Meltzer-Brody, S., Gartlehner, G., & Swinson, T. (2005). Perinatal depression: A systematic review of prevalence and incidence. *Obstetrics and Gynecology*, *106*(5), 1071–1083. doi:10.1097/01.AOG.0000183597.31630.db PMID:16260528

Gomez, B., Grønlie, A. A., Kristiansen, D. E., & Richardsen, K. (2014). *Implementering av Tidlig innsats for barn i risiko (TIBIR): Fra teori til praksis* [Implementation of Early Initative for Children at Risk: From theory to practice]. Oslo: The Norwegian Center for Child Behavioral Development.

Gravel, K., Légaré, F., & Graham, I. D. (2006). Barriers and facilitators to implementing shared decision-making in clinical practice: A systematic review of health professionals perceptions. *Implementation Science; IS*, *1*(1), 16. doi:10.1186/1748-5908-1-16 PMID:16899124

Hadjistavropoulos, H. D., Thompson, M., Ivanov, M., Drost, C., Butz, C. J., Klein, B., & Austin, D. W. (2011). Considerations in the development of a therapist-assisted internet cognitive behavior therapy service. *Professional Psychology, Research and Practice*, *42*(6), 463–471. doi:10.1037/a0026176

Haga, S. M., Drozd, F., Brendryen, H., & Slinning, K. (2013). Mamma Mia: A feasibility study of a web-based intervention to reduce the risk of postpartum depression and enhance subjective well-being. *JMIR Research Protocols, 2*(2), e29. doi:10.2196/resprot.2659 PMID:23939459

Johansson, R., & Andersson, G. (2012). Internet-based psychological treatments for depression. *Expert Review of Neurotherapeutics, 12*(7), 861–870. doi:10.1586/ern.12.63 PMID:22853793

Miller, W. R., & Rollnick, S. (2002). *Motivational interviewing: Preparing people for change* (2nd ed.). New York: Guilford Press.

Murray, E., May, C., & Mair, F. (2010). Development and formative evaluation of the e-Health Implementation Toolkit (e-HIT). *BMC Medical Informatics and Decision Making, 10*(1), 61. doi:10.1186/1472-6947-10-61 PMID:20955594

Norwegian Directorate of Health. (2004). *Kommunenes helsefremmende og forebyggende arbeid i helsestasjons- og skolehelsetjenesten: Veileder til forskrift av 3. april 2003 nr. 450* [Municipalities health promotion and prevention in well-baby clinics and schools: Guidelines to regulations April 3, no. 450]. Oslo: Norwegian Directorate of Health.

Norwegian Directorate of Health. (2005). *Retningslinjer for svangerskapsomsorgen* [Guidelines for prenatal care]. Oslo: Norwegian Directorate of Health.

Norwegian Directorate of Health. (2013). *Nytt liv og trygg barseltid for familien. Retningslinje for barselomsorgen* [A new life and a safe puerperium for the family. Guidelines for postnatal care]. Oslo: Norwegian Directorate of Health.

Proctor, E. K., & Rosen, A. (2007). From knowledge production to implementation: Research challenges and imperatives. *Research on Social Work Practice, 18*(4), 285–291. doi:10.1177/1049731507302263 PMID:24089591

Shea, C. M., Jacobs, S. R., Esserman, D. A., Bruce, K., & Weiner, B. J. (2014). Organizational readiness for implementing change: A psychometric assessment of a new measure. *Implementation Science, 9*, 7. doi:; 10.1186/1748-5908-9-7

The Ministry of Health and Care Services. (2003). *Forskrift om kommunens helsefremmende og forebyggende arbeid i helsestasjons- og skolehelsetjenesten* [Regulations to the municipalities health promotion and prevention in well-baby clinics and schools]. Oslo: The Ministry of Health and Care Services.

Wisner, K. L., Sit, D. K. Y., Mcshea, M. C., Rizzo, D. M., Zoretich, R. A., Hughes, C. L., & Hanusa, B. H. et al. (2013). Onset timing, thoughts of self-harm, and diagnoses in postpartum women with screen-positive depression findings. *Journal of American Medical Association Psychiatry*, *70*(5), 490–498. doi:10.1001/jamapsychiatry.2013.87.Onset PMID:23487258

Yazici, E., Kirkan, T. S., Aslan, P. A., Aydin, N., & Yazici, A. B. (2015). Untreated depression in the first trimester of pregnancy leads to postpartum depression : High rates from a natural follow-up study. *Neuropsychiatric Disease and Treatment*, *11*, 405–411. doi:10.2147/NDT.S77194 PMID:25737636

KEY TERMS AND DEFINITIONS

Core Component: An essential part of implementation practice and the process of putting a program or intervention into routine care.

Guided Intervention: An internet-based, self-help program with regular, but minimal therapist-support or human involvement.

Guidelines: A set of standards or procedures by which to determine a specific set of actions to execute a plan or accomplish a goal.

Implementation: The process of putting a program, intervention, method, or similar, into practice.

Mamma Mia: An (un-)guided internet intervention designed to prevent pre- and postnatal depression and promote subjective well-being among pregnant and postpartum women.

Practitioner: A person trained in the delivery of a specific intervention and that directly interacts with service users to administer the program or intervention to their benefit.

Well-Baby Clinic: A universal service designed to deliver preventive healthcare and provide information about pregnancy, birth, and children 0–5 years.

Chapter 5
EHealth Interventions for People Suffering From Sleep Problems and Depressive Symptoms:
Qualitative Findings and Future Research Directions

Sitwat Usman Langrial
Sur University College, Oman

Päivi Lappalainen
University of Jyväskylä, Finland

ABSTRACT

This chapter highlights qualitative findings from two field studies that focused on supporting people with sleeplessness (Study 1) and moderate depression (Study II). Both the studies were designed to examine the prospective impact of reminders and rehearsal on the effectiveness of web- based eHealth interventions. The interventions were incorporated with Acceptance and Commitment Therapy. In this chapter, qualitative findings are reported with an aim to highlight issues that are at times overlooked. Further, the findings are expected to help researchers better understand eHealth interventions for mental health care. Results from the two studies uncover interesting contrasts. While the participants of the Study I (Sleeplessness) generally did not find reminders to be helpful, on the contrary, the participants of study II

DOI: 10.4018/978-1-5225-3241-5.ch005

(Moderate Depression) largely approved reminders especially in terms of task completion. In terms of rehearsal, participants from both the studies approved the virtual exercises in terms of learning desirable self-help behaviors. Finally, the chapter highlights some of the grey areas in the field of eHealth interventions for mental health care. The identified grey areas are expected to create opportunities for further research and advances in the field of mental health care.

1. BACKGROUND

A relatively under-studied area in the field of Mental Health Care is identifying the factors that contribute to continuous use of eHealth interventions for mental health care. In order to design and implement effective interventions, it is important to gain a richer insights about users' perspectives with a special focus on areas such as User-system feedback, Online support, Use of Reminders or prompts, Content of the interventions, Trust and Privacy. Despite bulk of published literature about Internet- and Mobile- based interventions for mental conditions, it appears that there is a lack of transparency as well as unified understanding on the part of system developers as well as researchers (Barak et al. 2009). In recent years, most of the studies in the area of mental health care have focused on areas such as adherence (Kelders et al. 2012), dropouts rates, perceived benefits (Drozd et al. 2012) and persuasiveness of eHealth interventions. Further, the overlap in terminologies as well as imprecise narratives (Langrial et al. 2012) have caused the field to become rather diffused and unnecessarily complex. Yet another issue in the area of mental health care is that there is more focus on technological aspects while designing the interventions and overlooking the significance of incorporating psychological content.

Technological advances have opened new opportunities to develop Internet- and Mobile- based Interventions that can support people suffering from mental conditions including but not limited to depressive symptoms, mild depression, acute depression, hypertension, stress, anxiety, trauma and sleeplessness. Both Internet- and Mobile- based interventions have shown promising results in supporting people with several mental conditions (Mohr et al. 2013). We propose that Internet- and Mobile- based eHealth interventions for psychological betterment is a step farther from more traditional behavior change interventions. Behavior change interventions have been studied and categorized differently; for example, Persuasive Technologies (PT), and Behavior Change Support Systems (BCSSs) (Langrial, 2012). However, we propose that designing an eHealth intervention is perhaps the easier part! The real challenge is to continuously monitor an intervention and make needed improvements by identifying the actual needs of users. In addition, involving users or in some cases their immediate caregivers would certainly help in re-shaping the very paradigm of Internet- and Mobile- based interventions for mental health care.

Information systems that are developed to support behavior and/or attitude change are often studied as digital interventions (Langrial, 2012). We cautiously argue that labeling behavior change technologies as digital interventions is a holistic approach. Research on eHealth interventions dates back to the early 90s where they were predominantly used for preventive medical area mostly through intermediations (paper- based and/or telephonic calls). A large number of studies have been carried out that aim to intervene health- related behaviors. For instance, Revere and Dunbar (2001) highlight that personalized digital interventions are moderately effective. Similarly, Langrial et al. (2014) propose that digital interventions have shown promise in supporting people's behavioral change process.

The research area of designing eHealth interventions that support people in improving mental health has received a great deal of attention (Eysenbach, 2000). Such interventions aim to support users in managing health- related disorders. Presently, different platforms are available for developing behavior change technologies i.e. Internet- and Mobile- based eHealth interventions delivered through portable devices and smart phones (Eysenbach, 2000). Still, the task of designing such interventions manifestly maintains its coherent challenges, for example, how would users interact with a given intervention and how would they process and experience the interaction (Or et al. 2011). Additionally, it is necessary that both researchers and system designers systematically understand how users anticipate benefiting from such technologies, what is their user experience (UX) and what are the factors that encourage them to continue using such interventions. The list of challenges in designing eHealth interventions aimed at supporting mental health care goes on like an endless loop.

Designing effective and engaging eHealth interventions is challenging for several reasons therefore designers need to concentrate on the actual needs and expectations of the users. Generally, there is a lack of understanding of theoretical paradigms that are aimed at changing or influencing human behavior (Benbasat, 2010) and, lack of emphasis on HCI- related methodologies being employed during the design process. According to Perkins et al. (2007), systems developed in the HCI discipline are neutral in nature however, this argument is subjective. On the contrary, bringing HCI into eHealth interventions can, for example, improve the aesthetics of the systems/ intervention and lead to prolonged interaction. One of the decisive objectives of designing therapeutic eHealth interventions is to effectively support and guide users to achieve enduring self- confidence that would lead to a feeling of self-control and empowerment. Effective strategies influence users and their perceptions when behavior change techniques are supported by Socio- psychological theories. It is for this reason that several researchers from Health Informatics and behavior change technologies have highlighted the importance of theory- driven design for behavior change technologies and interventions (Consolvo et al. 2009).

It is a promising to observe that researchers and system designers have recognized the significance of theories in the design process. For instance, Consolvo et al. 2009 have proposed Theory- driven approaches for designing behavior change interventions and have incorporated the Transtheoratical Model and Presentation of Self in Everyday Life (Consolvo et al. 2009). A detailed conception of Socio-psychological theories is essential in the design process nevertheless there is a technical side for developing and implementing eHealth interventions. As discussed by Andersson and Cuijpers (2009), technical support ought to be incorporated in such a way that the system (intervention) integrates seamlessly in users' everyday lifestyle.

Effectiveness of eHealth interventions that are incorporated with Cognitive Behavioral Therapy (CBT)- based techniques are emphasized in available literature (Seligman & Ollendick, 2011). Practicality of CBT- based interventions for mental well-being is also supported by (Forman et al. 2010). It is frequently proposed that these treatments are superior to other forms of available treatments. Incorporation of psychological components in behavior change interventions has shown promising outcomes. While there are several studies that highlight the practicality of traditional behavioral therapies, Acceptance and Commitment Therapy (ACT)- based interventions are fairly understudied (Lappalainen et al. 2014) despite the fact that Acceptance and Commitment Therapy is recognized for its positive influence on psychological flexibility (Hayes & Strosahl, 1999).

This chapter presents qualitative findings from two field studies that focused on supporting people with sleeplessness (Study I) and moderate depression (Study II). Both the studies were designed to examine the prospective influence of reminders and rehearsal on the efficacy of the web- based interventions that were developed by employing selected persuasive software features and incorporated with Acceptance and Commitment Therapy- based exercises/modules. Sleeplessness and moderate depression were chosen because first, they are interrelated and, second, they are essential for an individual's mental health. Quality of life depends on different factors, and both sleeplessness and depression, if not attended, can lead to serious negative consequences. In this chapter, qualitative findings are reported with an aim to highlight underlying issues that are at times overlooked. The findings are expected to help designers better understand the dynamics of eHealth interventions that are developed for mental health care. For data collection, we used semi- structured interviews and Likert- scale questionnaires. Although, we used SPSS V. 20 to perform statistical analyses on pre- and post- study psychological measures for both Study I and II, however in this chapter only qualitative findings are reported. This is because in the context of healthcare- related research, qualitative methodologies have been promoted as a practical approach. The results from the two studies reveal interesting differences. While the participants of the Study I (Sleeplessness) did not generally find reminders to be helpful, on the contrary, participants of study II (Moderate Depression) largely approved reminders, especially in terms of task completion. In terms of rehearsal, participants from both the studies approved the virtual exercises (ACT- based modules) in terms of learning desirable self- help behaviors. Based on the qualitative findings, we have identified six emerging themes that are expected to open further research opportunities for mental health care researchers.

1.1 Sleep Deprivation

Suitable amount and quality of sleep is necessary for healthy minds. Sleeplessness or insomnia is among serious mental disorders however this area is rather understudied (Langrial et al. 2014; Alhola & Polo-Kantola, 2007). Available literature suggests that sleep deprivation and insomnia are negatively correlated with an individual's intellectual performance (Water & Bucks, 2011; Durmer & Dinges, 2005; Aloha & Polo-Kantola, 2007). According to van Starten and Cuijpers (2009), physical fatigue, mood disorders, emotional anxiety and psychological stress are among the consequences of sleeplessness. It is generally argued that the consequences of sleeplessness and related disorders are alarming (Orzel-Gryglewska, 2010). For example, people who suffer from sleep deprivation face a higher risk of cardiovascular diseases, diabetes, despair and obesity (Faubel et al. 2009). There is a decent amount of litrature that focuses on promoting healthy diet and regular exercise with an aim to improve people's sleeps behaviors (Tang et al. 2010; Purpura et al. 2011; Albanina et al. 2009). However, it is surprising that less focus has been paid on managing sleeplessness and related disorders. It is essential that mental health care researchers accept the stern challenge of designing effective eHealth interventions that have the potential to provide novel health care solutions. The potential effect of Internet- and Mobile- based interventions when combined with Cognitive Behavioural Therapy (CBT) has been fairly well studied and encouraging findings have been reported for people suffering from Insomnia (Ong et al. 2012; Ritterband et al. 2009). Such findings highlight the potential of eHealth interventions that support people with sleeplessness and moderate depression.

1.2 Moderate Depression

Another major mental disorder is that of depressive thoughts, mild and/or moderate depression. It is well-known that sleeplessness and depression are positively correlated (Benca & Peterson, 2008). Depression whether mild or moderate, is among the most widespread mental disorders in modern day world (Johansson & Andersson, 2014; Kessler, 2012). It is a serious mental health condition that affects nearly 350 million people around the world (Lappalainen et al. 2015). Similar to sleeplessness, depression has been reported as a cause of high mortality rates, poor life quality, social isolation and even restlessness (Aromaa et al. 2011; Galatzer-Levy & Bonanno, 2014). Depression has also been correlated with tendency to commit suicide, alcoholism and social stigma (Langrial et al. 2014). Depressive disorders have been estimated to increase the ailment problem substantially by the year 2030 (Kleine-Budde et al. 2013). Health Information Systems (HIS) and Behavioural Psychology are well-studied research areas and provide ample openings for developing novel eHealth interventions for mental disorders such as depression especially by incorporating Cognitive Behavioural Therapies (Aromaa et al. 2011). Current literature underlines that eHealth interventions that are developed for mental health care can be improved when augmented with Cognitive Behavioural Therapy (CBT) (Meyer et al. 2009; Warmerdam et al. 2008).

It is worth noting that various hindrances have been identified that prevents people from using online or more traditional treatments both for sleeplessness and depression. Some of the deterring reasons include but are not limited to low motivation, difficulty in finding psychological experts, lack or absence of professional services, unwillingness to discuss personal matters, high treatment costs and humiliation (Langrial et al. 2014). It is however encouraging to observe that researchers have been working on developing eHealth interventions (both Internet- and Mobile- based) that could help overcome the said limitations. Further, there is substantial evidence in the existing literature about the effectiveness of e Health interventions that employ Cognitive Behavioural Therapy (CBT) (Andrews et al. 2010; Andersson & Cuijpers, 2009). However, interventions that employ Acceptance and Commitment Therapy (ACT) are relatively uncommon (Lappalainen et al. 2015).

2. RELATED LITERATURE

According to Oh et al. (2005) computing technologies provide an appropriate medium to deliver healthcare solutions. This is particularly true because computing technologies support cost effective delivery of innovative methods and practices to promote sustainable healthcare solutions (Kuonanoja et al. 2015). Ritterband and Tate (2009) point out that healthcare interventions that are delivered over the Internet have shown promise mainly in terms of scalability and reduced costs. As a result, Internet- based healthcare interventions have received growing attention (Kraft & Yardley, 2009). Carefully designed eHealth interventions for mental health care can offer innovative solutions that are convenient for people who either cannot reach healthcare professionals or, are not motivated enough to discuss psychological problems in person (Kuonanoja et al. 2015, Langrial et al. 2014). Accessible literature also supports the effectiveness of Internet- based psychological interventions that are integrated with Cognitive Behavioural Therapy (CBT) (Andersson & Cuijpers, 2009). There is an obvious support for the effectiveness of CBT- based interventions for mental health care (Seligman et al. 2011). While Cognitive Behaviour literature underscores substantiation pertaining to the usefulness of CBT- based eHealth interventions, it is remarkable to observe that a few studies have focused on exploiting Acceptance and Commitment Therapy (ACT), which is the latest wave of CBT (Hayes et al. 2005). What makes Acceptance and Commitment Therapy (ACT) an effectual tool is that it is known to improve an individual's psychological flexibility and is therefore positively correlated with improved mental health (Lappalainen et al. 2015; Hayes et al. 2005). Research efforts have been made to comprehend the particulars of eHealth interventions that are developed to support people with mental health conditions including insomnia, depression, stress and anxiety. Researchers from the fields of Information Systems and Human Computer Interaction (HCI) have also developed and evaluated the efficacy of selected software features and their likely impact on task completion (Mohr et al. 2014), user satisfaction (Kelders et al. 2011), task adherence and overall psychological outcomes (Langrial et al. 2014).

HCI researchers have emphasized on designing eHealth interventions/information systems that simplify the process of behavior change. For an instance, Consolvo et al. (2009) support the use of Theory- driven design for such interventions. On the other hand, Choe et al. (2011) propose that information systems, eHealth interventions and technological innovations have the potential to improve mental health care. They further add that designing such interventions is a challenging task therefore there is a need for deeper understanding of different aspects including cultural sensitivities, privacy issues, trust, user perceptions as well as individual drives and routines. While design strategies and broad agendas for theorizing and developing eHealth interventions for improved mental health care are frequently found in available literature, nevertheless it is manifest that the prospective influence of credible software features either in a selected combination or isolation have been generally ignored (Langrial et al. 2014). Reminders and cues have been among the most commonly reviewed software features that can be defined as prompts or triggers (see Masthoff et al. 2013) in the form of text messages, email- based messages, nudges or instant feedback that is delivered to users during their interaction with a given intervention (Lappalainen et al. 2015; Patrick et al. 2009; Neff & Fry, 2009). The effect of reminders could be further enhanced if they were to be supplemented by tailored content, appropriate timing and meaningful content. This could lead to more effective reminders designed for task completion (Schneider et al. 2013).

In contrast to reminders as a software feature, rehearsal/practicing has previously been used mostly in the area of Cognitive Behavior studies. Billet (2010) highlights that channelled learning practices when repeatedly exercised could help formation of new behaviours. Although Billet's work is focused on learning in the context of workplaces, however, we cautiously deduce that appropriate design and employment of learning methods, individuals' enthusiasm to learn and well-designed strategies could lead to the development of new skills and behaviours. Scholars from the field of Psychology have acknowledged cognitive progresses through performance- based processes (Thorpe et al. 1987). The basic idea of rehearsal could possibly be related with "learning through practice". According to Billet (2010), practice (rehearsal) pertains to routine exercise of a given skill, ability or vocation. It is further proposed that learning through practice is not only limited to developing an individual's faculties but equally to enable the user in dealing with existing or new tasks. Hence, we propose that exercising or practicing is related with rehearsal as a technique to learn new skills and behaviours. We have observed that there is little research in the area of mental health care that explores the prospective effect of rehearsal as a software feature. This research gap was identified and helped us in setting the tone for the two field studies concentrating on sleeplessness and moderate depression respectively.

Building upon Fogg's influential work (2002), several researchers have come up with their own theories and models. The Persuasive Systems Design Model (Oinas-Kukkonen & Harjumaa, 2009) is among one of them. Oinas-Kukkonen and Harjumaa (2009) propose that persuasive information systems should encourage users through reminders to perform desired behaviors. They further underline the use of virtual rehearsal as a software feature for assisting users in changing behaviors. Similarly, Fogg (2002) argues that rehearsal is a mean of providing a setting where people can rehearse and learn new behaviours. We propose that the concept of rehearsal as a method to learn new behaviours can be grounded on the Social Cognitive Theory (SCT) (Bandura, 1986). Bandura (1986) proposed that learning process is, "an information processing activity in which information about the structure of behaviour and about environmental events is transformed into symbolic representations that serve as cognitive guides for the construction of complex modes of behavior" (Bandura, 1986, p.51).

A persistent issue in e-Health interventions is low task completion and high dropout rates as pointed out by Eysenbach (2005). However, we have shifted away from a relatively well-studied area such as attrition rates and have focused more on task completion (by analysing the possible effect of reminders) and learning new behaviors (through the use of rehearsal). We propose that task completion is a distinctive phase of interaction that could lead to prolonged user commitment hence reducing dropout rates. Literature highlights valuable information about task completion, however, by emphasizing on the use of material rewards, admiration or social approval, and positive feedback (Volpp et al. 2008). We argue that it is vital for healthcare researchers not to confuse adherence with low attrition or high drop out rates. For example, dropouts generally pertain to participants of a given intervention who do not fulfil the entire research protocol (Kelders, 2013). Eysenbach (2005) describes adherence as the extent to which participants of a given intervention "experience" the content. Adherence has also been reported as the extent to which participants' behaviours balance with the guidance and suggestions enthused by an intervention (Aronson, 2007). These interpretations provide a better understanding of a fairly overlapping phenomenon. However, we propose that task completion can be improved by developing engaging interventions that are supplemented with consequential and meaningful content. In other words, task completion is more about forming compliance, completing anticipated tasks and it could be the first step in overcoming lack of devotion and high drop out rates in the area of eHealth interventions for mental health care. We also propose that both researchers and system developers need to pay meticulous attention to psychological theories in order to recognise causal accounts for high dropouts. Further, it is our conjecture that task completion can not only decrease high dropout rates but can also helps users reach a state of higher self- efficacy leading to self- confidence in learning new skills and performing desired actions. The following part of the chapter highlights our attempts to examine the above-mentioned issues particularly. This is because low task adherence and complications in learning new skills remain a challenge when it comes to mental health care (Mohr et al. 2010).

2.1 The Field Studies

Both the studies were carried out using a mixed- method research approach, which is occasionally known as triangulation and is applied in various disciplines (Östlund et al. 2011; Brewer & Hunter, 1989). In addition, mixed- method approach helps researchers explore research problems by using a blend of qualitative and quantitative methods (Onwuegbuzie & Leech, 2005; Wood et al. 1999). The different methods complement each other by revealing exhaustive results. According to Kaplan and Duchon (1988), mixing qualitative and quantitative methodologies offer a greater understanding for inferring and authenticating research conclusions. Applying qualitative research method is known to be constructive as it helps in reducing uncertainties about analytical views and themes. In other words, it could be taken as a developmental approach that advances the overall understanding of a research problem and helps in gaining expressive responses (Sofaer, 1999). Qualitative research becomes particularly valuable for performing research analyses as it elucidates participants' experiences, behaviours, interactions and their social interactions (Strauss & Corbin, 1990). In the context of mental health care research, qualitative methodology has been highlighted as a constructive approach.

3. PROCEDURES

3.1 Recruitment

Study I was conducted between October 2013 and November 2013. Participants were enrolled through newspaper advertisements. The advertisements elucidated that we were seeking people who were suffering from sleep problems. The eligibility criteria were: 1) Access to Internet, 2) Having an email account, 3) Access to telephone, 4) Not being part of a therapy for sleep disorders in parallel, 5) and aged 18 years or over. In response, 122 individuals contacted the university clinic (Department of Psychology, University of Jyväskylä, Finland) for initial screening process. From the 122 individuals, 14 were excluded, as they did not meet the inclusion criteria. Another 22 were excluded from the study because of limited research resources. Accordingly, the final number of participants for Study I was eighty-six (N=86).

Study II was carried out between September 2012 and January 2013. Participants were recruited through newspaper advertisements that described that we were seeking individuals who felt depressed. The inclusion criteria were: 1) Self-reported depressive symptoms, 2) Depressed mood, 3) No parallel therapy for depression, 4) Access to Internet, 5) Having an email account and 6) Age 18 years of over. In response, a total of 42 individuals contacted the university clinic (Department of Psychology, University of Jyväskylä, Finland) for initial screening. After initial screening, measurement packages and informed consent forms were sent out to the selected participants. One participant dropped out before the screening process and another two did not meet the inclusion criteria therefore the final number of the participants was Thirty-nine (N=39).

3.2 Ethical Approval

Because both the studies included people with sleep- related issues and depressive symptoms, the studies followed the Declaration of Helsinki and the Research. Further, Ethical Approval was officially obtained from the Ethical Committee at the University of Jyväskylä, Finland and the Central Finland Healthcare District (Diary no: 15U/2012).

3.3 Randomization Process

Randomization for Study II was performed on the 13th of September 2012. The participants were divided into two groups: (1) Intervention group 1 (n=19) that received the measurements, automated reminders and complete access to the weekly rehearsal modules, and (2) Intervention group 2 that first served as a waiting list control group and had to wait for a period of six-weeks before they could access the complete intervention. Although the Intervention group 2 had access to the weekly rehearsal modules, however, they did not receive automated weekly reminders. A total of 28 (71.8%) females and 11 (28.2%) males with an average age of 51 years comprised the total sample. Upon completion of the six weeks from Intervention group 1, login credentials for the intervention were sent to the participants of the Intervention group 2. For Study I, randomization was performed using a randomization tool (https://www.random.org/lists) on the 9th of October 2013. Again the participants were divided into two groups: (1) Intervention group (n=43) that received the measurements, and had complete access to the intervention supplemented with two automated weekly reminders, and (2) Wait-list control group (n=43). For ethical reasons, the Wait-list group received access to the complete intervention but no reminder were sent out. A total of 31 (72.1%) females and 12 (27.9%) males comprised the Intervention sample aged between 24 to 73 years.

3.4 Designing the Web- Based Interventions

The Web- based interventions were designed and developed in partnership between research groups from the Department of Information Processing Science, University of Oulu and Department of Psychology, University of Jyväskylä, Finland. A research team from the University of Oulu was responsible for implementing the software features whereas a research group from the University of Jyväskylä developed ACT-based rehearsal modules for both the studies. Rehearsal as a software feature was used to improve mindfulness, acceptance skills, value- based actions, and psychological flexibility with the help of vigilantly created metaphors, experiential exercises and behavioural activation (Hayes et al. 2006). Table 1 and 2 exhibit an outline of the modules that were used for the rehearsal content for Study II and I respectively.

Table 1. Acceptance and commitment therapy modules for rehearsing to overcome moderate depression

Week	Acceptance and Commitment Therapy Modules Used for Rehearsal
1	Creative hopelessness and values
2	Value-based actions
3	Contact with the present
4	Cognitive defusion
5	Self as context
6	Acceptance

Table 2. Acceptance and commitment therapy modules for rehearsing to improve sleeplessness

Week	Theme	Content
1	Values and value-based actions	Knowing what matters the most for an individual in users' life and acting in accordance
2	The present moment	Living in the present moment (mindfulness)
3	Cognitive defusion	Understanding that an individual's thoughts could be different
4	The observer stance	Learning to view one's thoughts and feelings from an observer's stance
5	Acceptance	Accepting one's feelings, and thoughts and admitting that one cannot change things
6	Summary	Rehearsing ACT exercises from the past five weeks

3.5 Qualitative Data Collection

Upon completion of the Study II, the participants were asked questions about system usefulness, influence of reminders on task completion, effect of rehearsal on learning new behaviors, impact of rehearsal on self-confidence and their intent to practice newly learnt (if any) skills in future. The questionnaire used Five-point Likert-type scale ranging from 1 = Strongly agree to 5 = Strongly disagree. In addition, the participants were interviewed in a post- intervention sitting where their experiences and overall observations were recorded, coded and analyzed. In Study I, participants' experiences with the intervention and its general practicality was evaluated by employing Likert-scale (Likert, 1932) questionnaires at the beginning and end of the intervention. The questions focused on participants' anticipations and perceived practicality of the system (pre- study) while their actual experiences, system usefulness, ease of use, influence of reminders on task completion, effect of rehearsal on self-confidence and impact of rehearsal module to improve sleep behaviors (post- study). Finally, the participants were interviewed (exit interview) in a post- intervention satisfaction survey where their experiences and interpretations were recorded, coded and analyzed.

4. RESULTS

4.1 Moderate Depression

In Study II, email- based reminders were sent to Intervention Group I only, in order to assess how the participants perceived the influence of reminders on task completion. A high majority of the participants (83.3%) approved the reminders and gave encouraging comments that; for example, it is easy to forget important tasks in a chaotic world. Some of the descriptive remarks are listed below:

P1: *Reminders assured me to remember doing the assignments (weekly modules); I use my email very often.*
P2: *They (reminders) reminded me of doing my homework (weekly modules) and I found the link (URL to the system) very handy.*
P3: *Reminders give you a feeling that you are not alone. They encouraged (me) and gave a boost for replying to the (weekly) assignments (modules).*
P4: *In addition to email-based reminders, SMS could be beneficial.*
P5: *Add supportive criticism, enveloping criticism in a way that it won't depress the person.*

Participants from the intervention group that did not receive reminders however they pointed out that reminders would have been useful in helping them completing important tasks. Some of the representative quotes are as below:

P6: *...If one has a tendency towards forgetting things that need to be done (reminders would have helped a great deal).*
P7: *Yes (reminders would have been useful), because I forgot since there were no reminders, the due dates were hard to remember.*

There were some varied comments and a few representative quotes are stated below:

P8: *I did not need to be reminded. I was already committed to the program (intervention).*
P9: *I would try to make the reminders and rehearsal (exercise modules) less demanding.*

Majority of the participants acknowledged the effect of rehearsal in helping them to learn new skills. Some of the representative comments are listed below:

P10: *Exercises (weekly rehearsal modules) were good. All in all, the interaction (experience) was excellent.*
P11: *Weekly themes (modules) were very good. They brought me in touch with my (core) values and I learned to be consciously present in the moment.*
P12: *I found the rehearsal (content) to be supportive. It kept me on track.*
P13: *I think the weekly rehearsal (modules) improved my understanding about life.*

4.2 Sleeplessness

In Study I, 41 out of the 43 participants gave comments about reminders. Some of the representative statements are listed below:

P1: *Reminders worked fine. Adding SMS – based reminders would have been better.*
P2: *The system was good. I found the reminders and rehearsal to be beneficial.*
P3: *I expected a little more from the system. The rehearsals were good and so were the reminders (they were much needed).*

Participants generally appreciated the rehearsal feature as well as its content. Some of the representative quotes are listed below:

P4: *I go to know myself (better) and now I have new (better) viewpoints (about my life).*
P5: *I had no problems with the systems. It was (indeed) a positive experience. The entire program was well built (designed) both technically and content wise.*
P6: *There was a lot of new information. The program provided broad (comprehensive) approaches towards (tackling) sleep problems, it was engaging. Although my sleep problems are still the same, I will continue to rehearse.*
P7: *Rehearsals were easy to use and reasonable (logical). It was (indeed) an interesting experience. Now I can sleep and breathe better.*
P8: *It was a positive experience. Working the exercises (rehearsals) has improved my situation.*
P9: *It was a surprising and exciting experience. I committed myself to the program (intervention) and I learnt new skills.*
P10: *The system (rehearsal modules) taught me to listen, breathe and mediate well. It helped me accept that there are bad times. Thank you.*

Some mixed remarks were also noted. Some of the representative quotes are stated below:

P11: *A little more interaction (prolonged study period) would have been better (desirable).*
P12: *The program (intervention) did not help me. The study period should have been longer.*
P13: *I expected more from the system (intervention). However, my own laziness influenced my learning process.*

4.3 Identified Themes

Based on the collected responses and criticisms, we identified six themes for researchers in the area of mental health care using eHealth interventions:

- **Provision of Positive Feedback:** Participants of a given eHealth intervention appreciate receiving positive feedback. The process of providing the participants with constructive feedback can lead to improved interaction between the users and the intervention. It is generally accepted that positive feedback improves the learning process (Mitrivic et al. 2013). It has also been observed that positive feedback improves the overall interactivity and engagement (Schubart et al. 2011). The effect of positive feedback through technological interventions can motivate participants to develop what could be termed as a reciprocal relationship. If this stands true, enhanced adherence could be achieved (Mohr et al. 2011; Ritterband et al. 2009) Therefore, it is important that interventions for mental health care and support offer carefully crafted feedback (content) to the participants.
- **Provision of Constructive Criticism:** People with mental conditions are usually sensitive towards criticism however, some might benefit from it by focusing on the constructive content of the feedback. However, such a strategy would perhaps best suit those individuals who are willing to receive criticism and have the motivation to benefit from it for individual progress (Bergner, 1995). The significance of a balance between using positive and negative feedback (criticism) is also highlighted in several studies (Iwashita, 2003; Cinquin & Demongeot, 2002) This could be an interesting area for further research in the research field of mental health care eHealth interventions.
- **Use of SMS to Supplement Email-Based Reminders:** Email- based reminders could be supplemented with short messaging service (SMS). The use of SMS- based reminders has been recommended for e-Health interventions (Pop-Eleches et al. 2011). The role of SMS- based prompts has also been supported by researchers in the area of mental health care as well as in behavior change (Sims et al. 2012; Neff & Fry, 2009). It is argued that mobile phones are like constant partners therefore making it easier for the reminders to be sent. This could be particularly useful for people who do not have access to computers or they rarely check their emails.
- **Adding Supportive Content to the Reminders:** It is important that people suffering from mental conditions such as depressive symptoms, stress, anxiety and trauma are not left in a situation where they feel secluded. One of the key themes identified from the interviews was that participants emphasized on the need for adding supportive content to the reminders. We therefore propose

that when developing the content of reminders, carefully crafted aspects of support and compassion should be incorporated. By adding the element of empathy, we can redesign the interventions that are more of supporting in nature and could lead to desired outcomes including higher adherence or lower dropout rates (Mohr et al. 2011). By virtue, human beings are social animals and the significance of social relationships can never be overlooked. It is hence argued that social relationships are highly significant for mental wellbeing. Sharma and colleagues (2015) also advocate use of proactive thinking in terms of designing supportive and empathetic interventions.

- **Reminding People of Their Core Values:** An intervention should be designed in a way that it prompts people and reminds them of their core values. Further, eHealth interventions for mental health care should assist the users to reflect upon their values (Ploderer et al. 2014). The content of the interventions should be designed in a way that it helps people to recognize what is really important for them, what are their aims and beliefs (Powers et al. 2009). Once people identify their core values, they are more likely to take actions to overcome challenging and impulsive circumstances hence making life easier for them (Kuonanoja et al. 2015). The use of behavioural therapies especially Acceptance and Commitment Therapy underscores the importance of core values in various studies in the area of mental health care (Lappalainen et al. 2014; Räsänen et al. 2016).
- **Engage Users by Developing Logical Content:** Mental health care eHealth interventions should be designed with an aim to provide participants with a rich and engaging user experience (Hefferman et al. 2016). In other words, the content of eHealth interventions for mental health should be meaningful and affective. By adding logical content, it would be easy to involve users emotionally because user engagement depends on elements that include but are not limited to behavioural actions, cognition and threads of logical arguments (O'Brian, 2010). In addition, logical content could perhaps be related with rich user experience (UX). While there is an array of definitions about UX, we propose that UX under the umbrella of Human Computer Interaction could support users in achieving desired goals as well as adhering with the entire period of the intervention. Andersson and Kjerrman (2013) support our proposition by underlining the significance of pragmatic and logical arguments and their influence on task adherence.

5. DISCUSSION

The main objective of the chapter is to highlight qualitative findings from two field studies that focused on two mental conditions namely moderate depression and sleeplessness. In this chapter, participants' subjective considerations about web- based interventions' effectiveness, influence of reminders on task completion, effect of rehearsal on learning new skills and behaviors, and participants' general experiences with the interventions have been underscored with an aim to identify budding themes that could help researchers in designing efficient eHealth interventions for mental health care. It is noted that the participants of both studies generally regarded reminders as being useful. However, a noteworthy finding was the there was a lack of influence of the reminders on the overall psychological outcomes.

Yet, reminders supported participants in completing their weekly tasks (rehearsal modules). Rehearsal on the other hand, markedly enhanced participants' self-efficacy by subsiding cognitive burden and perplexity. The moderately lower influence of reminders could be attributed to the rich, engaging and logical content of the ACT-based rehearsal modules because the participants reported them as highly beneficial and effectual. Yet another reason could be the intrinsic motivation of the participants. This is because notwithstanding the distress from stern mental conditions, they volunteered to partake the studies without any financial enticements. This suggests that people have a natural propensity to look for and try out different means that can help them manage and perhaps overcome mental health care issues.

Whereas lack of effect for reminders was spotted, it is worth noting that some of the participants felt that while receiving the reminders, they were being treated on an individual basis. This is an exciting observation and opens up further research occasions to develop and evaluate tailored reminders. In terms of rehearsal, it was observed that nearly all participants from both the studies not only favoured but also found it as a positive method to learn new skills leading to improved state of self-confidence. This observation is not only supported by the post- study questionnaires and interviews but also by obvious decline in the severity of depression and sleeplessness. Therefore, we cautiously propose that while patients with mental conditions is largely dealt in face-to-face therapeutic sessions, however, vigilantly devised eHealth interventions with no or minimal face-to-face contact can be as effective in treating such conditions. In both the studies, we observed noteworthy improvements in post- study psychological measurements where participants felt better mental state and improved self- confidence to manage such conditions. However, reporting the psychological measurements and their outcomes is beyond the objective and scope this chapter.

6. LIMITATIONS

Presented work has its limitations. First, an effort has been made to combine the qualitative findings from two field studies with slightly different research settings. The number of participants for the studies are not the same, however, it should be considered that the basic building block of the interventions for both the conditions was Acceptance and Commitment Therapy (ACT) that provides a solid ground to combine the qualitative findings. Second, the entire focus has been paid to qualitative comments and interpretations because reporting the quantitative and psychological measurements was outside of the objective and beyond the scope of this chapter. Further, even though presented work combines two field studies with real patients of moderate depression and sleeplessness, yet the overall sample size is rather small therefore it is hard to generalize the results.

7. CONCLUSION AND RESEARCH IMPLICATIONS

Presented chapter highlights qualitative findings from two field studies that examined the efficacy of reminders and rehearsal in web- based eHealth interventions for sleeplessness and moderate depression. The interventions were incorporated with Acceptance and Commitment Therapy (ACT), which is the latest wave of Cognitive Behavioural Therapy (CBT). Reminders were studied to observe their possible influence on task completion that is proposed to be a way forward to solve the established drawback of high dropout rates in health care interventions. Rehearsal was assessed to find out whether it could improve participants' self-efficacy and self-belief to manage mild to moderate mental conditions. The descriptive quotes underline participants' experiences with the interventions and offer notable insights that can have substantial implications for researchers in the area of mental health care. The chapter contributes to available literature relating with task completion and improved self- confidence and highlights the prospective usefulness of web- based eHealth interventions as a medium to deliver novel solutions for mental health care.

8. FUTURE RESEARCH AGENDA

Worldwide dissemination and acceptance of computing technologies have paved the way for developing novel eHealth solutions that can have a positive impact on the mental health of people suffering from a range of mental conditions. Irrespective of the economic conditions of a country, public access to eHealth interventions has already become a phenomenon. Hundreds of Web- and Mobile- based interventions / applications are available designed to promote general and mental health. However, from researchers' point of view, we argue that the field of eHealth interventions (web- and mobile- based) have various areas that need further investigation. These include the lack of clarity, biased designers' intent, overlapping terminologies, lack of communication between health care researchers, lack of collaborative efforts, overlooking the significance of privacy and ethical issues, and other issues such as continuous monitoring of the interventions, understanding users' expectations, involving users in the design process and trust in eHealth interventions. In future, we are planning to design an eHealth intervention for children's psychological wellbeing in collaboration with psychologists as well as prospective users for their feedback. We also aim to study various constructs especially "Perceived Concerns about Privacy", "Soft Trust", "User Experience" and "User Involvement in the Design Process". We are hopeful that our future studies will lead to advancements in the area of eHealth interventions of mental health and make scientific advances.

ACKNOWLEDGMENT

The authors would like to thank Professor Harri Oinas-Kukkonen, Professor Raimo Lappalainen, the OASIS Research Group (University of Oulu, Finland) and the Research Team from the Department of Psychology (University of Jyväskylä, Finland) for their contribution to the previously published studies. Further, the authors would like to mention that the present chapter is developed from the studies that were supported by the SalWe Research Program for Mind and body (Tekes - The Finnish Funding Agency for Technology and Innovation Grant 1104/10).

REFERENCES

Alhola, P., & Polo-Kantola, P. (2007). Sleep deprivation: Impact on cognitive performance. *Neuropsychiatric Disease and Treatment*, *3*(5), 553. PMID:19300585

Andersson, G., & Cuijpers, P. (2009). Internet-based and other computerized psychological treatments for adult depression: A meta-analysis. *Cognitive Behaviour Therapy*, *38*(4), 196–205. doi:10.1080/16506070903318960 PMID:20183695

Andersson, G., & Cuijpers, P. (2009). Internet-based and other computerized psychological treatments for adult depression: A meta-analysis. *Cognitive Behaviour Therapy*, *38*(4), 196–205. doi:10.1080/16506070903318960 PMID:20183695

Andersson, J., & Kjerrman, V. (2013). Patient Empowerment and User Experience in eHealth Services: A Design-Oriented Study of eHealth Services in Uppsala County Council.

Andrews, G., Cuijpers, P., Craske, M. G., McEvoy, P., & Titov, N. (2010). Computer therapy for the anxiety and depressive disorders is effective, acceptable and practical health care: A meta-analysis. *PLoS ONE*, *5*(10), e13196. doi:10.1371/journal.pone.0013196 PMID:20967242

Aromaa, E., Tolvanen, A., Tuulari, J., & Wahlbeck, K. (2011). Personal stigma and use of mental health services among people with depression in a general population in Finland. *BMC Psychiatry*, *11*(1), 52. doi:10.1186/1471-244X-11-52 PMID:21453504

Aronson, J. K. (2007). Compliance, concordance, adherence. *British Journal of Clinical Pharmacology*, *63*(4), 383–384. doi:10.1111/j.1365-2125.2007.02893.x PMID:17378797

Bandura, A. (1986). *Social foundations of thought and action*. Englewood Cliffs, NJ: Prentice Hall.

Barak, A., Klein, B., & Proudfoot, J. G. (2009). Defining internet-supported therapeutic interventions. *Annals of Behavioral Medicine*, *38*(1), 4–17. doi:10.1007/s12160-009-9130-7 PMID:19787305

Benbasat, I. (2010). HCI research: Future challenges and directions. *AIS Transactions on Human-Computer Interaction*, *2*(2), 1.

Benca, R. M., & Peterson, M. J. (2008). Insomnia and depression. *Sleep Medicine*, *9*, S3–S9. doi:10.1016/S1389-9457(08)70010-8 PMID:18929317

Bergner, R. M. (1995). Promoting Constructive Modes of Self-Criticism. In Pathological Self-Criticism (pp. 107-129). Springer US. doi:10.1007/978-1-4757-2410-3_7

Billett, S. (2010). *The practices of learning through occupations* (pp. 59–81). Springer Netherlands. doi:10.1007/978-90-481-3939-2_4

Brewer, J., & Hunter, A. (1989). *Multimethod research: A synthesis of styles*. Sage Publications, Inc.

Choe, E. K., Consolvo, S., Watson, N. F., & Kientz, J. A. (2011, May). Opportunities for computing technologies to support healthy sleep behaviors. In *Proceedings of the SIGCHI Conference on Human Factors in Computing Systems* (pp. 3053-3062). ACM. doi:10.1145/1978942.1979395

Cinquin, O., & Demongeot, J. (2002). Positive and negative feedback: Striking a balance between necessary antagonists. *Journal of Theoretical Biology, 216*(2), 229–241. doi:10.1006/jtbi.2002.2544 PMID:12079373

Consolvo, S., McDonald, D. W., & Landay, J. A. (2009, April). Theory-driven design strategies for technologies that support behavior change in everyday life. In *Proceedings of the SIGCHI Conference on Human Factors in Computing Systems* (pp. 405-414). ACM. doi:10.1145/1518701.1518766

Drozd, F., Lehto, T., & Oinas-Kukkonen, H. (2012, June). Exploring perceived persuasiveness of a behavior change support system: a structural model. In *Proceedings of the International Conference on Persuasive Technology* (pp. 157-168). Springer Berlin Heidelberg. doi:10.1007/978-3-642-31037-9_14

Durmer, J. S., & Dinges, D. F. (2005, March). Neurocognitive consequences of sleep deprivation. *Seminars in Neurology, 25*(1), 117–129. doi:10.1055/s-2005-867080 PMID:15798944

Eysenbach, G. (2000). Recent advances: Consumer health informatics. *BMJ: British Medical Journal, 320*(7251), 1713–1716. doi:10.1136/bmj.320.7251.1713 PMID:10864552

Eysenbach, G. (2005). The law of attrition. *Journal of Medical Internet Research, 7*(1), e11. doi:10.2196/jmir.7.1.e11 PMID:15829473

Fogg, B. J. (2002). Persuasive technology: Using computers to change what we think and do. *Ubiquity, 2002*(December), 5. doi:10.1145/764008.763957

Forman, E. M., Herbert, J. D., Moitra, E., Yeomans, P. D., & Geller, P. A. (2007). A randomized controlled effectiveness trial of acceptance and commitment therapy and cognitive therapy for anxiety and depression. *Behavior Modification, 31*(6), 772–799. doi:10.1177/0145445507302202 PMID:17932235

Galatzer-Levy, I. R., & Bonanno, G. A. (2014). Optimism and death predicting the course and consequences of depression trajectories in response to heart attack. *Psychological Science*. PMID:25298294

Hayes, S. C., Luoma, J. B., Bond, F. W., Masuda, A., & Lillis, J. (2006). Acceptance and commitment therapy: Model, processes and outcomes. *Behaviour Research and Therapy, 44*(1), 1–25. doi:10.1016/j.brat.2005.06.006 PMID:16300724

Hayes, S. C., Strosahl, K. D., & Wilson, K. G. (1999). *Acceptance and commitment therapy: An experiential approach to behavior change*. Guilford Press.

Heffernan, K. J., Chang, S., Maclean, S. T., Callegari, E. T., Garland, S. M., Reavley, N. J.,... & Wark, J. D. (2016). Guidelines and recommendations for developing interactive eHealth apps for complex messaging in health promotion. *JMIR mHealth and uHealth, 4*(1).

Iwashita, N. (2003). Negative feedback and positive evidence in task-based interaction. *Studies in Second Language Acquisition, 25*(01), 1–36. doi:10.1017/S0272263103000019

Johansson, R., & Andersson, G. (2014). Internet-based psychological treatments for depression. *Expert Review of Neurotherapeutics*. PMID:22853793

Kaplan, B., & Duchon, D. (1988). Combining qualitative and quantitative methods in information systems research: A case study. *Management Information Systems Quarterly, 12*(4), 571–586. doi:10.2307/249133

Kelders, S. M., Bohlmeijer, E. T., & Van Gemert-Pijnen, J. E. (2013). Participants, usage, and use patterns of a web-based intervention for the prevention of depression within a randomized controlled trial. *Journal of Medical Internet Research, 15*(8), e172. doi:10.2196/jmir.2258 PMID:23963284

Kelders, S. M., Kok, R. N., Ossebaard, H. C., & Van Gemert-Pijnen, J. E. (2012). Persuasive system design does matter: A systematic review of adherence to web-based interventions. *Journal of Medical Internet Research, 14*(6), e152. doi:10.2196/jmir.2104 PMID:23151820

Kelders, S. M., Van Gemert-Pijnen, J. E., Werkman, A., Nijland, N., & Seydel, E. R. (2011). Effectiveness of a Web-based intervention aimed at healthy dietary and physical activity behavior: a randomized controlled trial about users and usage. *Journal of Medical Internet Research, 13*(2), e32.

Kleine-Budde, K., Müller, R., Kawohl, W., Bramesfeld, A., Moock, J., & Rössler, W. (2013). The cost of depression–a cost analysis from a large database. *Journal of Affective Disorders, 147*(1), 137–143. doi:10.1016/j.jad.2012.10.024 PMID:23164461

Kraft, P., & Yardley, L. (2009). Current issues and new directions in Psychology and Health: What is the future of digital interventions for health behaviour change?

Kuonanoja, L., Langrial, S., Lappalainen, R., Lappalainen, P., & Oinas-Kukkonen, H. (2015). Treating depression with a behavior change support system without face-to-face therapy. *AIS Transactions on Human-Computer Interaction, 7*(3), 192–210.

Langrial, S. (2012). From digital interventions to behavior change support systems: Understanding persuasive systems' development and evaluation process. *Proceedings of IRIS '12* (pp. 1–16).

Langrial, S., Lehto, T., Oinas-Kukkonen, H., Harjumaa, M., & Karppinen, P. (2012, July). Native Mobile Applications For Personal Well-Being: A Persuasive Systems Design Evaluation. In PACIS (p. 93).

Langrial, S., Oinas-Kukkonen, H., Lappalainen, P., & Lappalainen, R. (2014). *Influence of Persuasive reminders and Virtual Rehearsal on Information Systems for Sleep Deprivation* (p. 228). PACIS.

Langrial, S., Oinas-Kukkonen, H., & Wang, S. (2012). Design of a Web-Based Information System for Sleep Deprivation–A Trial Study. In *Exploring the Abyss of Inequalities* (pp. 41–51). Springer Berlin Heidelberg. doi:10.1007/978-3-642-32850-3_4

Lappalainen, P., Granlund, A., Siltanen, S., Ahonen, S., Vitikainen, M., Tolvanen, A., & Lappalainen, R. (2014). ACT Internet-based vs face-to-face? A randomized controlled trial of two ways to deliver Acceptance and Commitment Therapy for depressive symptoms: An 18-month follow-up. *Behaviour Research and Therapy, 61*, 43–54. doi:10.1016/j.brat.2014.07.006 PMID:25127179

Lappalainen, P., Langrial, S., Oinas-Kukkonen, H., Tolvanen, A., & Lappalainen, R. (2015). Web-based acceptance and commitment therapy for depressive symptoms with minimal support a randomized controlled trial. *Behavior Modification, 39*(6), 805–834. doi:10.1177/0145445515598142 PMID:26253644

Likert, R. (1932). A technique for the measurement of attitudes. *Archives de Psychologie.*

Masthoff, J., Langrial, S., & van Deemter, K. (2013, April). Personalizing triggers for charity actions. In *Proceedings of the International Conference on Persuasive Technology* (pp. 125-136). Springer Berlin Heidelberg. doi:10.1007/978-3-642-37157-8_16

Meyer, B., Berger, T., Caspar, F., Beevers, C., Andersson, G., & Weiss, M. (2009). Effectiveness of a novel integrative online treatment for depression (Deprexis): Randomized controlled trial. *Journal of Medical Internet Research, 11*(2), e15. doi:10.2196/jmir.1151 PMID:19632969

Mitrovic, A., Ohlsson, S., & Barrow, D. K. (2013). The effect of positive feedback in a constraint-based intelligent tutoring system. *Computers & Education*, *60*(1), 264–272. doi:10.1016/j.compedu.2012.07.002

Mohr, D., Cuijpers, P., & Lehman, K. (2011). Supportive accountability: A model for providing human support to enhance adherence to eHealth interventions. *Journal of Medical Internet Research*, *13*(1), e30. doi:10.2196/jmir.1602 PMID:21393123

Mohr, D. C., Burns, M. N., Schueller, S. M., Clarke, G., & Klinkman, M. (2013). Behavioral intervention technologies: Evidence review and recommendations for future research in mental health. *General Hospital Psychiatry*, *35*(4), 332–338. doi:10.1016/j.genhosppsych.2013.03.008 PMID:23664503

Mohr, D. C., Duffecy, J., Jin, L., Ludman, E. J., Lewis, A., Begale, M., & McCarthy, M. Jr. (2010). Multimodal e-mental health treatment for depression: A feasibility trial. *Journal of Medical Internet Research*, *12*(5), e48. doi:10.2196/jmir.1370 PMID:21169164

Mohr, D. C., Schueller, S. M., Montague, E., Burns, M. N., & Rashidi, P. (2014). The behavioral intervention technology model: An integrated conceptual and technological framework for eHealth and mHealth interventions. *Journal of Medical Internet Research*, *16*(6), e146. doi:10.2196/jmir.3077 PMID:24905070

Neff, R., & Fry, J. (2009). Periodic prompts and reminders in health promotion and health behavior interventions: Systematic review. *Journal of Medical Internet Research*, *11*(2), e16. doi:10.2196/jmir.1138 PMID:19632970

OBrien, H. L. (2010). The influence of hedonic and utilitarian motivations on user engagement: The case of online shopping experiences. *Interacting with Computers*, *22*(5), 344–352. doi:10.1016/j.intcom.2010.04.001

Oh, H., Rizo, C., Enkin, M., Jadad, A., Powell, J., & Pagliari, C. (2005). What is eHealth (3): A systematic review of published definitions. *Journal of Medical Internet Research*, *7*(1), e1. doi:10.2196/jmir.7.1.e1 PMID:15829471

Oinas-Kukkonen, H., & Harjumaa, M. (2009). Persuasive systems design: Key issues, process model, and system features. *Communications of the Association for Information Systems*, *24*(1), 28.

Ong, J. C., Ulmer, C. S., & Manber, R. (2012). Improving sleep with mindfulness and acceptance: A metacognitive model of insomnia. *Behaviour Research and Therapy*, *50*(11), 651–660. doi:10.1016/j.brat.2012.08.001 PMID:22975073

Onwuegbuzie, A. J., & Leech, N. L. (2005). On becoming a pragmatic researcher: The importance of combining quantitative and qualitative research methodologies. *International Journal of Social Research Methodology*, *8*(5), 375–387. doi:10.1080/13645570500402447

Or, C. K., Karsh, B. T., Severtson, D. J., Burke, L. J., Brown, R. L., & Brennan, P. F. (2011). Factors affecting home care patients acceptance of a web-based interactive self-management technology. *Journal of the American Medical Informatics Association*, *18*(1), 51–59. doi:10.1136/jamia.2010.007336 PMID:21131605

Orzeł-Gryglewska, J. (2010). Consequences of sleep deprivation. *International Journal of Occupational Medicine and Environmental Health*, *23*(1), 95–114. doi:10.2478/v10001-010-0004-9 PMID:20442067

Östlund, U., Kidd, L., Wengström, Y., & Rowa-Dewar, N. (2011). Combining qualitative and quantitative research within mixed method research designs: A methodological review. *International Journal of Nursing Studies*, *48*(3), 369–383. doi:10.1016/j.ijnurstu.2010.10.005 PMID:21084086

Patrick, K., Raab, F., Adams, M., Dillon, L., Zabinski, M., Rock, C., & Norman, G. et al. (2009). A text message-based intervention for weight loss: Randomized controlled trial. *Journal of Medical Internet Research*, *11*(1), e1. doi:10.2196/jmir.1100 PMID:19141433

Perkins, M. B., Jensen, P. S., Jaccard, J., Gollwitzer, P., Oettingen, G., Pappadopulos, E., & Hoagwood, K. E. (2007). Applying theory-driven approaches to understanding and modifying clinicians behavior: What do we know? *Psychiatric Services (Washington, D.C.)*, *58*(3), 342–348. doi:10.1176/ps.2007.58.3.342 PMID:17325107

Ploderer, B., Reitberger, W., Oinas-Kukkonen, H., & van Gemert-Pijnen, J. (2014). Social interaction and reflection for behaviour change. *Personal and Ubiquitous Computing*, *18*(7), 1667–1676. doi:10.1007/s00779-014-0779-y

Pop-Eleches, C., Thirumurthy, H., Habyarimana, J. P., Zivin, J. G., Goldstein, M. P., De Walque, D., & Ngare, D. et al. (2011). Mobile phone technologies improve adherence to antiretroviral treatment in a resource-limited setting: A randomized controlled trial of text message reminders. *AIDS (London, England)*, *25*(6), 825–834. doi:10.1097/QAD.0b013e32834380c1 PMID:21252632

Powers, M. B., Zum Vörde Sive Vörding, M. B., & Emmelkamp, P. M. (2009). Acceptance and commitment therapy: A meta-analytic review. *Psychotherapy and Psychosomatics*, *78*(2), 73–80. doi:10.1159/000190790 PMID:19142046

Räsänen, P., Lappalainen, P., Muotka, J., Tolvanen, A., & Lappalainen, R. (2016). An online guided ACT intervention for enhancing the psychological wellbeing of university students: A randomized controlled clinical trial. *Behaviour Research and Therapy*, *78*, 30–42. doi:10.1016/j.brat.2016.01.001 PMID:26848517

Revere, D., & Dunbar, P. J. (2001). Review of Computer-generated Outpatient Health Behavior Interventions Clinical Encounters in Absentia. *Journal of the American Medical Informatics Association*, *8*(1), 62–79. doi:10.1136/jamia.2001.0080062 PMID:11141513

Ritterband, L. M., & Tate, D. F. (2009). The science of internet interventions. *Annals of Behavioral Medicine*, *38*(1), 1–3. doi:10.1007/s12160-009-9132-5 PMID:19816750

Ritterband, L. M., Thorndike, F. P., Cox, D. J., Kovatchev, B. P., & Gonder-Frederick, L. A. (2009). A behavior change model for internet interventions. *Annals of Behavioral Medicine*, *38*(1), 18–27. doi:10.1007/s12160-009-9133-4 PMID:19802647

Schneider, F., de Vries, H., Candel, M., van de Kar, A., & van Osch, L. (2013). Periodic email prompts to re-use an internet-delivered computer-tailored lifestyle program: Influence of prompt content and timing. *Journal of Medical Internet Research*, *15*(1), e23. doi:10.2196/jmir.2151 PMID:23363466

Schubart, J. R., Stuckey, H. L., Ganeshamoorthy, A., & Sciamanna, C. N. (2011). Chronic health conditions and internet behavioral interventions: A review of factors to enhance user engagement. *Computers, Informatics, Nursing*, *29*(2), 81–92. doi:10.1097/NCN.0b013e3182065eed PMID:21164337

Seligman, L. D., & Ollendick, T. H. (2011). Cognitive-behavioral therapy for anxiety disorders in youth. *Child and Adolescent Psychiatric Clinics of North America*, *20*(2), 217–238. doi:10.1016/j.chc.2011.01.003 PMID:21440852

Sharma, D., Clune, S., & Blair, L. (2015). Radicalising the designer: Combating age-related loneliness through radical-digital interventions.

Sims, H., Sanghara, H., Hayes, D., Wandiembe, S., Finch, M., Jakobsen, H., & Kravariti, E. et al. (2012). Text message reminders of appointments: A pilot intervention at four community mental health clinics in London. *Psychiatric Services (Washington, D.C.)*, *63*(2), 161–168. doi:10.1176/appi.ps.201100211 PMID:22302334

Sofaer, S. (1999). Qualitative methods: What are they and why use them? *Health Services Research, 34*(5 Pt 2), 1101. PMID:10591275

Strauss, A., & Corbin, J. (1990). *Basics of qualitative research* (Vol. 15). Newbury Park, CA: Sage.

Tang, M. F., Liou, T. H., & Lin, C. C. (2010). Improving sleep quality for cancer patients: Benefits of a home-based exercise intervention. *Supportive Care in Cancer, 18*(10), 1329–1339. doi:10.1007/s00520-009-0757-5 PMID:19834744

Thorpe, G. L., Hecker, J. E., Cavallaro, L. A., & Kulberg, G. E. (1987). Insight versus rehearsal in cognitive-behavior therapy: A crossover study with sixteen phobics. *Behavioural Psychotherapy, 15*(4), 319–336. doi:10.1017/S0141347300012714

Volpp, K. G., John, L. K., Troxel, A. B., Norton, L., Fassbender, J., & Loewenstein, G. (2008). Financial incentive–based approaches for weight loss: A randomized trial. *Journal of the American Medical Association, 300*(22), 2631–2637. doi:10.1001/jama.2008.804 PMID:19066383

Warmerdam, L., van Straten, A., Twisk, J., Riper, H., & Cuijpers, P. (2008). Internet-based treatment for adults with depressive symptoms: Randomized controlled trial. *Journal of Medical Internet Research, 10*(4), e44. doi:10.2196/jmir.1094 PMID:19033149

Waters, F., & Bucks, R. S. (2011). Neuropsychological effects of sleep loss: Implication for neuropsychologists. *Journal of the International Neuropsychological Society, 17*(04), 571–586. doi:10.1017/S1355617711000610 PMID:21554786

Wood, M., Daly, J., Miller, J., & Roper, M. (1999). Multi-method research: An empirical investigation of object-oriented technology. *Journal of Systems and Software, 48*(1), 13–26. doi:10.1016/S0164-1212(99)00042-4

KEY TERMS AND DEFINITIONS

ACT: Acceptance and Commitment Therapy.

CBT: Cognitive Behavioural Therapy.

Depression: Feeling of hopelessness, dejection and despondency.

eHealth Interventions: Healthcare solutions offered through technological platforms.

Persuasive Technology: Technologies developed with an aim to persuade people to adopt desirable behaviors.

Rehearsal: Software feature utilized in eHealth interventions to support users perform desired actions regularly.

Reminders: Software features utilized in eHealth interventions for reminding users to perform an action.

Sleeplessness: Lack of appropriate sleep.

Chapter 6
An Internet-Based Quantum Biofeedback and Neurotechnology Cybertherapy System for the Support of Transpersonal Psychology

Raul Valverde
Concordia University, Canada

ABSTRACT

Transpersonal psychology is the study of human nature and proceeds on the assumption that human beings possess potentials that exceed the limits of their ego and integrate the spiritual experience within a broader understanding of the human psyche and consciousness. Altered states of consciousness have been used as psychotherapy in transpersonal psychology for decades. A Cyberpsychotherapy system is proposed to support transpersonal psychotherapy. The system can be used to induce non-ordinary state of consciousness that can be used by transpersonal psychologists as a healing tool to cure his patients with psychological problems such as psychosis at a distance location with the help of Internet technologies. The Cyberpsychotherapy system uses quantum signal generator for the induction of altered states of consciousness based on the God's helmet of Persinger (1983). The Cyberpsychotherapy has integrated an EEG that serves as a biofeedback device

DOI: 10.4018/978-1-5225-3241-5.ch006

in order to assess if the patient has reached the desired level of consciousness and can be used it to adjust the frequencies of the signal generator in order to improve the psychotherapy experience of the patient if necessary. A sample of 10 patients was used to test the Cybertherapy system based on Neurotechnology and quantum biofeedback, data was collected and analyzed. Although the results show that the patients were not able to reach the desired level of consciousness for the psychotherapy, there is statistical significant evidence that the proposed system can help to raise the level of consciousness; this can help with future designs that will eventually assist to reach the desired level for the psychotherapy.

BACKGROUND

Cybertherapy is an Internet based computer-mediated system used to facilitate psychotherapy (Botella et al. 2009). This includes new applications of technology within psychology and healthcare, which utilize augmented and virtual reality components in order to facilitate psychotherapy (Botella et al. 2009). Although there are many Cybertherapy systems in the literature (Takacs, 2005), none of them addresses transpersonal psychotherapy and are based on quantum biofeedback. Transpersonal psychotherapy that is based on transpersonal psychology, considers that the psyche is multidimensional and there are several "levels of consciousness" and each has different characteristics and is governed by different laws. Transpersonal psychology is the study of human nature and development proceeds on the assumption that human beings possess potentials that exceed the limits of ego developed normally. A main goal of transpersonal theory is to integrate the spiritual experience within a broader understanding of the human psyche and consciousness (Grof, 1988).

The trend to explain consciousness by applying quantum theories has gained popularity in recent years and, although clearly disdained by neuroscientists, more and more researchers direct their steps this way up. Brian D. Josephson (1962) of the University of Cambridge, winner of the 1973 Nobel Prize in Physics for his studies on the quantum effects in superconductors (Josephson effect), proposes a unified field theory, quantum nature, that would explain not only the consciousness and its attributes, but also all the phenomenology observed to date in terms of psychological and mystical experiences.

The human being experiences different altered states of consciousness, that is, consciousness can be altered in different ways. Stanley Kripner (2000) defines altered states of consciousness as mental states that can be subjectively recognized by an individual or by an objective observer than the individual who experiences it as different in mental functions, the normal state of the individual, the alertness and the waking.

Altered states of consciousness have been used as psychotherapy in transpersonal psychology. One of these techniques is known as holotropic breath work that is produced by using hyperventilation making the individual breathing deeply and rapidly for several minutes. Grof (1988), with this technique, causes a crisis that leads to an altered state of consciousness and allows the study the consciousness of the individual from that new state. Stanislav Grof (1988) uses the experiential healing power of this new state of consciousness to cure his patients. Although holotropic breath work induces these altered states of consciousness, biofeedback and neurotechnology offer an alternative way to induce altered state of consciousness for transpersonal therapy that can be easily implemented with the use of quantum computer technology and used in combination with the internet to facilitate online transpersonal therapy (Valverde 2015a).

Quantum biofeedback uses sensors to monitor physiological relaxation indicators, as the temperature of the skin and muscle tension. It expands classical biofeedback by using galvanic skin response (GSR) together with modern computer technology to detect the response of the built-mind-spirit body (sometimes called the super-conscious) to a large array of stress indicators. Quantum Biofeedback is a sophisticated biofeedback technique based on advanced quantum scientific principles that promote a deeper understanding of health and healing. Seeing the body as a complex electrical circuit and the application of the principles of electrical engineering, who are able to analyze and balance the body electric.

Quantum Biofeedback interacts with all cellular matrix of the body, which allows communication with the conscious and unconscious reactions of the body. This is accomplished by establishing electrical communication using 12 electrodes are attached to the head, wrists, and ankles of the patient. A loop and cyber handshake between Quantum Biofeedback System and the patient using a calibration procedure is then created. By connecting in this way all 200 billion cells in the human body are included in the the exchange of information. On this basis, it is now possible to identify and prioritize the tensions and toxins that are a major concern and bring them into balance.

Classic Biofeedback is based on electrical measurements taken from the front (frontal cortex). In this information it is presented to the customer who then tries to consciously change their internal reactions to modify electrical results. Quantum Biofeedback uses your link to all body cell matrix interface, not only the conscious aspects, but also with the unconscious. This provides greater gain in the understanding of health, as our conscious perception of the world is limited by design to 17% of the stimulation we receive.

An application of quantum physics (neurotechnology) in the altered states of consciousness was carried out by Persinger (1983). Persinger (1983) was able to induce visions of God and other religious and mystical experiences in the laboratory by using a computer and with what he called the Koran helmet that has also the nickname of the God helmet. He found that the temporal lobes of the brain are the source of the most spiritual experiences and other alternate state of consciousness.

This God helmet is a device to induce altered states of consciousness using weak magnetic signals to direct brain activity that can induce spiritual experiences that helps with transpersonal exploration and transformation of many people that is able to heal because of these transpersonal experiences (Persinger 2000). It is suggested that altered states of consciousness such as sensed presence and out-of-body experience whether they are produced by magnetic, electric or other stimulations or circumstances can be most effectively explained as the changes of the relative contents and/or intensities of the test subjects' neural quantum entanglement with their surroundings including possibly spiritual environments or information (Hu & Wu 2012).

With the aid of quantum biofeedback and neurotechnology, people can discover hidden deep events and conflicts in their subconscious that can lead to healing experiences. The proposed research has the objective of creating a cyberpsychoterapy system that uses quantum biofeedback and neurotechnology to facilitate transpersonal psycho therapy by inducing altered state of consciousness over the internet.

The work has the intention to contribute to the existing literature in the application of quantum biofeedback and neurotechnology to psychology by suggesting a cyberteraphy system for the facilitation of transpersonal psychotherapy.

LITERATURE REVIEW

Quantum Consciousness

The trend to explain quantum consciousness by applying quantum theories has gained popularity in recent years (Valverde 2016), a character that has stood in defence of a theory quantum of consciousness was the physicist Roger Penrose (1994), famous for its friendly Stephen Hawking differences regarding certain cosmological aspects and a world authority with regard to the theories of relativity and quantum. Penrose (1994) attacks and almost ridicules those who argue that the artificial intelligence of computers can reproduce human attributes, including consciousness.

Penrose, based on the mathematical theorem of Gödel and based on subsequent his elaborations, concludes that no system deterministic, that is, which is based on rules and deductions, they can explain the creative powers of the mind and your judgment. This nullifies the claim of physics classic, computer, neurobiology, etc., to structure themselves into a complex phenomenon of consciousness. Penrose says that only the peculiar characteristics non-deterministic quantum physics could issue an approximate judgment on consciousness, within a theory that involved quantum phenomena, macro physical and conditions of non locality. At this point perhaps it would be interesting clarify that local conditions are not known in quantum physics those capabilities that either has a quantum system, communication instant between parts, ie, without there being time duration between communication of an event from one point to another system.

Albert Einstein called this peculiarity that occurs in the innermost parts of matter, the universe, "that mysterious action at a distance '. If some concepts explained at the time in the course of "Matter and Energy" understand the model proposed by Penrose relates to the concept of Universe "Nonlocal" to quantum levels, in the sense that everything that happens in a corner any of our cosmos is immediately 'felt', "meaning" for any another.

In his last conference Penrose ventures even indicate that probably It is in microtubules, microscopic tubes that form the skeleton of cells, including neurons, where the complicated interactions occur quantum kind that give their "magic" character, "mysterious" from the point of view of science, consciousness. Hameroff (1994), claims to have found evidence that loss of consciousness by providing anesthesia is due to some inhibition of the flow and movement of electrons within the microtubules. Hameroff argues that certain cellular elements such fluctuations occur quantum-relativistic that "somehow" do emerge consciousness. The major objection to this theory by neuroscientists is that all animals, including elementary, have microtubules in the cells which it seems to imply that they all possess consciousness. Hamenoff argues that such statement would be indefensible, but it is inevitable the observation of "some degree of apparent intelligence" in all animal species. There is still another favorable group to this explanatory theory of consciousness, which is headed by Dr. Ian N. Marshall (Marshall and Zohar 1997) who through empirical testing system claims to have the key to the issue. Marshall and Zohar (1997) showed that conscious thought emerges from quantum effects. Indeed, it has been found that the ability of subjects to carry out work simple while they are connected to an electroencephalogram (EEG).In general, we can say that the Achilles tendon of this group of theories lies in the extreme conditions in which the quantum interactions are observable, for example, the effect of local not manifested in conditions close to absolute zero temperature is absolutely clear that they are not exactly those of our brains. However, supporters of quantum school, as expected, they find answers to these problems and many other objections, in which are indistinguishable from the other schools that obviously do the same to defend their ideas.

Neurotechnologies

Interest in neutechnological devices has grown strongly since the release of 1986's classic text of Michael Hutchison "Megabrain" (1986). Besides neurotechnological machines, the industry has developed a range of related devices including peripherals-tapes, subliminal tapes, hypno-peripheral processing, sound meditation devices and altered state induction software programs for personal computers, etc. It seems like neurotechnology combined with contemporary psychology may seem to be revolutionary but its roots are much older as humanity has made many attempts in the past to involve consciousness with technology. The flashing LEDs in a light and sound machine can be traced back to the old practice of starting a fire in order to induce trance. Sound recordings of brain entrainment undoubtedly have their roots in the ritual singing and shamanic use of wind instruments.

This current era of neurotechnology was born from the experiments made in biofeedback that resulted in the work of some researchers of consciousness as Masters & Houston (1966) that created the AVE (an abbreviation of Audio Visual Environment) that is one of the first electronic brain entrainment devices. The AVE was the first device to use visual and auditory stimuli as a means of altering consciousness. Not much different that many of audiovisual devices of today, the AVE consisted of a wrap-around screen and headphones to bomb the sense in these two stimuli.

These signals generated by AVE devices and detectable by electroencephalogram (EEG) tests at specific frequency ranges; seem to vary from one state of consciousness to another for their users. The products of neurotechnology appear to make possible to "tune" the brain to these different alternating frequencies, and in turn achieve new psychological states. When you "tune" into these frequencies at a slower pace, our thought processes and central nervous system are altered, causing the brain to fall into a deep level of activity. In addition, when one is tuned to a frequency faster and a higher range, the wave activity can have a highly stimulating effect on the brain.

Altered states of consciousness have been used as a therapy for modern psychological paradigms as transpersonal psychology (Valverde, 2015). Although there are several techniques such as holotropic breathing used to induce these altered states of consciousness, terotechnology offers an easier to control alternative to the transpersonal therapies.

The area called Neuro includes all types of technology that any it contributes to the advancement of knowledge related to the brain. Despite that neurotechnology is relatively old, its most significant advances occurred in the last 30 years. The 90s were even proclaimed by the US government American as the "Decade of the Brain". Much of the responsibility for this development exacerbated is due to the advent and popularization of brain imaging techniques, including MRI, CT, PET

(Positron Emission Tomography), among others. With technological advances, some of these techniques at first provided only structural information from the brain but now it allows us to study the brain dynamics.

Experimentation and published research on the altering of brain activity has been going on for decades. A vast amount of applicable data has been collected by researchers and scientists concerning the manipulation and influencing of brain waves and states of consciousness. One effect discovered by German scientists in the 1930's is called the Ganzfield effect (Hyman 1985). It is an effect in which the eyes are exposed to a totally uniform visual field, with no edges, color changes, or movement. This effect can be achieved by looking up at the sky on a clear, cloudless day or with very specially constructed illuminated glasses. It affects the circuitry in the brain, which normally is constantly scanning the visual field for edges and movement. The eye responds primarily to changes, and with visual sensations shut off and the brain finding absolutely nothing, the subject cannot tell if his eyes are open or closed. This is an example of an altered state of consciousness resulting from the shift in brain waves to the theta state.

The effects of flickering light stimulation have been known for centuries. Ancient shamans used flickering lights to achieve a trance state, a key component in the development of the spiritual practices of a wide variety of ancient cultures. In the literature of the common era, Ptolemy noted around 200 A.D. that the flickering of sunlight seen through the spokes of a spinning wheel could cause patterns and colors to appear to the observer, producing a feeling of light headedness and euphoria. The onset of modern times, (1940's and 50's) brought the research of neuroscientist W. Gray Walter (Walter and Walter 1949). Walter used a strobe light to create flickering light stimulation, noting that the brain wave pattern of the cortex—just the area associated with vision—was changed. Ever since the adrenaline rush brought about by dancing around the tribal fire, the intent of scientists, researchers, and ancient religious practitioners has been to create relaxation and altered states by affecting the vibrational frequency of the brain waves. The use of technology is a modern day attempt to create desired changes in the brain's functioning, bringing about states of well-being and health.

Robert Monroe, one of the most prominent people in neurotechnology in particular in the field of sound with neurological efficiency, devised the method HEMI-SYNC: (Synchronization of the cerebral hemispheres by means of sounds). Like a glass resonates when a pure tone is emitted, the brain resonates when receives certain frequencies of waves, being synchronized with these, (similar to the previous with the flashes of light) effect is known as FFR Frequency Following Response (Response a frequency tracking).

Machines created based on FFR began to be popular, the typical machine based on the principle of Monroe using stereo headphones that are used are separately sent sound to each ear signals, for example 2 signs of 300 and 304 Hz. In one ear will be heard only 300 Hz signal and the other only 304, but since the sounds are combined in the brain, this will hear a third signal of 4 Hz which is the difference between the two sound impulses.

This third sign is not an audible sound, but an electrical signal that can only be created by the cerebral hemispheres acting in unison, and may go unnoticed, producing as a result, the two hemispheres are focused simultaneously on the same state of consciousness, increasing and brain power.

The Monroe Institute was created based on the principles of Monroe. This institute was founded by Robert A. Monroe, who began studying the effects of sound on accelerated learning in the 50's.The work is the result of thousands of hours of laboratory sessions.

Participants listen volunteer's specific combinations and sequences of sound patterns and simultaneously are reporting their experiences; while electronic instruments measure the effects on the activity of their brain waves.

W. Grey Walter (1964) conducting experiments in which strobe devices used to send rhythmic flashes of light in the eyes, watched amazed that the flickering light could alter the activity of the entire cerebral cortex, rather than exclusively associated areas with vision. The subjective experiences of those who received the flashes were even more curious reported seeing "lights like comets, ultra fantastic colors, color mental". Moreover, Walter discovered that certain visual stimuli of a certain frequency could cause the brain to respond quickly adjusted to the same frequency of the stimulus it received.

In 1982 a psychiatrist Denis Gorges created a machine called brain wave synchronized energized, patented and sold by his company, Synchro-Tech Inc which applies the latest technology in the first device designed optical-acoustic stimulation. This is able to promote as its inventor claimed, "an increase in the capabilities and functions of the human mind" unleashed a wave of unprecedented research and experimentation, catalyzed by M. Hutchinson (1986) through his famous book Megabrain that is being developed in and outside universities around the world.

Studies on this type of equipment is underway in North American universities, in areas including education and training, substance abuse, gerontology, pharmacology and physiology as well as pain reduction. In Europe, at the University of Vienna, it has created a special subject for further study of these devices. The neurological investigations in the last 15 years have shown that our cerebral hemispheres work independently. Each hemisphere collects the same information that its sensors (eyes, ears, taste, touch, smell) and processed differently. Our scheme of thought is influenced by the predominance of left hemisphere, logical and analytical thinking. Right hemisphere, creative thinking, visualization, and which carries out a holistic synthesis.

On the back of the brain is where the intuitive thought (Subconscious). Obviously use one of the two hemispheres or either of the Brain regions severely limits our abilities. The optimal functioning of our brain, is given by the synchronization of the two hemispheres: By left-right and front-back alternating stimulation occurs almost simultaneously, an issue of brain wave amplitude and frequency identical. It is that how you might think with our whole brain.

Neurotechnology are typically used for process brainwave entrainment to tune brainwaves any range brainwave. With these machines, you may experience theta waves, alpha, delta or including combinations of ranges using frequencies layered that mix several ranges brainwave in a brainwave pattern synergistic as pattern brainwave.

Hemi-Sync is a patented process sound pulses to create the same electric waves in frequency and amplitude simultaneously in both hemispheres of the brain for specific purposes.

Our brains have a hemisphere left and right. The left brain is linear, logical, practical, and time -oriented. The right hemisphere seems to be much more nonlinear, abstract, creative, holistic, and not logic. We tend to use one hemisphere at a time, or better said, will favor hemispheres particular in terms of what we're doing. An accountant probably uses less of his right hemisphere that an artist would during the course of their workday.

If the person is doing math, the staff would be using more of your left hand. If the person is going to paint a picture, the person would have the activity hemispheric more right. Both hemispheres are constantly interacting and both can be in use simultaneously. By merging both hemispheres, a person is allowed to work together and with this the person can increase his or her ability mental and improve his or her performance cognitive in general. Basically it's like having a computer processor faster able to work at faster speeds. The greater integration creates better performance.

The mind machines that help the brain synchronizes naturally to balance hemispheric activity and adjusts the activity of brain waves to match the carrier frequencies embedded brainwaves. This hemispheric coherence induced audio produces an optimal state of comprehensive synergy of the entire brain.

These hemispheres are connected by the corpus callosum. It serves as a conduit or a bridge between both sides. This bridge literally be exercised and strengthened until it is physically larger and more capable of transmitting data, ideas and feedback between the hemispheres.

The advance occurs when you use this principle to synchronize our brain wave frequencies chosen with the help of specific mental machines. We can do this easily by using technology binaural beat audio and ringtones monophonic. This phenomenon is called trailing phenomenon.

The scientific principle of drag can be used to resonate, or synchronize your brain to tune specific frequencies. The drive is quite simple. If you have two tuning forks of the same pitch, if you strike one and hold it near the other, which both resonate at the same frequency. Given this fact and the fact that our brains function as a resonating chamber. Oscillating pulses and patterns of neural excitation ripple through our brains like endless waves on a pond of subtle dynamic electric field.

The creation process frequency binaural beat - brainwave entrainment is very simple to explain. First, you create two audio tones two frequencies slightly different (ie 100 Hz and 107 Hz). When playing a tone in the ear left and the other tone in his right ear, the brain reacts to the stimulus audio by resonance brain activity to the difference between these two tones. His brain waves adjust to match this frequency differential.

For example, if you play a frequency of 100 Hz in the ear and left 107 Hz in the right ear, your brain tune the 7 Hz differential (107 Hz - 100 Hz = 7 Hz). This frequency tracking response makes your brain to resonate at 7 Hz frequency falls within the range of brainwaves theta. This guide psychoacoustics state of the art can create phenomenal results.

The electrical activity of neurons is changing patterns of electrical potential through all cell membranes. Each cell generates in the membrane potential can be detected in about one micrometer of the cell but large sets of brain cells that can work in harmony to generate potential of few micro volts, that can be detected through the skull and scalp using electrodes. The variation of the electrical potential around the scalp is the basis of operation of the electroencephalogram. This method of recording the electrical activity of the brain, digitized maps produces the electrical activity of brain.

The state in which the two hemispheres are synchronized, that is, showing similar activity in both hemispheres, sometimes known as “whole brain” naturally occurring randomly for short periods. Stimulation through the differential tone makes it possible to sustain this state for longer periods.

EEG based on data collected in the laboratory of Gateway Institute, it is clear that after a brief period of use of frequencies of Hemi-Sync, it can be demonstrated the benefits of the technology without the use of external sources.

The Hemi-Sync process has already been tested and implemented in many ways for:

- Sleep better
- Reduce tension or stress
- Control pain
- Accelerate learning
- Study and concentration
- Enhance creativity
- Find solutions to problems

Light and Sound Machines have the purpose to create a relaxed state through the use of sound and light stimulation. It was discovered in the 1930's that repetitive light stimulation (strobing) caused brain waves to follow and pulse at the same frequency (Walter & Walter 1949). This discovery had profound implications for the human condition, giving rise to an entire industry that explores the possibilities in using outside stimulation to provide a functioning aid to the workings of the brain. The devices on the market today are set at predetermined frequencies of 1 to 40 Hz. The user is then free to experiment on just how these vibrational frequencies influence their affect on the mind's eye. Most users report patterns of colors that pulse in synch with the frequency of the beats. The patterns are often quite psychedelic and geometrical.

Light and sound machines are often used for meditation assistance, or to aid the learning process. The technologies are referred to as audio-visual stimulation systems, light and sound machines, or mind machines.

Varying patterns of light and sound are used to create different states of awareness, attention, relaxation, creativity, and receptivity to information. Most systems are controlled by a microprocessor. The sound and music sometimes comes on a CD, with the frequency patterns embedded in the music.

A typical system is made up of three components: a light/sound synthesizer, stereo headphones, and stimulation glasses with pulsating lights. A carefully composed sequence of rhythmic light and sound patterns direct the stimulation synthesis, creating light and or sound sessions for the desired effect. Some systems connect to your music CD player, or have one built in. The process employs a technology called an audio strobe system, which creates inaudible, high frequency beats that drive a light/sound system. Other systems have computer interface capabilities that allow the user to vary the tone, frequency, pitch and other parameters to tailor the program to individual needs. Some metaphysical technology companies have downloadable programs that allow for even more growth, variety, and individual tailoring. A few make a point of offering customer service where the company provides you with specifics that are designed to individual needs (Dumit 1995).

The light and sound systems are designed to blank out the visual and auditory stimulation that the mind generally receives, and replaces it with very simple, rhythmic stimulation. Some light systems come with glasses that block certain colors so that the brain focuses on others to create the desired stimulation. The basic rhythms of light and sound cause the mental processes to change in response. Thus, the rate of brain waves adjusts to the desired vibrational rate.

Another technology designed to create specific body changes is biofeedback. Biofeedback is a non- invasive, painless, non-pharmaceutical method of teaching you to become aware of your body processes and help you learn to change them. Electrodes are placed on the skin and feed information into a small box attached to your computer via a serial port. The equipment feeds information back to you about your body. The feedback is usually auditory, a soft beep, and, by concentrating on this sound, the user can focus on specific bodily processes and learn to relax in very specific ways. The process is designed to provide the individual with an ongoing progress report as to how their body is responding to their own internal controls. In this way, one can learn to change heart rate, skin temperature, muscle tension, and certain brain wave patterns (Turnbull & Ritvo 1992). Biofeedback information is used to teach the patient what are the brain regions responsible for a certain behavior and thus be able to learn to control these areas and monitor the progress of the training.

The difference between the two technologies is that light and sound machines provide direct stimulation that affects the rate of brain waves, whereas biofeedback places the impetus on the individual to control their body's processes themselves. The goal of biofeedback is to train oneself to respond to intrinsic cues, which contrasts to the light sound stimulation machine's purpose of matching one's brain frequencies to outside stimulation.

Neurothecnology is for healing, and affecting one's mental and physical state in a positive way. However, in order to best apply the technologies to one's personal circumstances, diagnostic processes may be needed in regards to one's individual circumstances. One such diagnostic tool is called Kirlian Photography.

This process was discovered in 1939 when Semyon Kirlian (1973) found that if a living object on a photographic plate is subjected to a high-voltage electric field, an image is created on that plate. The image looks like a colored halo or coronal discharge. This process captures what the spiritual community refers to as the "aura," and the scientific community calls the "Meissner" field. This field is the area of gas ionization that is produced when electricity enters a living object. The image of the moisture is transferred from the subject to the emulsion surface of the photographic film. The field is visible to the photographic process because of the exchange of photons, or light particles, which takes place as our cells communicate through the chemical process with each other and with the surrounding environment. The light particles the body produces carry information in the same way that fiber optics carry information from one point to the next.

The color and densities that appear on the photo will vary due to the variances of energy output as a result of the different quantities and balances of acids and alkalis the body gives off as it attempts to optimize its chemical processes. The appearance of this gas ionization process on film varies in ways that are consistent. Thus, diagnosis of one's chemical balance can be inferred from the colors and densities that appear on the film.

Therefore, a good interpreter can detect specific energy imbalances from the color variances in the field surrounding the image of the body. Pulsed electromagnetic fields—which induce measurable electric fields—have been demonstrated to be effective for treating slow-healing fractures and have shown promise for a number of other conditions. This has opened up a huge effort to market a wide variety of magnetic products to assist with the healing process. A whole range of products is available for what is referred to as "magnetic therapy." Small spot magnets can be used at the point of pain on the body. There are wraps, belts and pads, which are held on the body in some fashion. In addition, there are mattress pads that claim to balance the body's energies while one sleeps. Various types of jewelry incorporate magnets into their design, including a wide variety of bracelets and necklaces. Many magnetic necklaces, bracelets, and earrings are formed from silver and gold-rich magnetic alloys and are promoted as both fashionable and therapeutic. One catalog claims that magnetic earrings "stimulate nerve endings that are associated with head and neck pain," and magnetic bracelets "act upon the body's energy field" and "correct energy imbalances brought by electro-magnetic contamination or atmospheric changes" (Vallbona, C., & Richards 1999).

The broadest explanation of the use of magnets in treating physical ailments was presented by Dr. Kyochi Nakagawa of Japan (Nakagawa, 1976). Dr. Nakagawa claims that many of our modern ills result from "Magnetic Field Deficiency Syndrome." The earth's magnetic field is known to have decreased about 6 percent since 1830, and indirect evidence suggests that it may have decreased as much as 30 percent over the last millennium. He argues that magnetic therapy simply provides some of the magnetic field that the earth has lost. Magnetic therapy is also prominent in the treatment of thoroughbred racehorses. The incentive to try "alternative medicine" to supplement mainstream veterinary treatment is considerable; an injured racehorse represents potential loss of a substantial investment. Magnetic pads, magnetic blankets, magnetic hoof pads, and more are used for a variety of leg problems. All get ringing endorsements from many horse trainers, and even some veterinarians. One marketer of magnetic products for humans reports that he first became convinced of their effectiveness when he used them on his llama. Some argue that the placebo effect might be taking place in these circumstances, but the psychological aspects of the healing treatments are obviously not happening with the animal. However, magnet therapy enthusiasts forget that it may influence the human who is interpreting the effect of magnetic therapy on the animal.

Clinical studies report between 75-85% of patients experience relief using magnetic therapy. Whether or not the placebo effect is taking place is always part of the debate. One point of contention in the argument is that the magnetic back braces used by many senior golfers may help ease their back pains through providing mechanical support, through localized warming, and through constant reminder to the aging athletes that they are no longer young and should not overexert their muscles. All these effects are helpful with or without magnets. One British study of pulsed-field bone-growth stimulators, which were approved decades ago by the FDA, found that they were equally successful when the devices were not activated. It concluded that their effectiveness resulted from the enforced inactivity associated with their use rather than from the pulsed magnetic fields. The logical conclusion is that with circulation increased, the body's natural healing mechanism can work more efficiently. Some doctors believe that the magnetic field affects the iron component of blood, hemoglobin, thereby increasing circulation to the area where magnets are applied. Another theory is that the magnetic field energizes and oxygenates the white corpuscles in the blood stream, and these white corpuscles are nature's healing agents. In this regard, the charged ions increase the blood flow, which provides increased oxygenation to the blood. This increased oxygenation is the prevalent factor to enhancing your body's natural healing powers, and the results are less pain, decreased inflammation, and the possibility of increased energy levels. Other specialists believe that, since nervous signals travel via tiny electromagnetic charges, an electromagnetic field may actually tune out "false" signals. The actual pain relief mechanism of magnetic energy may never be truly understood, since it operates within the tissues at such a microscopic level. What is clear, however, is that belief is necessary for effective healing.

Studies of magnetic therapy practices and results are more common in Eastern Europe and Asia where there is less access to pharmaceutical drugs. There is evidence that magnetic therapy does improve circulation and oxygenation in the bloodstream, and thus it would serve the purpose of facilitating healing for areas of the body recovering from injury or weakened by age or disease.

One property of magnetic energy is that it has no measurable mass. This is also true for another kind of energy relevant to this course, Orgone energy. Orgone energy was objectified and scientifically demonstrated by Dr. Wilheim Reich (1951). Reich built on Freud's early work, which strongly suggested that emotions and sexuality were expressions of a tangible energetic "something." It was Reich who provided the clearest evidence that the Freudian libido was a real energy, discharged during emotional expression and sexual orgasm. Reich discovered that this same discharging energy was present in a single cell, which apparently caused him to question whether that energy could be collected and harnessed.

In 1940 Reich discovered a way to accumulate that energy, and labelled it Orgone Energy. His work was not taken seriously at the time. There was no social context providing an atmosphere of acceptance for the idea of energy from repressed sexuality. However, a simple Internet search reveals 23 published articles on the treatment of a wide variety of ailments, from cancer to rheumatoid arthritis, by the application of Orgone energy. However, despite being used to treat specific ailments since at least 1971, there are numerous qualifiers in the dialogue on its applications. The point is frequently presented that science and society will have to go through some significant changes before its use will be accepted by the general public. Orgone energy is the primordial life energy, the fundamental creative force long known to people who are in touch with nature. Perceived as "chi" by acupuncturists, Orgone energy is accumulated naturally in biological organisms by food, water, breathing, and through the skin. In 1940 Reich discovered a way to collect or "accumulate" Orgone energy from the atmosphere. Reich's research revealed that energy is attracted to and absorbed by organic substances, but is attracted to and instantly re-radiated by metallic substances. He developed a special enclosure resulting from his experiments with the Faraday cage, a device built in 1836 by Michael Faraday to exclude energy. Reich's accumulator was made from layers of organic materials which absorb and hold the energy, and inorganic materials which attract and then rapidly repel Orgone energy. He found that the inside of a metal-lined enclosure that is layered with organic and inorganic materials contained a higher concentration of Orgone energy which was detectable by a higher temperature reading inside the accumulator.

Reich's device allowed him to isolate Orgone radiation from its environment, and then accumulate the energy within his device. Orgone radiation is not foreign to the body. The Orgone energy in the atmosphere is just another form of the same Orgone energy within the human body. The accumulator concentrates that energy and helps the body to help itself. Reich discovered that the energy moves in the direction of a magnetic field. Thus, when a person with their own energy field comes into contact with an accumulating device, the two fields make contact and excite each other. This creates a stronger excitation called "lumination." This strong, orgonotic charge has been found to be very beneficial to living systems. It may help to strengthen the immune system, improve circulation, and raise one's energy level. Investigations have shown that contact with energy from the accumulator stimulates the body's parasympathetic nervous system, inducing relaxation and a feeling of expansion.

Modern research has found ways to manipulate and focus the energy, thus resulting in applications to the medical field. The motion is a pulsating expansion and contraction, and a flow normally along a curved path. Inside an accumulator, the energy is emitted as a spinning, pulsating wave. A wide range of devices, and even blankets, are available on the market that makes use of this technology.

Another use of technology that has its roots in Asia is the adaptation of modern technology to the ancient art of acupuncture. Electro-acupuncture is the application of a pulsating electrical current to acupuncture needles as a means of stimulating the acupoints. The acupoints connect the individual's body to the universal, cosmic energy that connects us all. The stimulation of these points has been an ancient healing tradition that reaches back through the millennia. In 1934, according to Subhuti Dharmananda (2003), the Director of the Institute for Traditional Medicine in Portland, Oregon, Chinese healers added electronic stimulus to the process as an extension of hand manipulation of the acupuncture needles. The process is described, though only briefly, in most comprehensive texts of acupuncture. The procedure for electro-acupuncture is to insert the acupuncture needle as would normally be done, attain the qi reaction by hand manipulation, and then attach an electrode to the needle to provide continued stimulation. The idea was to help ensure that the practitioner, who may otherwise pause due to fatigue, gives the patient the amount of stimulation needed. It was also thought that Electro-acupuncture could produce a stronger stimulation without causing tissue damage associated with the twirling and thrusting of a needle.

The stronger stimulus provided by the electronic current is better for treating more difficult cases of paralysis. Positive results have also been seen from treating patients with the chronic pain and spasms associated with neurological diseases. The application of modern day electronic technology to an ancient healing art was developed to reduce total treatment time by providing a specific continued stimulus. The assumption was that it would be easier to control the frequency of the stimulus and the amount of stimulus than with hand manipulation of the needles. An added benefit was that it would free the practitioner to attend to other patients. However, the subsequent inattention to the patient receiving the electro-acupuncture limits the opportunities to respond to changes that are taking place during treatment. In addition, the literature cautions against using the technique on patients with serious cardiac diseases. It is generally recommended to avoid placing electrodes near the heart, as the heart can respond adversely to electrical impulses.

Another use of electrical impulses in the healing arts is Cranial-Electro Stimulation machines (Gilula & Kirsch 2005). The use of these machines involves placing sensors under the ears to send a minute electrical impulse. A slight tingling sensation on the skin is felt. The stimulation has the affect of tricking the brain into releasing the body chemical serotonin. Serotonin is a neurotransmitter that plays an important role in the biochemistry of depression, migraine headaches, bipolar disorders, and anxiety. There is also evidence that its presence or absence in the body influences sexuality and the appetite. The serotonin released can help relieve anxiety, tension, and the feeling of being "on edge."

There are portable versions of this machine, powered by a 9 Volt battery, that are small enough to put in a pocket. The sensors are placed on the neck below the ears, and can be used while walking or using the computer. They are designed to be used once a day in response to feelings of anxiety. It generally provides adjustments to the body chemistry and the ensuing relief from anxiety within 5 to 10 minutes. Another device in the category of neuro technology facilitates lucid dreaming. Lucid dreaming is being aware of the fact that you are dreaming while you are doing so. This allows the dreamer to gain insight into the purpose and symbolic meanings behind the dream, thus facilitating their analysis and the ensuing psychological healing process.

The technology for this process was developed by Stephen LaBerge, Ph.D. (1990), during twenty years of research at Stanford University. Dr. LaBerge developed a device called the NovaDreamer, a mask-like device that detects the time that one is in REM sleep, the state of rapid eye movement that one experiences when dreaming.

The device gives cues, such as flashing lights or specific sounds, that remind one to realize he or she is dreaming. In other words, one "wakes up" while still in the dream. The purpose is to give the dreamer detachment from the dreaming process during the course of the dream. This provides the impetus for the analytical process of dream interpretation to take place during the course of the dream. Users have reported that having lucid dreams have allowed them to make spontaneous choices that enable them to learn from, and even guide, the dream to constructive ends. Anecdotal evidence of these choices includes suddenly deciding to fly away from situations, empowering the dreamer to feel safer and have more free choice. There are also reports of incidents of making an old friend appear and talking to that person about consequential matters or resolving conflicts. Dreamers report being able to feel textures, hear sounds and smell odors in the dreamscape. The users reported that these sensations were as real as any in the physical world, and they were able to make conscious decisions and choices.

The entire process of lucid dreaming gives the spiritual sojourner tools and techniques, developed deep within the psyche, to explore and use their dreams for self-discovery, creativity, fantasy fulfillment, emotional healing, and profound spiritual insights.

Full Spectrum Lighting, another simple use of technology is the use of full spectrum lighting (Veitch et al. 1991). Full spectrum lighting is a process that uses specifically designed lighting fixtures that mimic the full spectrum of colors provided by our sun's rays. The purpose is to treat Seasonal Affective Disorder, a psychological malady that is brought on by the deprivation of light. This is generally a result of the changing of summer, with its bright sunshiny days, to the fall season, with its shorter and darker day-time periods. The onset of this change can result in depression and lack of energy (Veitch et al. 1991). The use of full spectrum lighting fixtures allows for the same kind of light energy that the sun offers.

The ultimate achievement so far in modern day development of neurotechnology is the Hemi-Sync device, or Holistic Sensory Response Audio. In 1956, Robert A. Monroe founded the Monroe Institute to study the effects of various sound patterns on human consciousness, including the feasibility of learning during sleep. Monroe was a highly successful businessman, the owner of several radio and television stations. In 1958 he began to have out of body experiences in which, while relaxing or attempting to fall asleep at night, he found himself hovering above his body. At the time, he thought he was having some kind of health problem, but was reticent to discuss it openly for fear it would interfere with his dealings with a very conservative business community. Monroe soon began to quietly but thoroughly examine the circumstances of his experiences. The discoveries made in exploring this phenomenon were validated later by the work of Dr. Melvin Morse and others in their work exploring Near Death Experiences. But as the work continued, and technology was developed to stimulate out of body experiences, the information gathered was to have a profound affect on the whole of our collective perception of the nature of reality (Monroe 1977).

In 1976 Monroe was issued an original patent for technology that altered brain states through sound. Hemi-Sync produced binaural beats, which are a series of barely audible tones which play in the background of soft music, barely noticeable beneath the music. The beats are at one rhythm in one ear, and a different rhythm in the other, producing a combination that takes the brain to a specific output rate of brain waves. The two hemispheres of the brain act in unison to "hear" a third signal—the difference between the two tones. The tones counter balance each other in a way that forms an anchor, or a signal which helps you quickly and easily re-enter the trance state when your unconscious mind begins to hear them in the background. The tones begin by synchronizing with the brain waves associated with the normal awakened state of the mind, and then slowly changing them to assist the listener in reaching the "alpha" level. The signal can only be perceived within the brain by both brain hemispheres working together. The result is a focused, whole-brain state known as hemispheric synchronization, or "Hemi-Sync." This relaxed level was the exact state of mind, it was discovered, to facilitate not only healing, but out of body experiences (Monroe 1977).

The process has been subjected to decades of research and thousands of lab sessions, and has been refined with over 40 years of research and development. Ongoing experimentation, data collection, and analysis are conducted at the institute's laboratory facilities to demonstrate the correlations between subjective experiential reports and objective electronic measurements. Healing benefits have been extensively documented, ranging from enhanced alertness to relief from insomnia and the myriad of circumstances that fall between.

There are also testimonials regarding profound healing experiences. One woman with an undiagnosed brain injury suffered in a car accident reports using Hemi-Sync to reverse a very frustrating condition. After being released from the hospital the same day of an accident that totaled her car, she noticed a severe change in her ability to concentrate. After many months of forgetting how to cook, getting lost, and "losing her train of thought" in a middle of a conversation, she began using Hemi-Sync to produce a state of relaxation. Within weeks, she became aware of regaining her sense of humor. From there she noticed a gradual regaining of her ability to concentrate (Monroe 1977).

The device, which looks like a bulky set of headphones, is designed to move one's consciousness past the limitation of being within a body. The spectacular success this device has had in facilitating astral travel has been documented in Omni magazine, amongst others, and experienced by thousands. The most profound research for the Hemi-Sync device was done by the founder of the Monroe Institute himself. Monroe said, "The greatest illusion is that mankind has limitations." This implies that we have limitless possibilities.

The work of the Monroe Institute, with its profound breakthroughs in the use technology for spiritual exploration, has the potential of enabling vital specifics in the evolution of humankind. Despite Monroe's death in 1995, his institute continues to attract and change forever the visitors to its campus as well as the thousands who have visited the virtual reality of its web site.

The implications of Monroe's work developing the Hemi-Sync device take on a whole new meaning when viewed as to the potential for learning from other times, places, and species. The development of this technology, a technology that enables astral travel and contact with guides and other beings with purposes that are highly relevant to both personal and planetary evolution, brings focus and significance to the whole idea of pursuing the potential ramifications of neuro technologies.

Royal Rife is the inventor of the Rife Machine (Hess 1996), it is said that "one day Royal Rife will be acknowledged as one of history's greatest medical geniuses." In 1902 he discovered the human cancer virus with a microscope that he had to invent himself, since no microscope at the time was powerful enough to detect it. Through endless and exhaustive experimentation and laboratory testing, he discovered that this virus could be killed using certain frequencies that were emitted from a prototype machine he created. He was then successful at destroying cancer in patients who sat within 10 feet of the machine. His legend built from there, and by 1931 he was the most honored among the medical society for his track record of being able to cure cancer almost 100% of the time. The cure for cancer has been found long ago! However, by 1939 these same doctors and scientists who so highly praised him denied that they had ever met Royal Rife. A violent attack was set upon Rife by unseen forces, but they could most likely be identified as the drug companies (through the American Medical Association) who had the most to lose from the Rife Machine, and a miffed Morris Fishbein who tried to buy the rights to Rife's work unsuccessfully. After that, people who worked with him were harmed and poisoned, Rife's papers were mysteriously lost, and his labs were destroyed by arson.

He was shortly indicted and taken to trial for "fraudulent medical practices," and for the most part, his life was undone. He became a ruined man. All the doctors who were associated with him lost their medical licenses if they did not stop using Rife's invention, even though they were having incredible success at curing people of cancer. Rife became an alcoholic in order to deal with the terrible turn of events his life has taken. Rife himself was later killed in 1971 by a very lethal dose of valium at a hospital which some do not believe was an accident.

For a long time, Rife's work lay dormant. However, it has been recently re-visited. Others are picking up where he left off. It has been discovered that far more than just the cancer virus can be killed with the Rife technology. Any virus can be killed. It just has to be identified and the right frequency that kills it must be found.

Others have begun to catalog this list. Work on cataloging viruses and the frequencies that kill them has begun again. There are now thousands of viruses that can be addressed using the Rife Machine. It is not that expensive, either, compared to what the medical costs of drugs, doctor's visits, surgeries and hospitalizations would cost. A Rife Machice could be purchased for anywhere between $500 and $5000, depending on how many bells and whistles you want it to come with. If you do an internet search on Rife Machine, there will be plenty of results to peruse, but the only place you will be able to purchase one is from overseas. It is still illegal to use them in the United States. Almost all other countries in the world allow the use of the Rife Machine, at least for personal purposes or experimental purposes, if not for the public. This does seem quite strange.

A Rife Machine works by generating a field of frequency, or frequencies, and anything within that field that it has been discovered to kill will be killed. It works one of two ways. Some of the less expensive machines entail two metal, or glass, cylinders that you grasp in your hands while frequencies pulse through them, and thus into your body. Some of the more expensive machines entail detailed digital readouts and the ability to diagnose your condition by finding out which viruses are present. You also do not have to hold onto cylinders and you are able to go about your business in the room as the machine generates the frequency field that addresses the virus (Hess 1996).

Kilner (1965) proposed a device that is a way for the naked eye to see the first three layers of the human aura. The device consists of two plates of glass with a dycanin dyed liquid between them. Dicyanin is a coal tar dye. Some say that a subject's aura can be seen through the screen, while others say that one must look at a bright light first, and then look at the subject through the screen. There have been several doctors in the past years who have used this technology for discerning illnesses in their patients and diagnosing their condition.

Transpersonal Psychology

Transpersonal psychology integrates the spiritual experience within a broader understanding of the human psyche. It is with the study of states of consciousness and the full potential of man, that transpersonal psychology assumes that humans can achieve harmony and transcend through spiritual development. Transpersonal is something that exceeds the range of human's own experience or personal history. Transpersonal refers to that which is beyond of the person who is the essential being.

Transpersonal psychotherapist Anthony Sutich (founder and first editor of the Journal of Transpersonal Psychology) provides one of the first formal definitions of transpersonal psychology in 1969 at the inaugural edition of the *Journal of Transpersonal Psychology:*

"The emerging Transpersonal Psychology refers specifically to the empirical, scientific study, and the responsible application of relevant results, becoming meta-needs individual and species-wide, the final values, conscience unitive, peak experiences, values, ecstasy, mystical, amazing experience, being, self, essence, joy, wonder, ultimate meaning, transcendence of self, the spirit, unity, cosmic consciousness, synergy of individual and species level, maximum interpersonal encounter, sacralization of everyday life, transcendental phenomena, self-cosmic humor and joy maximum sensory awareness, responsiveness and expression; and concepts, experiences and activities " (Sutich, 1969).

Stanislav Grof, co-founder of transpersonal psychology with Abraham Maslow, defines transpersonal psychology as "The psychology that respects the entire spectrum of human experience, including holotropic states, and all domains of the psyche - Biographical, perinatal and transpersonal "(Grof, 2000).

Transpersonal psychology covers a multitude of experiences and behaviors produced by spontaneous or altered states of consciousness, impulses into higher states of being, and extraordinary spiritual practices induced. Transpersonal phenomena include the meditative experiences, dreaming, drug-induced psychedelia, peak experiences, cosmic consciousness, enlightenment, mysticism, out of body experiences, channeling trance, near death experiences, memories reincarnations, extrasensory awareness, archetypal phenomena, accelerated learning, exceptional state of health and well-being, the mind-body healing and miraculous cures. Parapsychological phenomena are important for the reduction of science and spirit implications.

Altered States of Consciousness and Transpersonal Psychology

Ludwig (1966) defines an "altered state of consciousness" as any mental state(s) for various manoeuvres of physiological, psychological or pharmacological agents, which can be recognized subjectively by the same (or an objective observer of the individual person induced) as representing a sufficient deviation in the subjective experience or psychological functioning of certain general rules for that individual during alert awareness. This deviation can be sufficiently represented by a greater concern than usual with internal sensations or mental processes, changes in the formal characteristics of thought, and the deterioration of the test of reality to varying degrees.

The cognitive approach to altered states of consciousness has revealed that similar features that are characteristic of many altered states of consciousness including alterations in thinking, sense of disturbed weather, loss of control, change in emotional expression, change of body image, perceptual distortions,change in the meaning or importance, sense of the ineffable and feelings of rejuvenation(Ludwig, 1966).

By applying the disruptive force requirement for the basic state of consciousness (either through some physiological action, such as drugs or deployment of attention and meditation), the current organization of cognitive subsystems is destabilized until a new force patterns (such as mental set, setting, expectations, drug effects) is applied to shape the subsystems in a whole new system, the production of a new discrete state of consciousness with its own stabilization processes.

Cognitive awareness approach has helped differentiate transpersonal psychologists' grades waking state of consciousness. Awareness, for example, is not one homogenous thing, but varies and changes as the colors of the rainbow. It is possible to stratify and states order to raise awareness of alert and focused relaxed concentration and spread the cosmic consciousness. A range of altered states of consciousness have been identified as drug-induced states, hypnosis, biofeedback, daydreaming, night dreaming, sensory deprivation, and paranormal experiences. With each state consisting of many levels and functions, in each region or area of consciousness, individuals are able to process different types of information at different levels of control (Goleman &Davidson, 1979; Ornstein, 1972).

Transpersonal psychologists tend to see the experiences of "mystical union", "enlightenment", "nirvana", and related experiences as natural and beneficial non-ordinary states of consciousness that may be subject to effects of state-dependent learning. The idea that the experience of the sacred can be interpreted as altered states of consciousness arose from the observation of twice that (a) psychedelic drugs have been used through the centuries and cultures to induce religious experiences and (b) reports from some drug experiences are phenomenologically (descriptively or experiential) indistinguishable from accounts of natural mystical experiences (Smith, 1964).

Transpersonal psychologist Charles T. Tart has examined the altered states of consciousness from a cognitive perspective in terms of changes in the configuration and operation of the underlying mental processes (Tart, 1971; 1976; 1983; 1992). A state of consciousness involves cognitive functioning following subsystems: exteroceptors (receives sensory information), interoceptors (kinesthetic receives input), input processing (working memory), the subconscious processes, sense of identity, evaluation and decision making, emotions, space / time sense, long term memory, the motor output (behavior) plus latent functions. These 10 subsystems (more possible latent functions) define any discrete state of consciousness. The particular configuration of the subsystems in a given time is shaped and limited by the deployment of attention, the body's energies, characteristics of the structures themselves and the particular social and cultural environments in which they operate.

Grof (1988) suggested that the term "altered states of consciousness" cover transpersonal experiences; however, there are certain types of altered states of consciousness that do not meet the criteria for being transpersonal (involving an expansion or extension of consciousness beyond the limits of the usual and limitations time and space). For example, a living and complex childhood memory occurs in an altered state of consciousness (e.g., hypnosis or psychedelic sessions), but do not meet the criteria for being transpersonal.

The cultural context of the 1960s and 1970s provided fertile ground for the emergence of transpersonal studies as an independent field of study in psychology. The infusion of ideas Eastern contemplative traditions of Zen, Advaita, Vedanta and Taoism, along with the institutionalization of the humanist revolution in academic psychology, and the growing interest in consciousness and altered states of consciousness that are triggered by the widespread use of psychedelics, paved the way for the birth of transpersonal psychology movement in California in the late 1960s (Ferrer, 2002).

Since the 1970s, transpersonal psychology, as the humanist movement that preceded it, has been divided into three different groups; the first group represented by the ideas of Grof (1988) that believes that transcendence can only occur in the presence of an altered state of consciousness. This group produces conceptual models of non-ordinary states of consciousness. The second group, led by Wilber (1975), include those trying to assign internal states of consciousness and identify with the monistic and perennial philosophy of Aldous Huxley. Wilber believes that all expressions of the highest state of consciousness in each tradition are the same as the psychopathic conditions occurring at the bottom, the normal waking reality in the middle and meditative states of higher consciousness in the top. The third and by far the largest segment of the transpersonal movement has no identifiable bearer, it sees the self as getting up and go to work in the morning, the higher consciousness is sweeping the floor, washing dishes, and raking leaves. The lighting is doing everything we are supposed to be doing at this minute. There is a preconceived thing; is not an altered state of consciousness, it is simply the deep philosophy, which is to be found most clearly in the mundane.

Altered states of consciousness answer the question "who we really are?" The answer to this question is that we are a part of God and that humans are spiritual beings having human experiences that somehow reveal the direction of our full identity of our cosmic status.

Brain Waves

Our brain works primarily with bioelectrical energy. Although the power of electricity that handles our neurons is low (measured in mill volts), this power processes, manage, distribute and use vast amounts of information and generates multiple answers (almost infinite in possibilities). So by using micro electricity, we can conclude that the brain is a machine of low frequencies. Our brain, in addition to process information that comes by the senses, is capable of emitting extra-sensory information received via similar "electromagnetic waves", but with lower intensity similar to the frequencies of a radio transmitter-receiver. Our brain can act as a radio station, similar to numerous species of birds that in their migrations are guided by a genuine receiver of terrestrial magnetism located in the pituitary gland. With this receiver, they know where they have to fly and in what direction. It's like having a real compass incorporated into the brain. The mind could be defined as the "sense" of the brain (like sight is the sense of the eye).

A German psychiatrist, Hans Berger (1843-1941), demonstrated that a device "amplifier" that was called later electroencephalograph could capture electrical potential (voltage fluctuations) in the human brain. Before him, the English physician Richard Caton (1842-1926) showed similar potential in dogs. The first types of brain frequencies that were discovered were the "alpha" and "theta". Later, these findings were complemented by research in the range frequencies captured by the electroencephalograph. Each type of wave results in a different neuropsychological state. That is, our mind, our body and our physical and physiological activity are completely different in each of these states or frequencies. The type of neuro-chemicals and hormones substances discharged into the blood flow varies depending on frequency and as much as the presence and quantity of such substances as the mood we have, interact to produce a physiological-mental-physical-end that involves a mental state. A level of consciousness is conscious thought that is always thinking even in moments of apparent inactivity, but trivial ideas continually pass by consciousness. Most of the thoughts are accompanied by reactions in behavior, and small involuntary movements. When you're not actively thinking then you're probably dreaming, according Signer and Streiner (1966) a person has throughout the day about 200 daydreams. Therefore, consciousness is the sum of all the different perceptions. The most common consciousness are wakefulness and sleep; however, changes in expressing both cerebral and psycho states change according to conscious or subconscious feelings of each person are distinguished. These changes are directly related to the electrical activity of the brain. This activity can be measured by the number of oscillations per second (Hz) that are linked to different states of consciousness in the brain: our brain only perceives a limited range of frequencies indispensable to operate with ease in this three-dimensional medium. 20 to 20,000 vibrations per second are perceptible by our ears, the colors perceived by our eyes range from red to violet (although extending beyond, up and down), all possible smells and tastes (which are also vibrations) and the endless textures that we can distinguish with our skin. But the brain is not only receiver but also is sends vibrations. It has been proven thanks to the EEG that the brain emits waves of varying intensity and frequency depending on the mental state of the person being observed. These waves are classified into those shown in Table 1.

The alpha state is when, if we would connect to an electro encephalogram, our brains would work between 7.5 to 14 cycles per second. When "operate" in this state, we rank among the border of the conscious and the unconscious. Is the gate between both states of consciousness and this makes "alpha state" therefore a special status because it allows us, on the one hand, still have a conscious activity of our mind and body, that is, we realize what we think and happening around us? On the other hand, since the "lift" of consciousness in the "lower floors" of the mind, gives us access to information and own subconscious states, can use all the wealth of the 90% of "power" mental residing in the subconscious. This state is a "being comfortable" in inner peace and happiness, in deep relaxation. Greatly increases the power of suggestion and auto-suggestion, that is, anything that we suggest alpha, will be more easily accepted and less "filters" by our conscious rationality.

Magnus & Van der Holst (1987) speak of frequencies whose frequency ranges from 3.5 to 7.5 cycles per second. They are associated with the states of creative and decisive hallucination. During its broadcast, the person can discover events deeply hidden in the recesses of your subconscious, as well as conflicts and personality

Table 1. Types of brainwaves

Types of Brain Waves	States of Consciousness
BETA WAVES: 14 Hz to 30 Hz	This type of waves is recorded when the person is awake in a state of normal activity. Correspond to states of conscious attention, anxiety, surprise, fear, stress.
GAMMA WAVES: 25 and 100 Hz	They express pathological conditions of maximum tension, excitement and the individual enters a state of STRESS in which the coordination of ideas and normal physical activity are seriously altered.
DELTA WAVES: 1 Hz to 3 Hz	It arises mainly in the states of deep sleep and unconsciousness. Very rarely can be experienced being awake unless with a very hard training (Yoga, Meditation, Zen, Hypnosis, Self-hypnosis) or with a synchronizer of hemispheres. It corresponds to deep sleep, hypnotic trance, REM sleep. It corresponds to sleep without dream, trance, deep hypnosis. Delta waves are very important in the healing process and strengthening the immune system.
THETA WAVES: 3.5 Hz to 7 Hz	During sleep or in deep meditation, autogenous training, hypnosis, yoga (whenever the formations of the subconscious act). The state stimulates creative inspiration. Considered a state for maximum capacity of learning. Fantasy, imagination. Hypnagogic images.

in particular. Is the wave of imagination and dynamic contact with other possible "dimensions psi" offering you the opportunity to research our personality and deep in our psychology?

METHODOLOGY

The state of consciousness of someone can be measured by using possible physiological changes. Some physiological changes are typically associated with altered state of consciousness so measuring these physiological changes may provide evidence to more accurately determine the state of consciousness someone is in. Cade and Coxhead (1979) was able to map altered state of consciousness with alpha brain waves between 10 to 8 cycles.

This research uses EEG that was specifically designed to show the ephemeral patterns of the electrical signals from the two hemispheres of the cortex as they are happening (Cade & Coxhead 1979).

The EEG technology used for this research is the Emotiv 3D Brain Activity Map EEG software (Emotiv 2016) that works with the Emotiv EPOC neuroheadsets. The neuroheadset captures the users' brainwave (EEG) signals. After being converted to digital form, the brainwaves are processed, and the results are wirelessly transmitted to the USB receiver. The Emotiv 3D Brain Activity Map interprets these signals to displays mental activity in real time. The software displays brain activity in four significant brainwave frequency bands (Delta, Theta, Alpha, Beta) and uses the headset EPOC to read data. The software displays a colored gradient map showing the distribution of the indicated frequency band activity where red indicates the highest level of activity, falling away to orange, yellow, green, blue then black.

Figure 1, shows theta frequency bands with the highest level of activity indicating that the individual in this case indicating deep meditative states, daydreaming and automatic tasks. Emotiv 3D Brain Activity Map EEG software has data collection and replay functionalities that can be use to analyze the collected data.

An application of quantum physics (neurotechnology) in the altered states of consciousness was carried out by Persinger (1983). Persinger (1983) was able to induce visions of God and other religious and mystical experiences in the laboratory by using a computer and with what he called the Koran helmet that has also the nickname of the God helmet. He found that the temporal lobes of the brain are the source of the most spiritual experiences and other alternate state of consciousness.

This God helmet is a device to induce altered states of consciousness using weak magnetic signals to direct brain activity that can induce spiritual experiences that helps with transpersonal exploration and transformation of many people that is able to heal because of these transpersonal experiences (Persinger 2000). It is

Figure 1. 3D viewer

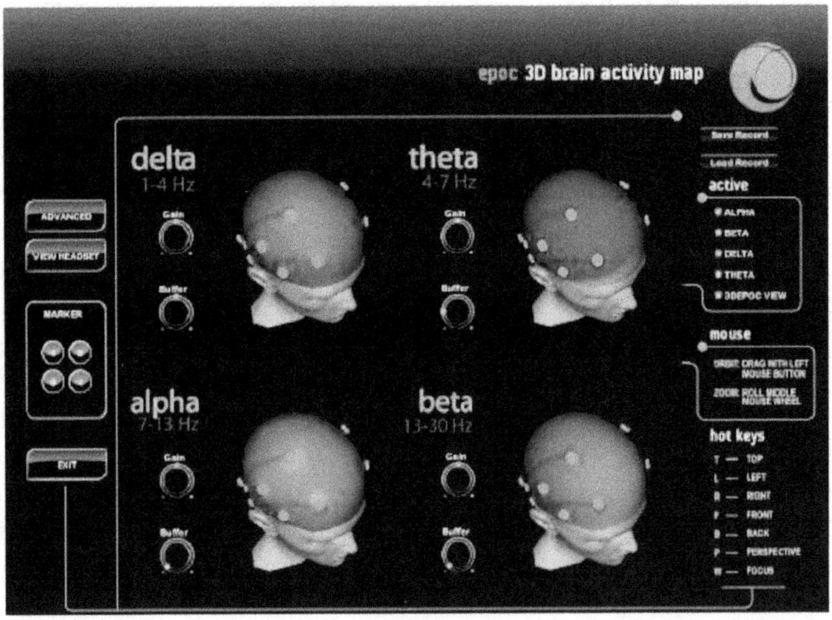

**For a more accurate representation of this figure, please see the electronic version.*

suggested that altered states of consciousness such as sensed presence and out-of-body experience whether they are produced by magnetic, electric or other stimulations or circumstances can be most effectively explained as the changes of the relative contents and/or intensities of the test subjects' neural quantum entanglement with their surroundings including possibly spiritual environments or information (Hu & Wu 2012).

Intense experiences are based in the temporal lobes (Persinger 1983), The sessions used in the research are intended for eliciting altered states of consciousness, and use the coils over the temporal lobes, which is understood to be the source of mystic experiences (Persinger 1983).

This research uses a product called Shakti (Shakti 2016) that is based on the Koran helmet of Persinger (1983). Shakti Software produces audio analogs to EEG signals. These are applied to the brain using modified commonly available magnetic coils. The magnetic signals are applied to the head at very low strength. The signals are short bursts, followed by intervals of silence. Each signal speaks a language that only one brain structure understands and responds. The brain has two hippocampi and two amygdalas, one on each side. Shakti is applied using the structures own signal, but only over the side of the head where it supports something positive. When these structures respond, they put the person in a positive altered state of consciousness (Shakti 2016).

The Shakti sessions that were used for this research are 'interhemispheric' (switching from both hemispheres to one) sessions, incorporating the same principles used in the study of Sculthorpe & Persinger(2003). In this last study, it was showed that the most effective sessions turned out to be two-phase sessions. This study applies the Modulated 40 Hz signal to both temporal lobes, followed by the amygdala signal to only the left temporal lobe as indicated in figures 2 and 3. This is the session design that comes closest to the sessions used in the "God Helmet" experiments (Shakti 2016).

Electromagnetic frequency emissions (EMF) emissions are varieties of radiation, and/or electrons. The Shakti helmet uses magnetic fields, which are neither radiation nor electrons. Electromagnetic radiation is composed of photons. Magnetic fields are not. Magnetic fields are not composed of the elementary particles than can interact with some organic compounds, nor are they composed of electrons, ions, or anything else that is encompassed by the word 'emission'. These are simple magnetic fields created by two poles, and are not composed of ions, electrons, or photons. Fields from an electromagnet are made of the same matter as the earth's magnetic field. These are 'made' of 'lines of force', and are not 'EM emissions'. These do not pose a health risk of any kind (Greenland et al 2000).

Figure 2. Left side of the session used

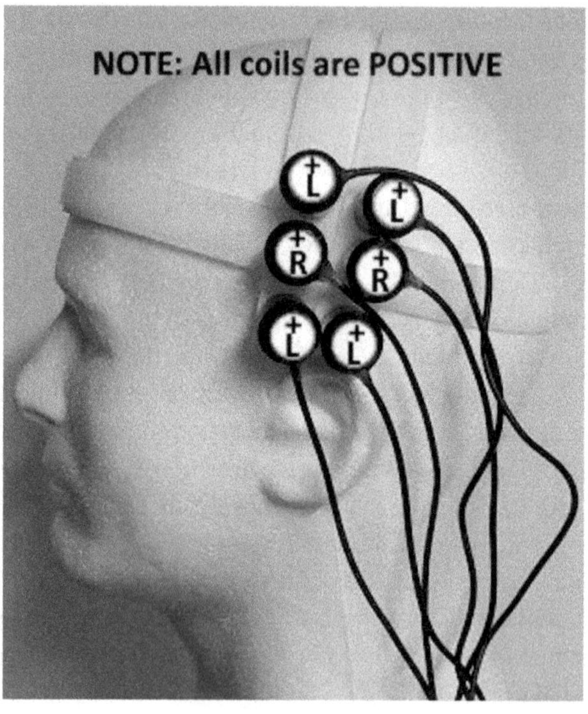

Figure 3. Right side of the session

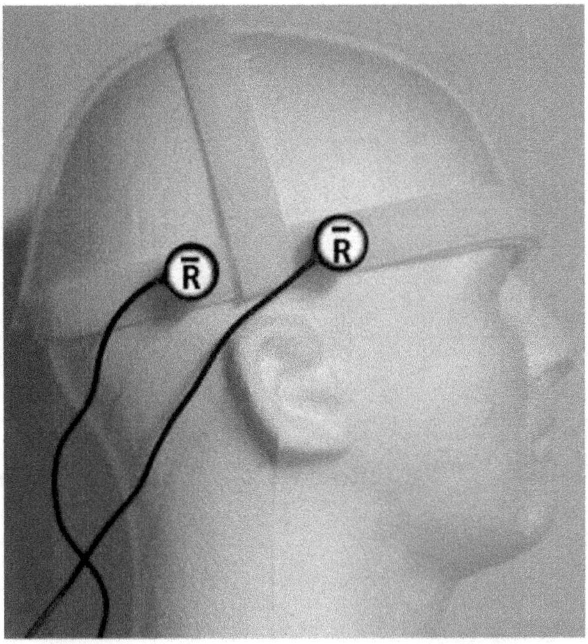

NOTE: Both Coils are NEGATIVE.

The Shakti helmet uses magnetic coils connected to a computer sound card. The output of a sound card is modulated DC. The polarity - one wire is positive and the other wire is negative - is always the same, no matter how the amplitude varies. A speaker or headphones uses a magnetic coil to move a diaphragm to make sound. Generally, the goal is to move the coil two ways to make sound. However, because of the springiness of the coil you only need one polarity. For example, a given voltage might push the coil. When the voltage drops lower, the voice coil will rebound and move the other way. EM fields reach deep inside the brain. Magnetic fields cannot be blocked (Hatch, G. P., & Stelter, R. E. 2001). The proposed helmet's magnetic signals reach deep inside the brain because there is nothing in or around the brain that can stop them (Persinger 1997).

The proposed architecture of the cybertherapy is depicted in Figure 4. The therapist computer has installed 3D activity map software and Skype. Skype is a telecommunications software that allows verbal and text communications with the patient, the 3D activity map software allows the therapist to visualize the states of consciousness of the patient by detecting the frequency band with the highest level of activity.

Figure 4. Proposed cybertherapy system

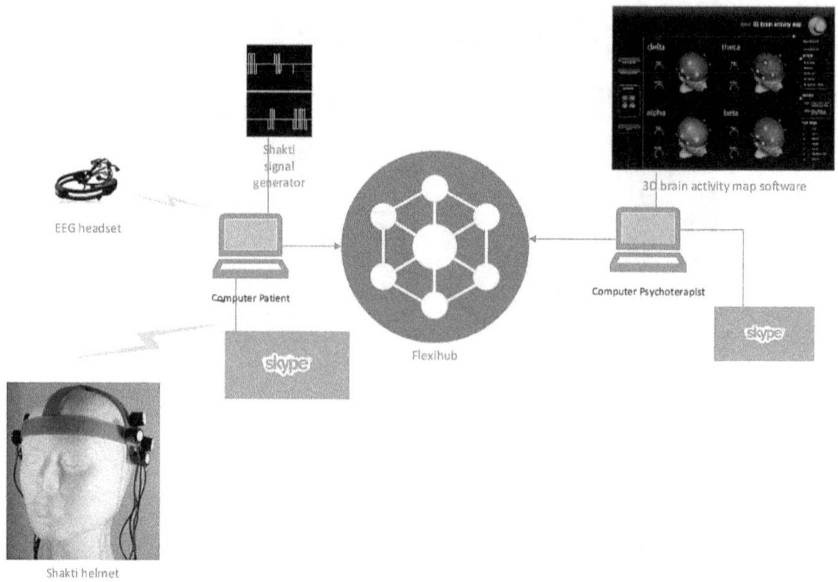

The therapist is able to access the EEG signals collected by the EEG headset wore by the patient. These digital signals are transmitted over the internet by using Flexihub software (Flexihub 2016), FlexiHub is a USB over IP software solution, it enables sharing access to USB devices over Internet. The EEG headset is connected to the USB of the patient's computer via a USB wireless adaptor. The Shakti helmet is worn by the patient and is meant to induce altered states of consciousness by receiving modulated 40 Hz signals to both temporal lobes from a signal generator installed in the patient's computer.

A sample of 10 patients was used to test the cybertherapy system and quantum biofeedback data collected and analyzed to confirm that the patients were able to reach a desired level of consciousness for the psychotherapy. Each patient was required to sit down and relax in a quiet room for a period of 40 minutes wearing an EEG headset without being exposed to the Shakti system (Figure 5), the therapist recorded the session during this 40 minute (pre-test). After, the patient was required to be exposed to the Shakti signals by wearing the Shakti helmet, the therapist also recorded the session for 40 minutes (post-test). Information about the difference between the two tests was not given to the patients in order to avoid bias in the measurements.

Each recording for each session displays the different frequency bands that represent each level of consciousness including alpha, beta, theta and delta. For

Figure 5. Patient during session

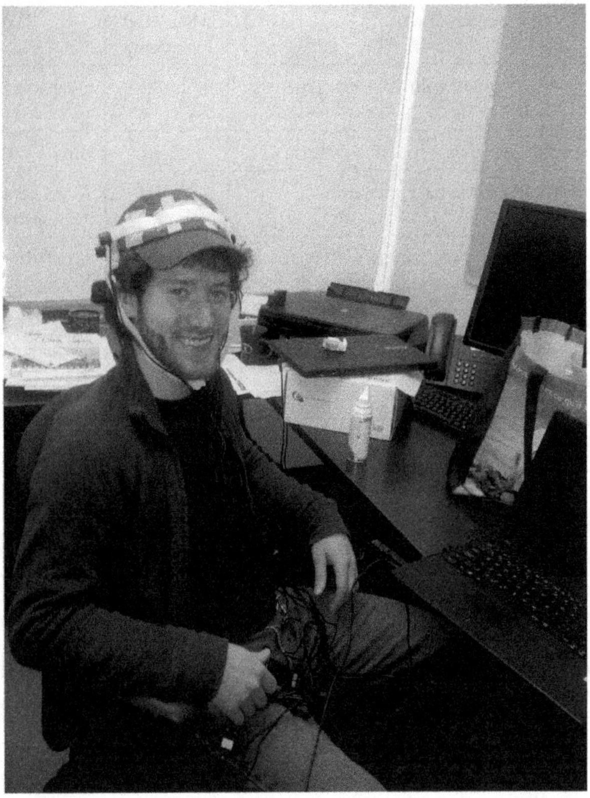

the analysis, we quantified the different states of consciousness according Cade and Coxhead (1979) that conducted EEG tests in 70 subjects and measured the ESR (electrical resistance of the skin) and with the application of its results to the work of Terry Lesh (1970) were able to build in the table below that represents the objective and subjective correlates of these states. The targeted level is 5 as this represents altered state of consciousness but it is expected that the average of the levels is under 5 as the patient needs go from 0 to 5 at different stages. However, it is expected that the post test average is higher than the pre-test as we want to probe that the cybertherapy system is capable of raising the level of consciousness.

A mean and standard deviation for these levels were calculated for each pre-test and post-test sessions for each patient. The mean values of pre-test and post-test results were compared to check if there is an improvement in state of consciousness with the use of the cybertherapy system. The mean values were tested using the t-Student test, and the t-values were calculated by using the following formula:

Table 2. States of consciousness and frequency measurements

Level	Consciousness	Measured Frequency	Types of Waves
0	Just he is beginning to relax with difficulty quieting the mind.	25-20	alpha and beta
1	Not very clear conscience or sense of anesthesia	20-16	Guests beta alpha continuous
2	Calm and relaxed with flash back memories	16-13	Alpha continues without beta theta intermittent
3	Well defined state. Feeling of floating with increased imagination and more concentration sustained	13-10	Alfa falling Continuous theta
4	Extremely vivid awareness of breathing heartbeat, or other bodily sensations. Living consciousness. Sometimes an alternation of internal and external awareness	10-8	alpha continuous theta falling Frequency
5	Awareness with satisfaction and deep intense alertness and calmness and detachment. Feeling of altered state lacking in previous levels 0 to 4.	8-5	Theta continuous alpha close to theta
6	New way of feeling by intuitive vision synthesis of opposites in a higher unity	below 4	Delta occasionally

t-value = (Mean of post-test – Mean of pre-test) / square root (Variance of post-test / Sample size of post-test + Variance of pre-test / Sample size of pre-test)

The Alpha level used was 0.05 of one tail test; with 18 degrees of freedom (sample size of pre test + sample size of post test – 2). According to the t-distribution significance table, the critical value is 1.734 for one tail test for this alpha and degrees of freedom. The Null Hypothesis is that there is no difference between the pre test and post test sample means for the states of consciousness because of the use of the cyberteraphy system.

ANALYSIS OF RESULTS

Table 3 shows the results of the study, a mean of the pre-test and post-test for each patient was calculated during the 40 minutes sessions for each patient because of the use of the cyberteraphy system. The levels of consciousness for each patient reached over time during each 40 minute pre-test and post test sessions are documented in the graphs included in the Appendix, each graph indicates the levels of consciousness reached at each second over the session. The results present that each patient had a different reaction to the use of the system, while some patients showed very little difference from the pre-test and post-test (e.g. patient 8) or even a decrease of the level of consciousness (e.g. patient 2) some patients observed a great level of improvement with the post-test session (e.g patients 3, 6 and 9). The mean of means for all the patients for the pre-test is 2 (Calm and relaxed) while the mean of means for all the patients for the post-test is 3 (Feeling of floating with increased imagination and more concentration sustained). While it seems that the cybetherapy system contributes to raise the level of consciousness, none of the patients were able to maintain an altered state of consciousness (level 5) during the sessions although this level was reached for few minutes by few patients.

Table 4 displays the standard deviation for the pre-test and post-test for all the patients, these results show that all the patients experienced variability of the states of consciousness during the sessions as expected but this variability was of not more than one level of consciousness. The standard deviation for the pre-test was calculated as 1.34 and the standard deviation for the post test is 1.108 for all the patients. The t-value for the sample is 1.75. Based on this last value, the null hypothesis can be rejected; this means that there is enough statistical evidence that the cybertherapy system is able to raise the level of consciousness. However, this is not enough to raise the level to an altered state of consciousness that is required to conduct transpersonal therapy.

The results suggest that although it seems that the proposed system is on the right track, the system should be enhanced by including other known means to reach altered states such as music therapy (Bonny 1975), guided meditations (Brown & Engler 1980) and channeling (Valverde 2015b).

Table 3. Results of the experiment

Patient	Mean Pre-Test	Mean Post-Test
1	2.82	3.19
2	2.73	2.48
3	2.45	3.55
4	2.73	3.00
5	1.73	3.55
6	1.45	2.95
7	0.91	2.18
8	2.27	2.36
9	1.64	3.27
10	1.36	3.18

Table 4. Standard deviations of the results

Patient	Standard Deviation Pre-Test	Standard Deviation Post-Test
1	1.53741223	1.569046
2	1.190874392	1.167007
3	1.213559752	0.687552
4	1.420627262	0.894427
5	1.489356176	1.29334
6	1.035725481	0.218218
7	0.301511345	0.873863
8	1.103712743	0.924416
9	1.361816968	0.64667
10	1.120064933	1.32802

DISCUSSION AND CONCLUSION

Inducing altered states of consciousness with neurotechnology is a relatively new concept and although there are serious studies, they are not incorporated into psychology or traditional medicine more than anything because of a lack of understanding of this technology.

This study introduces technologies that are based neurotechnology including quantum biofeedback, the latter has proven curative value much of particular diseases that seem to tend to be psychosomatic.

Transpersonal psychology was presented as a paradigm that recognizes the immortality of consciousness and relies on spiritual concepts that have roots in mystic religions as reincarnation and survival of consciousness brain death. The immortality of consciousness is based largely on the quantum theory explaining the origin of consciousness and its connection to the universe.

Neurotechnology explores the use of technologies of sound, light and radiofrequency to control the frequency of brain waves with the reason to induce altered states of consciousness. Altered states of consciousness have been proposed as therapies for healing in transpersonal psychology, these therapies recognize the spiritual essence of the individual and are based on the concept that psychological illnesses are rooted in the spirit and not in the brain. The patient to know the root of their problems, seem to find the answer to your anxieties and can self heal with these transpersonal experiences.

In this research, a cyberpsychoterapy system is proposed to support transpersonal psycho therapy. The system can be used to induce non ordinary state of consciousness that can be used by transpersonal psychologists as a healing tool to cure his patients with psychological problems such as psychosis at a distance location with the help of internet technologies. The proposed cyberpsychoterapy system uses quantum signal generator for the induction of altered states of consciousness and has integrated an EEG that serves as a biofeedback device in order to assess if the patient has reached the desired level of consciousness and can be used it to adjust the frequencies of the signal generator in order to improve the psychotherapy experience of the patient if necessary. A sample of 10 patients was used to test the cybertherapy system based on neurotechnology and quantum biofeedback, data was collected and analyzed.

The researched showed that with the aid of quantum biofeedback and neuroquantology, people can discover hidden deep events and conflicts in their subconscious that can lead to healing experiences. Although the results show that the patients were not able to reach the desired level of consciousness for the psychotherapy, there is statistical significant evidence that the proposed system can help to raise the level of consciousness, this can help with future designs that will eventually assist to reach the desired level for the psychotherapy.

The aim of this study is to open the eyes of the therapists about the potential of the covered technologies for this purpose and the ability of the use internet technology to be able to conduct transpersonal therapy at a different location than the therapist. Although the results do not probe that the presented technologies are effective to induce altered states, they show that there is potential for this as there is statistical significant evidence that they are able to aid to increase the level of consciousness.

The work contributed to the existing literature in the application of quantum computing to psychology by suggesting a cyberteraphy system that uses quantum biofeedback and neuroquantology for the facilitation of transpersonal psychotherapy. Although there are many cybetherapy systems in the literature (Takacs 2005, Wiederhold& Wiederhold 2004, Botello et. Al 2009), none of them addresses transpersonal psychotherapy and are based on quantum biofeedback and neurotechnology.

A recommendation for future research is the inclusion of supporting methods such as music therapy, guided meditations and breath work in the cybertherapy system in order to reach the desired state that can help the therapist to heal patients at distance with the use of transpersonal psychology. It seems that the use of neurotechnology alone is not enough to reach desired results but a combination of methodologies can be the solution for the creation of the altered states of consciousness induction machine.

REFERENCES

Bonny, H. L. (1975). Music and consciousness. *Journal of Music Therapy, 12*(3), 121–135. doi:10.1093/jmt/12.3.121

Botella, A. M., Banos, C., Zaragoza, R. M., & Guixeres, J. (2009). The Intelligent e-Therapy system: A new paradigm for telepsychology and cybertherapy. *British Journal of Guidance & Counselling, 37*(3), 287–296. doi:10.1080/03069880902957015

Brown, D., & Engler, J. (1980). The stages of meditation: A validation study. *Journal of Transpersonal Psychology, 12*, 143–192.

Cade, C. M., & Coxhead, N. (1979). *The Awakened Mind: Biofeedback and the Development of Higher States of Awareness*. New York: Delacorte Press.

Dumit, J. (1995). Brain-mind machines and American technological dream marketing: towards an ethnography of cyborg envy. In *The cyborg handbook* (pp. 347-362).

Emotiv. (2016). 3D-Brain. Retrieved from https://emotiv.com/store/product_74.html

Ferrer, J. N. (2002). *Revisioning transpersonal theory: A participatory vision of human spirituality*. Suny Press.

Flexihub. (2016). Flexihub software. Retrieved from http://www.flexihub.com/

Gilula, M. F., & Kirsch, D. L. (2005). Cranial electrotherapy stimulation review: A safer alternative to psychopharmaceuticals in the treatment of depression. *Journal of Neurotherapy, 9*(2), 7–26. doi:10.1300/J184v09n02_02

Goleman, D., & Davidson, R. J. (1979). *Consciousness: Brain, states of consciousness, and mysticism*. New York: Harper.

Grof, S. (1988). *The Adventure of Self-Discovery*. New York: State University of New York Press.

Grof, S. (2000). *Psychology of the Future: Lessons from modern consciousness research*. Albany, NY: State University of New York Press.

Hameroff, S. R. (1994). Quantum coherence in microtubules: A neural basis for emergent consciousness? *Journal of Consciousness Studies, 1*(1), 91–118.

Hatch, G. P., & Stelter, R. E. (2001). Magnetic design considerations for devices and particles used for biological high-gradient magnetic separation (HGMS) systems. *Journal of Magnetism and Magnetic Materials, 225*(1), 262–276. doi:10.1016/S0304-8853(00)01250-6

Hess, D. J. (1996). Technology and alternative cancer therapies: An analysis of heterodoxy and constructivism. *Medical Anthropology Quarterly*, *10*(4), 657–674. doi:10.1525/maq.1996.10.4.02a00140 PMID:8979243

Hu, H., & Wu, M. (2012). Scientific GOD: Michael Persinger & the GOD Experiments. *Scientific GOD Journal*, *3*(10).

Hutchison, M. (1986). *Megabrain: New tools and techniques for brain growth and mind expansion*. William Morrow & Company.

Josephson, B. D. (1962). Possible new effects in superconductive tunneling. *Physics Letters*, *1*(7), 251–253. doi:10.1016/0031-9163(62)91369-0

Kilner, W. J. (1965). *The human aura*. Citadel Press.

Kirlian, S. D., & Kirlian, V. (1973). *Photography by means of high-frequency currents. Galaxies of life*. New York: Interface.

Krippner, S. (2000). The epistemology and technologies of shamanic states of consciousness. *Journal of Consciousness Studies*, *7*(11-12), 93–118.

LaBerge, S., & Rheingold, H. (1990). *Exploring the world of lucid dreaming*. New York: Ballantine Books.

Lesh, T. V. (1970). Meditators Zen and the Development of Empathy in Counselors. *Journal of Humanistic Psychology*, *10*(1), 39–74. doi:10.1177/002216787001000105

Ludwig, A. (1966). Altered states of consciousness. *Archives of General Psychiatry*, *15*(3), 225–234. doi:10.1001/archpsyc.1966.01730150001001 PMID:5330058

Magnus, O., & Van der Holst, M. (1987). Zeta waves: A special type of slow delta waves. *Electroencephalography and Clinical Neurophysiology*, *67*(2), 140–146. doi:10.1016/0013-4694(87)90036-8 PMID:2439290

Marshall, I. N., & Zohar, D. (1997). *Who's Afraid of Schrödinger's Cat?* (p. 402). All the New Science Ideas You Need to Keep Up with the New Thinking.

Masters, R., & Houston, J. (1966). *The Varieties of Psychedelic Experience*. New York: Delta Books.

Monroe, R. A. (1977). *Journeys out of the body* (Vol. 79). Main Street Books.

Nakagawa, K. (1976). Magnetic field deficiency syndrome and magnetic treatment. *Japanese Medical Journal*, *2745*, 24–32.

Ornstein, R. E. (1972). *The psychology of consciousness*. New York: WH Freeman.

Penrose, R. (1994). *Shadows of the Mind* (Vol. 4). Oxford: Oxford University Press.

Persinger, M. A. (1983). Religious and mystical experiences as artifacts of temporal lobe function: A general hypothesis. *Perceptual and Motor Skills*, *57*(3f), 1255–1262. doi:10.2466/pms.1983.57.3f.1255 PMID:6664802

Persinger, M. A., Tiller, S. G., & Koren, S. A. (2000). Experimental simulation of experience and a elicitation haunt of activity by paroxysmal electroencephalographic transcerebral complex magnetic fields: Induction of a synthetic ghost. *Perceptual and Motor Skills*, *90*(2), 659–674. doi:10.2466/pms.2000.90.2.659 PMID:10833767

Reich, W. (1951). *Cosmic Superimposition: Man's Orgonotic Roots in Nature*. Wilhelm Reich Foundation.

Shakti. (2016). Shakti-Neuromagnetic signal generator. Retrieved from https://www.shaktitechnology.com/winshakti/rotating/

Singer, J. L., & Streiner, B. F. (1966). Imaginative content in the dreams and fantasy play of blind and sighted children. *Perceptual and Motor Skills*, *22*(2), 475–482. doi:10.2466/pms.1966.22.2.475

Sutich, A. J. (1969). Some Considerations Regarding transpersonal psychology. *Journal of Transpersonal Psychology*, *1*, 11–20.

Takacs, B. (2005). Special education and rehabilitation: Teaching and healing with interactive graphics. *Computer Graphics and Applications*, *25*(5), 40–48. doi:10.1109/MCG.2005.113 PMID:16209169

Tart, C. T. (1971). Scientific foundations for the study of altered states of consciousness. *Journal of Transpersonal Psychology*, *3*(1), 93–124.

Tart, C. T. (1975). *States of consciousness* (p. 206). New York: EP Dutton.

Tart, C. T. (1976). The basic nature of altered states of consciousness: A systems approach. *Journal of Transpersonal Psychology*, *8*(1), 45–64.

Tart, C. T. (1989). *States of consciousness*. El Cerrito, CA: Psychological Processes.

Tart, C. T. (1992). *Transpersonal psychologies*. Washington, DC: American Psychological Association.

Turnbull, G. K., & Ritvo, P. G. (1992). Anal sphincter biofeedback relaxation treatment for women with intractable constipation symptoms. *Diseases of the Colon and Rectum*, *35*(6), 530–536. doi:10.1007/BF02050531 PMID:1587169

Vallbona, C., & Richards, T. (1999). Evolution of magnetic therapy from alternative to traditional medicine. *Physical Medicine and Rehabilitation Clinics of North America, 10*(3), 729–754. PMID:10516987

Valverde, R. (2011). *Principles of Human Computer Interaction Design*. Germany: Lambert Academic Publishing.

Valverde, R. (2015). a. Neurotechnology as a Tool for Inducing and Measuring Altered States of Consciousness in Transpersonal Psychotherapy. *NeuroQuantology, 13*(4), 502–517. doi:10.14704/nq.2015.13.4.870

Valverde, R. (2015). b. Channeling as an Altered State of Consciousness in Transpersonal Psychology Therapy. *Journal of Consciousness Exploration & Research, 6*(7), 405–416.

Valverde, R. (2016). Possible Role of Quantum Physics in Transpersonal & Metaphysical Psychology. *Journal of Consciousness Exploration & Research, 7*(4), 303–309.

Veitch, J. A., Gifford, R., & Hine, D. W. (1991). Demand characteristics and full spectrum lighting effects on performance and mood. *Journal of Environmental Psychology, 11*(1), 87–95. doi:10.1016/S0272-4944(05)80007-6

Walter, V. J., & Walter, W. G. (1949). The central effects of rhythmic sensory stimulation. *Electroencephalography and Clinical Neurophysiology, 1*(1), 57–86. doi:10.1016/0013-4694(49)90164-9 PMID:18129183

Walter, W. G. (1964). Slow potential waves in the human brain associated with expectancy, attention and decision. *European Archives of Psychiatry and Clinical Neuroscience, 206*(3), 309–322. PMID:14345314

Wiederhold, B. K., & Wiederhold, M. D. (2004). The future of Cybertherapy: Improved options with advanced technologies.

Wilber, K. (1975). Psychologia Perennis: The Spectrum of Consciousness. *Journal of Transpersonal Psychology, 7*(2), 105–132.

APPENDIX: PATIENT RESULTS

Figure 6. Patient 1 pre-test results

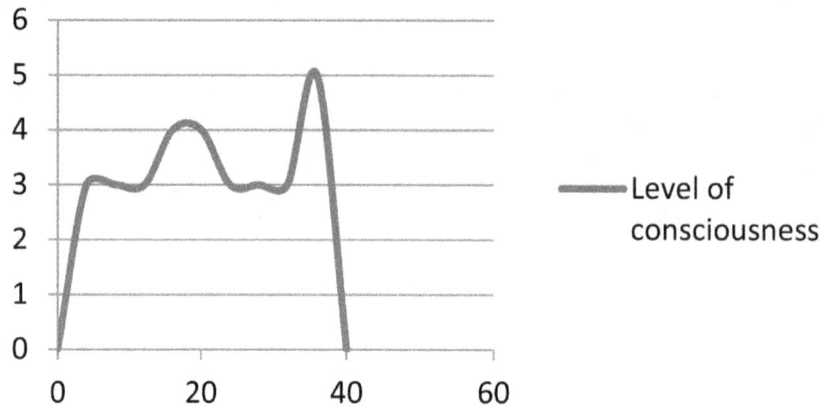

Figure 7. Patient post-test results

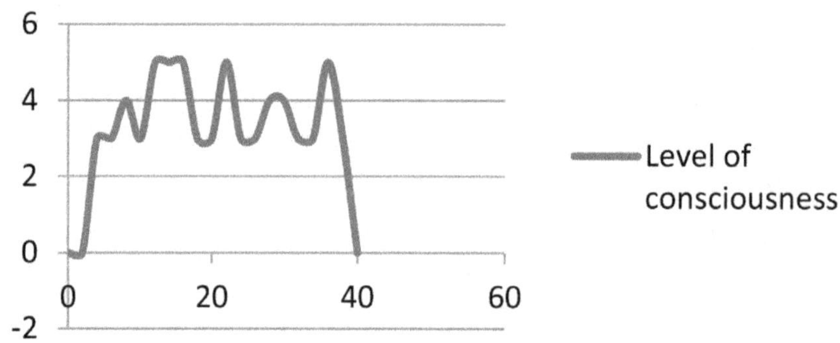

Figure 8. Patient 2 pre-test results

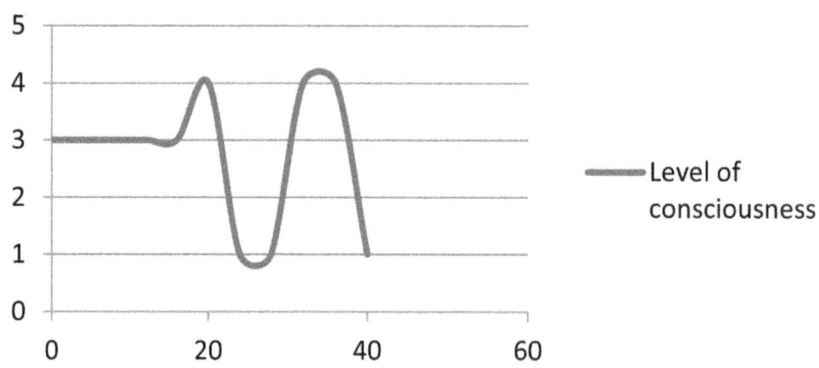

Figure 9. Patient 2 post-test results

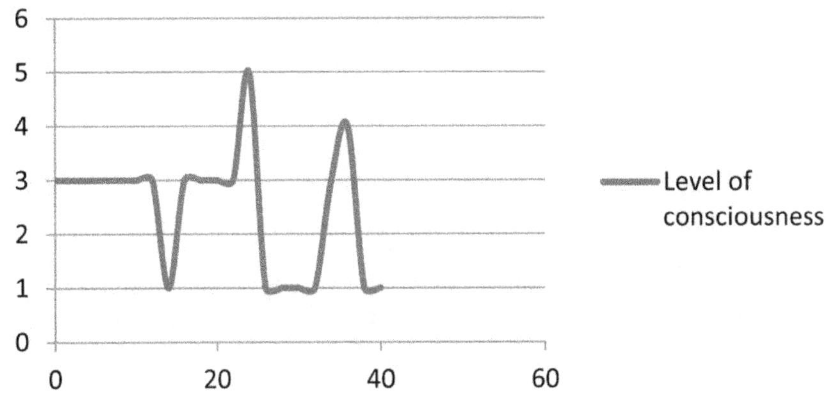

Figure 10. Patient 3 pre-test results

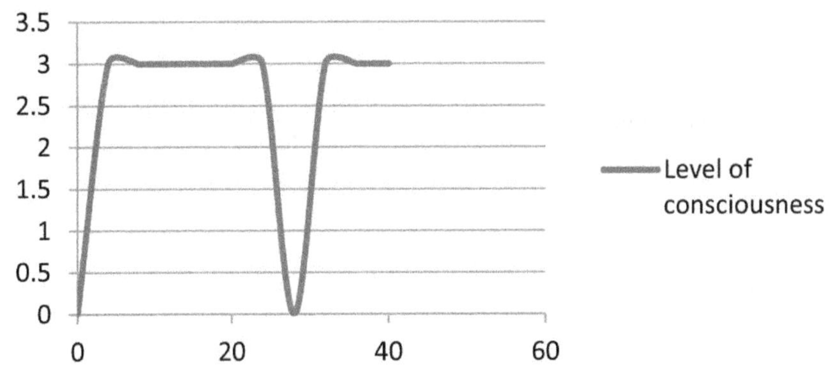

Figure 11. Patient 3 post-test results

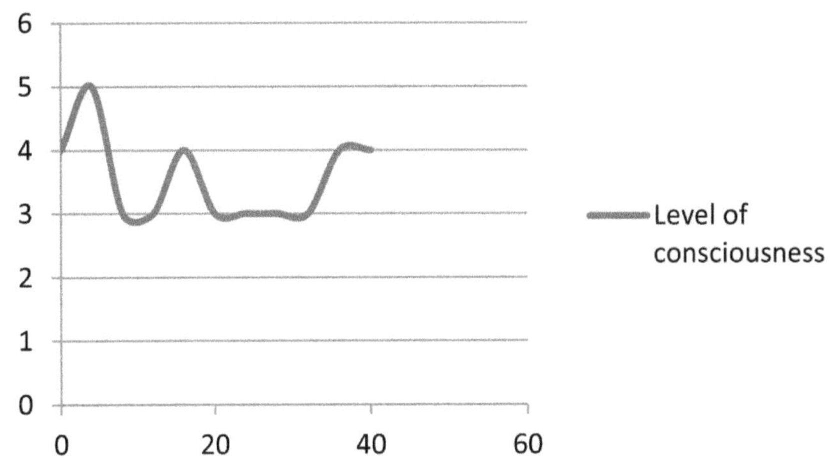

Figure 12. Patient 4 pre-test results

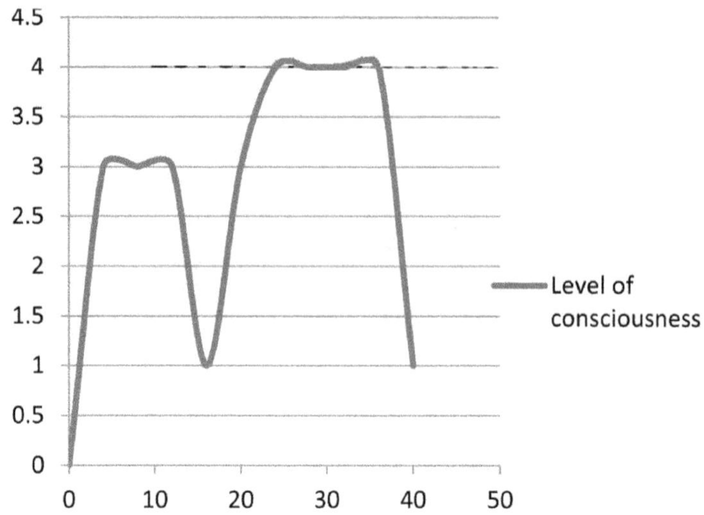

Figure 13. Patient 4 post-test

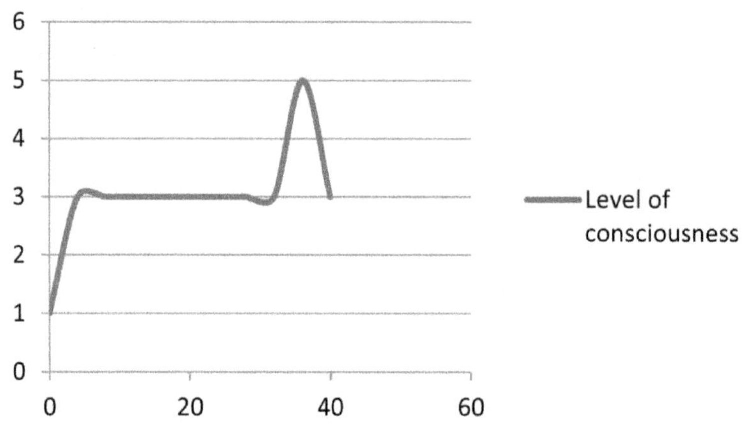

Figure 14. Patient 5 pre-test

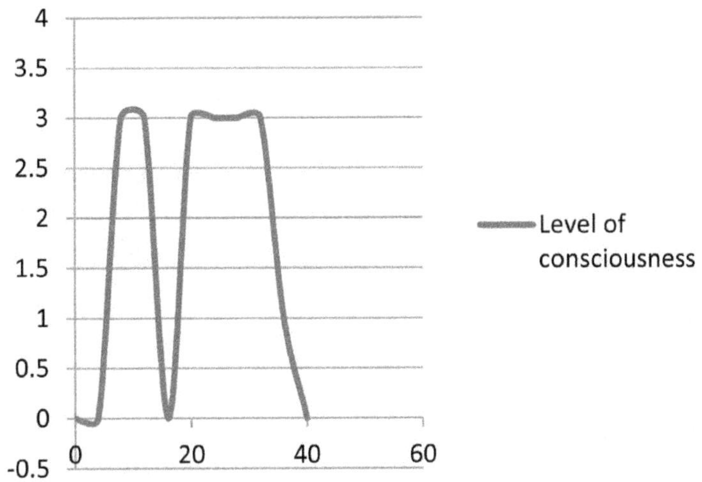

Figure 15. Patient 5 post-test

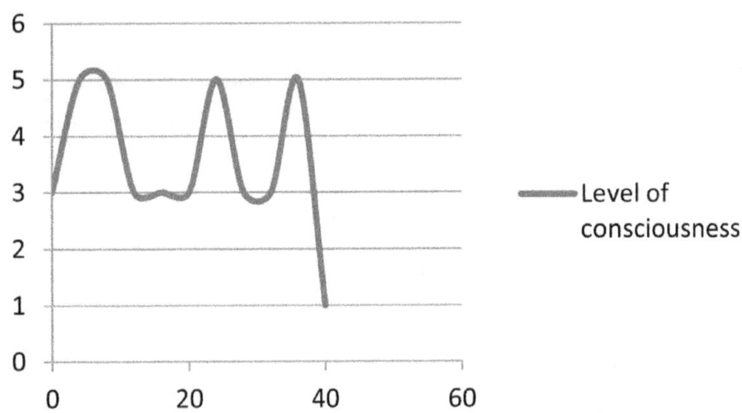

Figure 16. Patient 6 pre-test

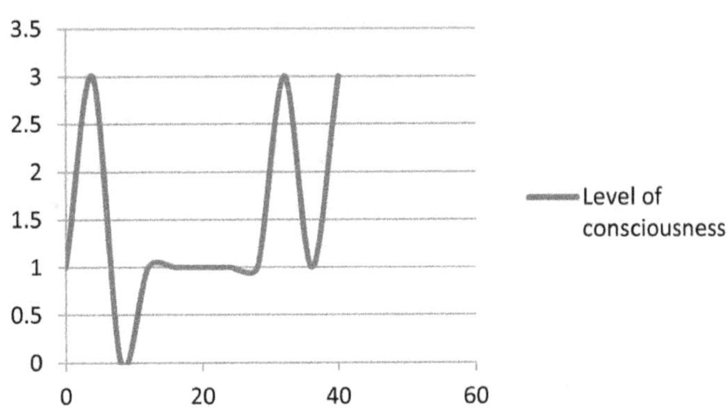

Figure 17. Patient 6 post-test

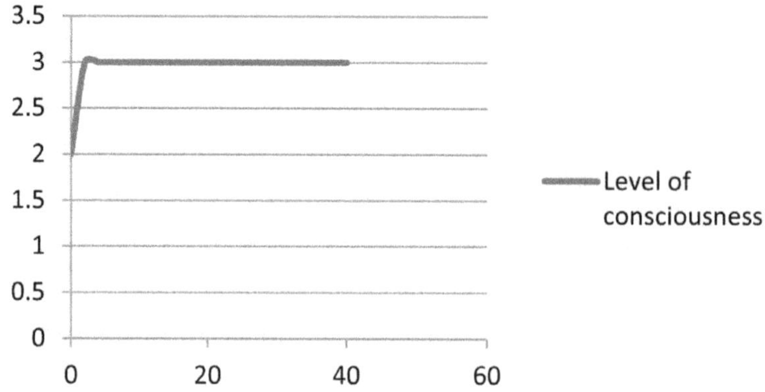

Figure 18. Patient 7 pre-test

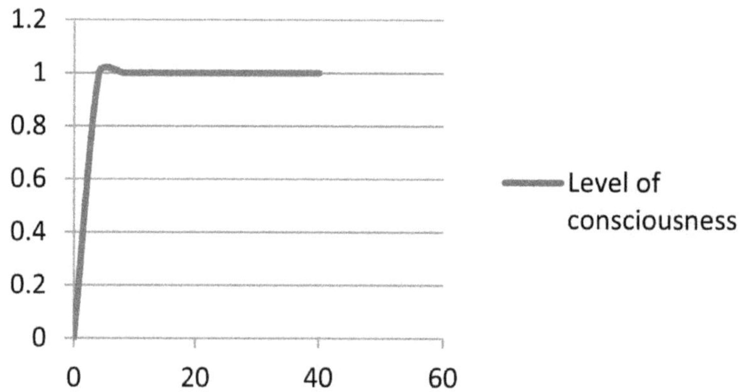

Figure 19. Patient 7 pro-test

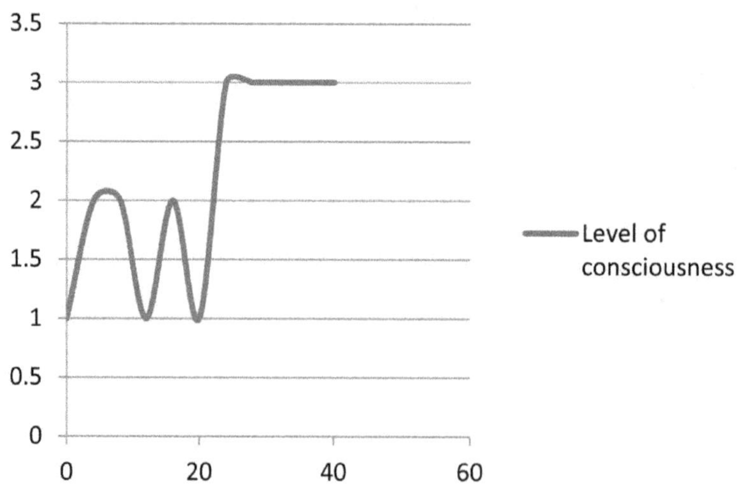

Figure 20. Patient 8 pre-test

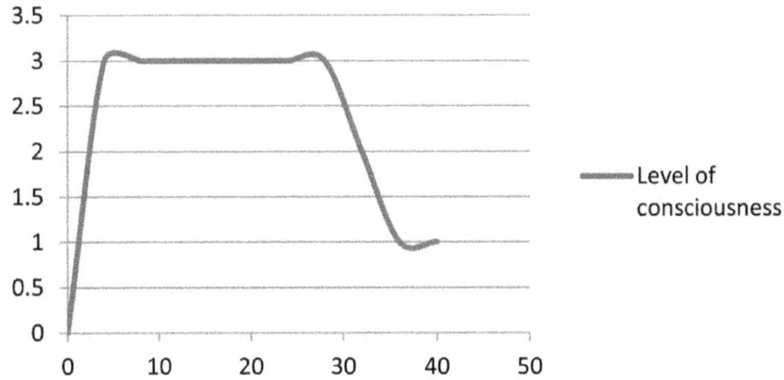

Figure 21. Patient 8 post-test

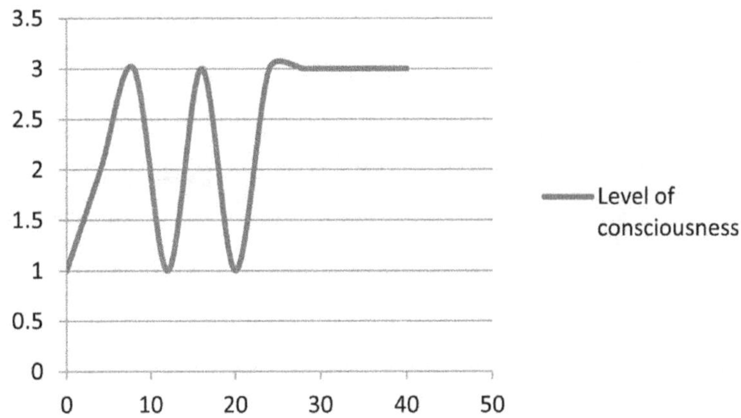

Figure 22. Patient 9 pre-test

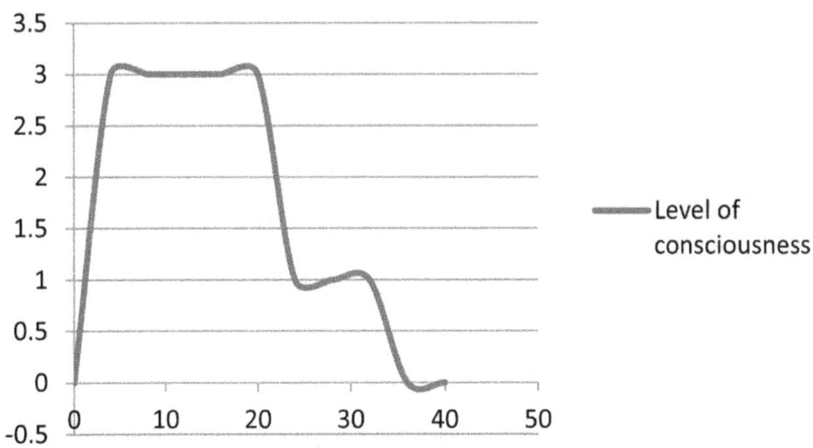

Figure 23. Patient 9 post-test

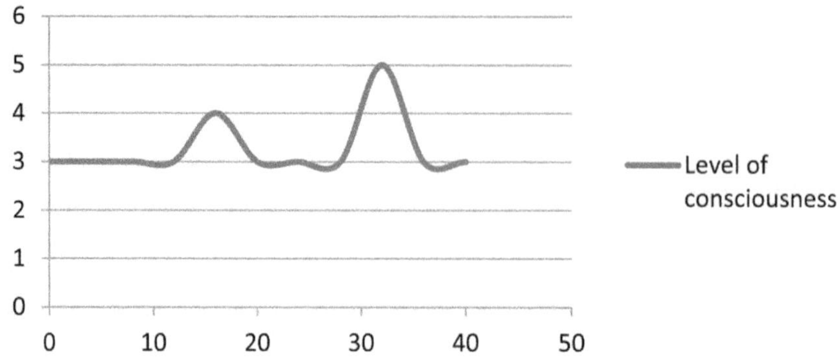

Figure 24. Patient 10 pre-test

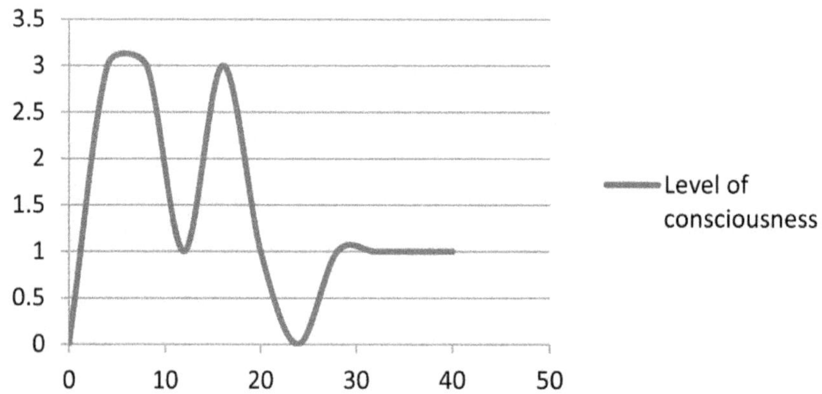

Figure 25. Patient 10 post-test

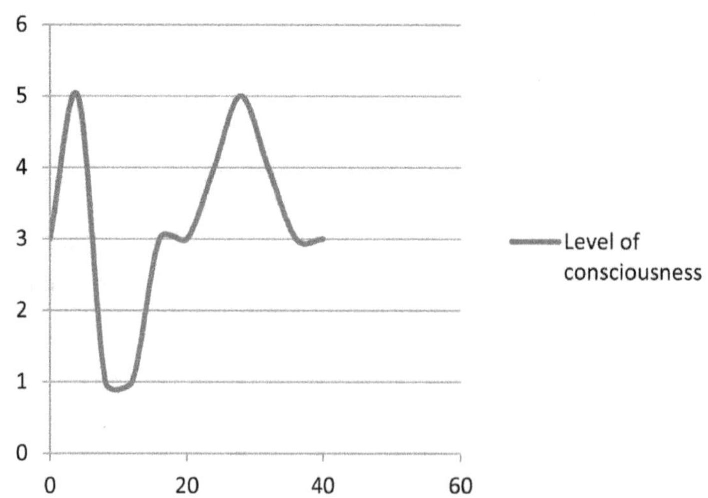

Chapter 7
Neurotechnology in the Development of Cyber-Psychotherapy Systems for Inducing and Measuring Altered States of Consciousness in Transpersonal Psychotherapy

Raul Valverde
Concordia University, USA

ABSTRACT

Transpersonal psychotherapy is based on transpersonal psychology and considers that the psyche is multidimensional and that there are several "levels of consciousness" and each has different characteristics and is governed by different laws. Transpersonal psychology is the study of human nature and proceeds on the assumption that human beings possess potentials that exceed the limits of their ego and integrate the spiritual experience within a broader understanding of the human psyche and consciousness. Altered states of consciousness have been used as psychotherapy in transpersonal psychology for decades. Although there are very well known techniques to induce

DOI: 10.4018/978-1-5225-3241-5.ch007

altered state of consciousness as holotropic breathwork, Neurotechnology offers an alternative way not only to induce these states for transpersonal therapy but also to measure the level of a state of consciousness. The objective of this chapter is to provide a review of the main concepts of Neurotechnology and the main technologies that can be used to induce and measure altered state of consciousness for transpersonal psychotherapy and propose an architecture for a Cyber psychotherapy system that uses these technologies.

INTRODUCTION

Cyber therapy is an Internet based computer-mediated system used to facilitate psychotherapy (Botella et al. 2009). This includes new applications of technology within psychology and healthcare, which utilize augmented and virtual reality components in order to facilitate psychotherapy (Botella et al 2009). Interest in Neurotechnological devices has grown strongly since the release of 1986's classic text of Michael Hutchison "Megabrain" (1986). Besides Neurotechnological machines, the industry has developed a range of related devices including peripherals-tapes, subliminal tapes, Hypno-peripheral processing, sound meditation devices and altered state induction software programs for personal computers, etc. It seems like Neurotechnology combined with contemporary psychology may seem to be revolutionary but its roots are much older as humanity has made many attempts in the past to involve consciousness with technology. The flashing LEDs in a light and sound machine can be traced back to the old practice of starting a fire in order to induce trance. Sound recordings of brain entrainment undoubtedly have their roots in the ritual singing and shamanic use of wind instruments.

This current era of Neurotechnology was born from the experiments made in biofeedback that resulted in the work of some researchers of consciousness as Masters and Houston (1966) that created the AVE (an abbreviation of Audio Visual Environment) that is one of the first electronic brain entrainment devices. The AVE was the first device to use visual and auditory stimuli as a means of altering consciousness. Not much different that many of audiovisual devices of today, the AVE consisted of a wrap-around screen and headphones to bomb the sense in these two stimuli.

These signals generated by AVE devices and detectable by electroencephalogram (EEG) tests at specific frequency ranges; seem to vary from one state of consciousness to another for their users. The products of Neurotechnology appear to make possible to "tune" the brain to these different alternating frequencies, and in turn achieve new psychological states.

When you "tune" into these frequencies at a slower pace, our thought processes and central nervous system are altered, causing the brain to fall into a deep level of activity. In addition, when one is tuned to a frequency faster and a higher range, the wave activity can have a highly stimulating effect on the brain.

Altered states of consciousness have been used as a therapy for modern psychological paradigms as transpersonal psychology (Valverde 2015). Although there are several techniques such as holotropic breathing used to induce these altered states of consciousness, Neurotechnology offers a more easy to control alternative to the transpersonal therapies.

In order to understand Neurotechnology, this review begins with an introduction to the technologies that made possible the modern Neurotechnology including biofeedback, quantum physics, quantum biofeedback, theory of consciousness, principles and applications of Neurotechnology for inducing altered states of consciousness in transpersonal therapies. Finally, the chapter proposes an architecture to conduct transpersonal therapy over the internet with the use of Neurotechnology in order to induce and measure altered states of consciousness.

BIOFEEDBACK

Biofeedback literally means, "responding to life". The work of Miller opened the doors to research processes in biofeedback. Miller (1978) constructed an apparatus equipped with sensitive electrodes connected to a monitor on which the patient could see how the skin temperature behaved, teaching patients to relax and concentrate to get it to relax the smooth vasculature of vessels peripheral blood in order to descend skin temperature.

Biofeedback is the process by which a person learns to influence involuntary body processes to receive physiological data from an electronic device that continuously monitors certain physiological parameters. It is a way of measuring the response to the physical, emotional, mental and spiritual stresses of life. Bodies under high stress are more prone to physical discomfort and even illness. The biofeedback response occurs when the body receives new information about their status (e.g. get 'feedback') and make healthy adjustments to reduce stress and tension. The result is a reduction of the nervous activity and increased vitality. Users of the feedback report a greater sense of well-being and joy.

Biofeedback Neurotechnology instruments measure muscle activity, skin temperature, electro-dermal activity (sweat gland activity), respiration, heart rate, heart rate variability, blood pressure, brain electrical activity and blood flow. These technologies are able to capture analog electrical signals from the body and translate those signals into meaningful information through complex algorithmic software that a technician can then decipher. Research shows that biofeedback, alone and in combination with other therapies is effective for treating a variety of medical and psychological disorders. Doctors, nurses, psychologists, counsellors, physical therapists, occupational therapists and other professionals currently use biofeedback. Computer scientists also use biofeedback in order to build human computer interactions (Valverde 2011).

Studies by Jonas and Levin (1999) show that biofeedback is ideal for patients that are looking for therapies that are softer, less toxic and less invasive. The biofeedback technique is applied in the field of psychology for treating phobias, neurosis, anxiety, depression and insomnia.

Quantum Physics

What we are able to perceive with our five senses is not reality. Quantum physics has shown that space and time are illusions of perception. Our body cannot really be a reality if it does not occupy most of the space it seems to occupy; an experiment made at the University of Manchester revealed the shape of the interior of an atom is almost entirely empty space. The question then became how we could possibly make the world around us see us if this is the case (Russell et al 1993).

Our true consciousness does not exist in our brains or in our bodies, but this illusion of our individual bodies along with the misinformation of our true origins has manifested the idea that we all think independently from one another. With this understanding, it seems possible to scientifically explain telepathy, clairvoyance, spiritual mediums related to the transfer of information between sources without physical means of communication phenomena. But when we understand that there is a common spiritual bond between all things in the universe and that we are all part of a divine intelligence, this simple understanding fills all the holes in modern religions and predictions about the future and literally every occurrence of events (Russell et al 1993).

According to quantum physics, the physical world and its reality, it's just a recreation of the observed. We created the body and reality, as we create the experience of our world in its different manifestations dimensional. In its essential state (atomic or cosmic sub quantum micro), the body is made of energy and information, not solid matter, this is only a meager level of perception. According to Tornell (2001), this is energy and information arising from the endless fields of energy and information spanning the entire universal creation. The quantum school explains consciousness by applying quantum theories and explains that consciousness has a quantum origin, is non local and creates our perceived reality from vibrating entities that can have multiple versions based on the observer's perception (Valverde 2016).

When looking at the electronic microscope, we are looking at our microcosm, we then can see how the quantum particles manifest virtually as a symphony and intelligent orchestration at speeds much higher than the visible light, this quantum view also represents the immutability of our macrocosm. In this reality, each individual inhabits a reality that is beyond all change, as more deep within us without the knowledge of our three-dimensional or physical outer senses. There is a core of being, an energy field that creates immortality in nature, and manifests as the physical body. This core is the essential being or soul, primordial seed, which is contained in an atom called seed. We are seeds of eternal essence at this stage of quantum eternity.

This is the seed based on new paradigms posed by Max Planck, J. Clark Maxwell, Faraday, Heisenberg, Schrodinger, Bohr, Einstein, S. Hawking, among many other pioneers of quantum mechanics. They understood that the way to see the world in their time was very wrong. Within the quantum paradigm, we are more than our physical body; our true self and personality are governed by the rules of the principle of cause and effect and are embedded into a body for the duration of human life. The field of human life is open and unlimited in its deeper quantum level, this means that we are immortal and timeless. Once we identify with the eternal reality that is consistent with quantum vision of the universe, we will enter the new paradigms of quantum consciousness. Everything that exists has a natural vibration to its atoms all the way up to the immensity of the universe to show a simple connection between land and our bodies.

Consciousness

Being aware is to realize everything that happens around you. It is as if in the previous moment you take an action, before acting you asking yourself: Is it right what I do? And someone who "is not you" answers only "yes" or "no" (Hawnser, 1997). Our mind before ordering an action to the physical body, studies the elements it has to do with the action: knowledge, physical strength, skill, etc. Consider the risks, the consequences, the material benefits that give us the results of the act, also any loss and damage and / or suffering that the action may bring to our selves or third parties (Hawnse, 1997).

Edelman and Tonomi (2000) think that the whole universe is actually one living organism with full conscious awareness of self. The consciousness of our universe is responsible for the form and purpose that all matter assumes. Carl Jung (1981) found that there is a collective unconscious connected to all humans. This means that all humanity shares a single mind with one another. This is evident in the world through accounts of shared mythology and symbols. This collectivity is a global example of the unconscious mind of the human body in which billions of cells share a similar signal. Human consciousness is an electromagnetic energy field; this could explain many paranormal phenomena such as telepathy and clairvoyance that seem to probe this.

Most Western scientists assume that consciousness is produced in some form by the brain. There is of course some evidence for that position. There is evidence of common sense in our daily lives. When we drink too much alcohol or takes a hard hit to the head, we do not think clearly. We also have more sophisticated tests of the relationship between the brain and consciousness. In fact all the theories of consciousness during the last century has been supported by psychologists who have been moving towards the materialism that characterized the nineteenth-century physics based on Newton's classical mechanics. These have been trying to show that consciousness is only the functioning of the physical brain. This materialistic psychology was supported by John Watson (1916), who wrote that psychology is a purely objective experimental branch of science that needs no consciousness in the same way that science does not need chemistry and physics. It is ironic that while Watson links psychology to the classical physical knowledge of Newtonian physics, there is overwhelming experimental evidence that the universe is related to quantum physics that could not be made without reference to consciousness.

John Lorber (1978) specialized in children with hydrocephalus, or water on the brain is a British neurologist. Children with this condition have an abnormal amount of cerebral spinal fluid accumulation in the cavities inside their brain compressing brain tissue that usually leads to mental retardation seizures, paralysis and blindness and if not treated to death. However, Lorber describes dozens of children and some adults with severe hydrocephalus but live normal lives. Indeed, in a sample of children with their cerebral space filled with ninety-five percent of spinal fluid in their skull leaving virtually no room for any brain tissue, half of them had a higher IQ than one hundred and thirty.

Some of the best evidence that consciousness can function independently of the brain come from near death experiences, profound experiences that some people report when they have been on the threshold of death. The near-death experiences are very short stories of people who have been clinically dead and then are resurrected or revived spontaneously after a brief interval with the memory of what they experienced during that period. According to Greyson (2010), many people with near death experiences reported vivid mental clarity exceptional sensory imagery and a clear memory of the experience and an experience that is more real, then in their daily lives.

Quantum Biofeedback

As the traditional biofeedback, uses sensors to monitor physiological relaxation indicators as the temperature of the skin and muscle tension, quantum biofeedback expands classical biofeedback by using galvanic skin response (GSR) and other similar devices together with modern computer technology to detect and measure the response of the built-mind-spirit body (sometimes called the super-conscious) to a large array of stress indicators. Quantum Biofeedback is a sophisticated biofeedback technique based on advanced scientific principles that promote a deeper understanding of health and healing. By seeing the body as a complex electrical circuit and by applying the principles of electrical engineering, wearable to analyze and balance the electric body. We usually think of the body as just anatomy and physiology; however, one of the easiest way to learn about the state of health of the body is by measuring electrical properties of the electric body.

Super-conscious makes adjustments to biological speeds to reduce internal tensions and sends 'back feedback' that allows the practitioner to focus the session on the parts of the body-mind-spirit more in need of relaxation. The result is a smooth passive relaxation session, still focused on those areas most in need of attention. When the body becomes so relaxed, the therapist can start the natural healing process. Many long-term stress cases can be reduced with biofeedback sessions. Quantum Biofeedback interacts with all cellular matrix of the body, which allows communication with the conscious and unconscious reactions of the body. This is accomplished by establishing electrical communication using 12 electrodes that are attached to the head, wrists, and ankles of the client. Classic Biofeedback is based on electrical measurements taken from the front (frontal cortex). This information is presented to the users who then try to consciously change his or her internal reactions to modify electrical results. Quantum Biofeedback uses people's link to all body cell matrix interface, not only the conscious aspects, but also with the unconscious, this provides greater gain in the understanding of health.

Users of this technology experience increases in physical health, strength and stamina, they can also display more confidence, they may find it easier to sleep, which can be more relaxed, and they may experience more happiness and satisfaction in a day-to-day basis (Health and Public Policy Committee 1985). Today, thousands of doctors and medical researchers worldwide are investigating electro medicine and biofeedback Neurotechnology devices as effective traditional methods of treatment alternatives. These pathways are new possibilities for the treatment of conditions such as spinal cord injury, muscular restoration, nerve regeneration, brain stimulation, bladder disorders, tumors, heart disease and other chronic diseases and disorders.

Transpersonal Psychology.

Transpersonal Psychology considers that the psyche is multidimensional. There are several "levels of consciousness" and each has different characteristics and is governed by different laws. Transpersonal psychology does not deny other schools of thought, as psychoanalysis does not arise as opposed; the right thing would be to say that attempts to go further. For transpersonal vision, Freud developments have been of fundamental value in the development of psychological science to include the idea of the unconscious in a discipline that was tied to the positivist rationalism. Certainly, psychoanalysis opened the possibilities of understanding the human psyche. Transpersonal psychology integrates the spiritual experience within a broader understanding of the human psyche. It is with the study of states of consciousness and the full potential of man, that transpersonal psychology assumes that humans can achieve harmony and transcend through spiritual development. Transpersonal is something that exceeds the range of human's own experience or personal history. Transpersonal refers to that which is beyond of the person who is the essential being.

Much of its discoveries and contributions come from the study of Eastern religions, and Christian mysticism. Transpersonal psychology is interested in the different forms of Buddhism, for meditation, for yoga, for mystical experiences, psychophysiological effects that all these phenomena, the limits of consciousness, etc. The ultimate goal of all this is to try to achieve an awakening that is the greater awareness that would raise the level of "being" that integrates psychology and spirituality.

Transpersonal psychotherapist Anthony Sutich (founder and first editor of the Journal of Transpersonal Psychology) provides one of the first formal definitions of transpersonal psychology in 1969 at the inaugural edition of the Journal of Transpersonal Psychology (Vol. 1, No. 1, Spring 1969). "The emerging Transpersonal Psychology refers specifically to the empirical, scientific study, and the responsible application of relevant results, becoming meta-needs individual and species-wide, the final values, conscience unitive, peak experiences, values, ecstasy, mystical, amazing experience, being, self, essence, joy, wonder, ultimate meaning, transcendence of self, the spirit, unity, cosmic consciousness, synergy of individual and species level, maximum interpersonal encounter, sacralisation of everyday life, transcendental phenomena, self-cosmic humor and joy maximum sensory awareness, responsiveness and expression; and concepts, experiences and activities " (Sutich, 1969).

Stanislav Grof, co-founder of transpersonal psychology with Abraham Maslow, defines transpersonal psychology as "The psychology that respects the entire spectrum of human experience, including holotropic states, and all domains of the psyche. - Biographical, perinatal and transpersonal "(Grof, 2000). Transpersonal psychology covers a multitude of experiences and behaviors produced by spontaneous or altered states of consciousness, impulses into higher states of being, and extraordinary spiritual practices induced. Transpersonal phenomena include the meditative experiences, dreaming, drug-induced psychedelia, peak experiences, cosmic consciousness, enlightenment, mysticism, out of body experiences, channeling trance, near death experiences, memories reincarnations, extrasensory awareness, archetypal phenomena, accelerated learning, exceptional state of health and well-being, the mind-body healing and miraculous cures. Parapsychological phenomena are important for the reduction of science and spirit implications.

Altered States of Consciousness and Transpersonal Psychology

Ludwig (1972) defines an "altered state of consciousness" as any mental state (s) for various manoeuvres of physiological, psychological or pharmacological agents, which can be recognized subjectively by the same (or an objective observer of the individual person induced) as representing a sufficient deviation in the subjective experience or psychological functioning of certain general rules for that individual during alert awareness. This deviation can be sufficiently represented by a greater concern than usual with internal sensations or mental processes, changes in the formal characteristics of thought, and the deterioration of the test of reality to varying degrees. The cognitive approach to altered states of consciousness has revealed that similar features that are characteristic of many altered states of consciousness including "alterations in thinking", "sense of disturbed weather", "loss of control", "change in emotional expression "," change of body image, "" perceptual distortions "," change in the meaning or importance "," sense of the ineffable," and " feelings of rejuvenation "(Ludwig, 1972).

By applying the disruptive force requirement for the basic state of consciousness (either through some physiological action, such as drugs or deployment of attention and meditation), the current organization of cognitive subsystems is destabilized until a new force patterns (such as mental set, setting, expectations, drug effects) is applied to shape the subsystems in a whole new system, the production of a new discrete state of consciousness with its own stabilization processes.

Cognitive awareness approach has helped differentiate transpersonal psychologists' grades waking state of consciousness. Awareness, for example, is not one homogenous thing, but varies and changes as the colors of the rainbow. It is possible to stratify and states order to raise awareness of alert and focused relaxed concentration and spread the cosmic consciousness. A range of altered states of consciousness has been identified as drug-induced states, hypnosis, biofeedback, daydreaming, night dreaming, sensory deprivation, and paranormal experiences. With each state consisting of many levels and functions, in each region or area of consciousness, individuals are able to process different types of information at different levels of control (Goleman & Davidson, 1979; Ornstein, 1972).

Transpersonal psychologists tend to see the experiences of "mystical union", "enlightenment", "nirvana", and related experiences as natural and beneficial non-ordinary states of consciousness that may be subject to effects of state-dependent learning. The idea that the experience of the sacred can be interpreted as altered states of consciousness arose from the observation of twice that (a) psychedelic drugs have been used through the centuries and cultures to induce religious experiences and (b) reports from some drug experiences are phenomenologically (descriptively or experiential) indistinguishable from accounts of natural mystical experiences (Doblin, 1991; Grinspoon & Bakalar, 1997; Smith, 1964).

Transpersonal psychologist Charles T. Tart has examined the altered states of consciousness from a cognitive perspective in terms of changes in the configuration and operation of the underlying mental processes (Tart, 1971, 1976, 1983, 1992). A state of consciousness involves cognitive functioning following subsystems: exteroceptors (receives sensory information), interoceptors (kinesthetic receives input), input processing (working memory), the subconscious processes, sense of identity, evaluation and decision making, emotions, space / time sense, long term memory, the motor output (behavior) plus latent functions. These 10 subsystems (more possible latent functions) define any discrete state of consciousness. The particular configuration of the subsystems in a given time is shaped and limited by the deployment of attention, the body's energies, characteristics of the structures themselves and the particular social and cultural environments in which they operate.

Grof (1988) suggested that the term "altered states of consciousness" cover transpersonal experiences; however, there are certain types of altered states of consciousness that do not meet the criteria for being transpersonal (involving an expansion or extension of consciousness beyond the limits of the usual and limitations time and space). For example, a living and complex childhood memory occurs in an altered state of consciousness (e.g. hypnosis or psychedelic sessions), but do not meet the criteria for being transpersonal. The cultural context of the 1960s and 1970s provided fertile ground for the emergence of transpersonal studies as an independent field of study in psychology. The infusion of ideas Eastern contemplative traditions of Zen, Advaita, Vedanta and Taoism, along with the institutionalization of the humanist revolution in academic psychology, and the growing interest in consciousness and altered states of consciousness that are triggered by the widespread use of psychedelics, paved the way for the birth of transpersonal psychology movement in California in the late 1960s (Ferrer, 2002).

Since the 1970s, transpersonal psychology, as the humanist movement that preceded it, has been divided into three different groups; the first group represented by the ideas of Grof (1988) that believes that transcendence can only occur in the presence of a altered state of consciousness. This group produces conceptual models of non-ordinary states of consciousness. The second group, led by Wilber (1980), include those trying to assign internal states of consciousness and identify with the monistic and perennial philosophy of Aldous Huxley. Wilber believes that all expressions of the highest state of consciousness in each tradition are the same as the psychopathic conditions occurring at the bottom, the normal waking reality in the middle and meditative states of higher consciousness in the top. The third and by far the largest segment of the transpersonal movement has no identifiable bearer, it sees the self as getting up and go to work in the morning, the higher consciousness is sweeping the floor, washing dishes, and raking leaves. The lighting is doing everything we are supposed to be doing at this minute. There is a preconceived thing; is not an altered state of consciousness, it is simply the deep philosophy, which is to be found most clearly in the mundane (Taylor, 1999).

Altered states of consciousness answer the question "who we really are?" The answer to this question is that we are a part of God and that humans are spiritual beings having human experiences that somehow reveal the direction of our full identity of our cosmic status (Valverde 2015).

Brain Waves

Our brain works primarily with bioelectrical energy. Although the power of electricity that handle our neurons is low (measured in mill volts), this power processes, manage, distribute and use vast amounts of information and generates multiple answers (almost infinite in possibilities). So by using micro electricity, we can conclude that the brain is a machine of low frequencies. Our brain, in addition to process information that comes by the senses, is capable of emitting extra-sensory information received via similar "electromagnetic waves", but with lower intensity similar to the frequencies of a radio transmitter-receiver. Our brain can act as a radio station, similar to numerous species of birds that in their migrations are guided by a genuine receiver of terrestrial magnetism located in the pituitary gland. With this receiver, they know where they have to fly and in what direction. It's like having a real compass incorporated into the brain. The mind could be defined as the "sense" of the brain (like sight is the sense of the eye).

A German psychiatrist, professor at the University of Vienna named Hans Berger (1.843-1941), demonstrated that a device "amplifier" that was called later electroencephalograph could capture electrical potential (voltage fluctuations) in the human brain. Before him, the English physician Richard Caton (1842-1926) showed similar potential in dogs. The first types of brain frequencies that were discovered were the "alpha" and "theta".

Later, these findings were complemented by research in the range frequencies captured by the electroencephalograph. Each type of wave results in a different neuropsychological state. That is, our mind, our body and our physical and physiological activity are completely different in each of these states or frequencies. The type of neuro-chemicals and hormones substances discharged into the blood flow varies depending on frequency and as much as the presence and quantity of such substances as the mood we have, interact to produce a physiological-mental-physical-end that involves a mental state. A level of consciousness is conscious thought that is always thinking even in moments of apparent inactivity, but trivial ideas continually pass by consciousness. Most of the thoughts are accompanied by reactions in behavior, and small involuntary movements. When you're not actively thinking then you're probably dreaming, according Signer and Streiner (1966) a person has throughout the day about 200 daydreams. Therefore, consciousness is the sum of all the different perceptions. The most common consciousness are wakefulness and sleep; however, changes in expressing both cerebral and psycho states change according to conscious or subconscious feelings of each person are distinguished. These changes are directly related to the electrical activity of the brain. This activity can be measured by the number of oscillations per second (Hz) that are linked to different states of consciousness in the brain: our brain only perceives a limited range of frequencies indispensable to operate with ease in this three-dimensional medium. 20 to 20,000 vibrations per second are perceptible by our ears, the colors perceived by our eyes range from red to violet (although extending beyond, up and down), all possible smells and tastes (which are also vibrations) and the endless textures that we can distinguish with our skin. But the brain is not only receiver but also is sends vibrations. It has been proven thanks to the EEG that the brain emits waves of varying intensity and frequency depending on the mental state of the person being observed. These waves are classified into:

The alpha state is when, if we would connect to an electro encephalogram, our brains would work between 7.5 to 14 cycles per second. When "operate" in this state, we rank among the border of the conscious and the unconscious. Is the gate between both states of consciousness and this makes "Alpha state" therefore a special status because it allows us, on the one hand, still have a conscious activity of our mind and body, that is, we realize what we think and happening around us. On the other hand, since the "lift" of consciousness in the "lower floors" of the mind, gives us access to information and own subconscious states, can use all the wealth of the 90% of "power" mental residing in the subconscious. This state is a "being comfortable" in inner peace and happiness, in deep relaxation. Greatly increases the power of suggestion and autosuggestion, that is, anything that we suggest alpha, will be more easily accepted and less "filters" by our conscious rationality.

Table 1. Type of brainwaves

Types of Brain Waves	States of Consciousness
BETA WAVES: 14 Hz to 30 Hz	This type of waves are recorded when the person is awake in a state of normal activity. Correspond to states of conscious attention, anxiety, surprise, fear, stress.
GAMMA WAVES: 25 and 100 Hz	They express pathological conditions of maximum tension, excitement and the individual enters a state of STRESS in which the coordination of ideas and normal physical activity are seriously altered.
ALPHA WAVES: 8 Hz to 13 Hz	Relaxation and rest, calm, reflective state. Reduction of bodily sensations. The subconscious begins to emerge: Abstraction, suggestibility. Assimilation of the study. Ease of visualization of mental images.
THETA WAVES: 3.5 Hz to 7 Hz	During sleep or in deep meditation, autogenous training, hypnosis, yoga (whenever the formations of the subconscious act). The state stimulates creative inspiration. Considered a state for maximum capacity of learning. Fantasy, imagination. Hypnagogic images.
DELTA WAVES: 1 Hz to 3 Hz	It arises mainly in the states of deep sleep and unconsciousness. Very rarely can be experienced being awake unless with a very hard training (Yoga, Meditation, Zen, Hypnosis, Self hypnosis) or with a synchronizer of hemispheres. It corresponds to deep sleep, hypnotic trance, REM sleep. It corresponds to sleep without dream, trance, deep hypnosis. Delta waves are very important in the healing process and strengthening the immune system.

Music is a very effective instrument of suggestion and production of alpha state made many instruments produce vibrations at that frequency. Hence, with relative ease, many people stay asleep at concerts or simply feel "moved" by the music to another dimension. If we put them to an electroencephalograph, most of those attending a concert in an auditorium would be running on alpha. The contemplation of the sea, the rolling waves and the sound they produce is a good inducer of alpha state. The tone of individuals things like music, prayer, smells, certain types of images (especially of nature, certain types of painting, Tibetan mandalas symbols or own) can be used to put ourselves in this special state of the mind, that makes us touch our innermost and reach the "spiritual zone" of human beings. Therefore, as we see, there are many things that can induce this state.

Magnus & Van der Holst (1987) speak of frequencies whose frequency ranges from 3.5 to 7.5 cycles per second. They are associated with the states of creative and decisive hallucination. During its broadcast, the person can discover events deeply hidden in the recesses of your subconscious, as well as conflicts and personality in particular. Is the wave of imagination and dynamic contact with other possible "dimensions psi" offering you the opportunity to research our personality and deep in our psychology?

Neurotechnology Principles

Robert Monroe (1982), one of the most prominent people in Neurotechnology in particular in the field of sound with neurological efficiency, devised the method HEMI-SYNC: (Synchronization of the cerebral hemispheres by means of sounds). Like a glass that resonates when a pure tone is emitted, the brain resonates when receives certain frequencies of waves, being synchronized with these, this effect is known as FFR Frequency Following Response (FFR).

Machines created based on FFR began to be popular in the 80s, the typical machine based on the principle of Monroe used stereo headphones that are used to send sound signals to each ear, for example 2 signs of 300 and 304 Hz. One ear will hear only 300 Hz signal and the other only 304, but since the sounds are combined in the brain, this will hear a third signal of 4 Hz, which is the difference between the two sound impulses. This third signal is not an audible sound, but an electrical signal that can only be created by the cerebral hemispheres acting in unison, and may go unnoticed, producing as a result, the two hemispheres are focused simultaneously on the same state of consciousness, increasing the brainpower.

The Monroe Institute was created based on the principles of Monroe. The Neurotechnology of the Monroe Institute is a system that mixes and sequences sound patterns designed to evoke beneficial brainwave states for different human activities. Robert A. Monroe, who began studying the effects of sound on accelerated learning in the 50s, founded this institute. The work is the result of thousands of hours of laboratory sessions. Participants in these sessions listen to specific combinations and sequences of sound patterns and simultaneously report their experiences while electronic instruments measure the effects on the activity of their brain waves.

Walter (1964) while conducting experiments in which strobe devices used to send rhythmic flashes of light in the eyes, watched amazed that the flickering light could alter the activity of the entire cerebral cortex, rather than exclusively associated areas with vision. The subjective experiences of those who received the flashes were even more curious reported seeing "lights like comets, ultra fantastic colors, color mental". Moreover, Walter discovered that certain visual stimuli of a certain frequency could cause the brain to respond quickly adjusted to the same frequency of the stimulus it received. In 1982 a psychiatrist Denis Gorges created a machine called brain wave synchro-energizer, which applies the latest technology in the first device designed optical-acoustic stimulation. This is able to promote as its inventor claimed "an increase in the capabilities and functions of the human mind", this unleashed a wave of unprecedented research and experimentation, catalyzed by M. Hutchinson (1986) through his famous book Megabrain.

Our scheme of thought is influenced by the predominance of left hemisphere, logical and analytical thinking. Right hemisphere, creative thinking, visualization, and which carries out a holistic synthesis. On the back of the brain is where the intuitive thought takes place. Obviously use one of the two hemispheres or either of the brain regions severely limits our abilities. The optimal functioning of our brain, is given by the synchronization of the two hemispheres: by left-right and front-back alternating stimulation occurs almost simultaneously, an issue of brain wave of an identical amplitude and frequency. Neurotechnology is typically used for process brainwave entrainment to tune brainwaves. With these machines, we may experience theta waves, alpha, delta or including combinations of ranges using frequencies layered that mix several brainwave ranges in a synergistic pattern.

Hemi-Sync is a patented process sound that pulses to create the same electric waves in frequency and amplitude simultaneously in both hemispheres of the brain for specific purposes. Our brains have a hemisphere left and right. The left-brain is linear, logical, practical, and time -oriented. The right hemisphere seems to be much more nonlinear, abstract, creative, holistic, and not logic. We tend to use one hemisphere at a time, or better said, will favor hemispheres particular in terms of what we're doing. An accountant probably uses less of his right hemisphere than an artist would during the course of his workday. If the person were doing math, the staff would be using more of your left side. If the person were going to paint a masterpiece of art, the person would have the activity hemispheric more in the right. Both hemispheres are constantly interacting and both can be used simultaneously.

By merging both hemispheres we can make them to work together and with this we can increase our ability mental and improve our performance cognitive in general. Basically, it's like having a computer processor faster able to work at faster speeds. The greater integration creates better performance.

The mind machines that help the brain synchronizes naturally to balance hemispheric activity and adjusts the activity of brain waves to match the carrier frequencies embedded brainwaves. This hemispheric coherence induced audio produces an optimal state of comprehensive synergy of the entire brain. These hemispheres are connected by the corpus callosum that it serves as a conduit or a bridge between both sides. This bridge literally be exercised and strengthened until it is physically larger and more capable of transmitting data, ideas and feedback between the hemispheres.

The advance occurs when you use this principle to synchronize our brain wave frequencies chosen with the help of specific mental machines. We can do this easily by using technology of binaural beat audio and monophonic ringtones. This phenomenon is called trailing phenomenon.

The scientific principle of drag can be used to resonate, or synchronize our brain to tune specific frequencies. The drive is quite simple. If we have two tuning forks of the same pitch, if we strike one and hold it near the other both resonate at the same frequency. Given the fact that our brains function as a resonating chamber, oscillating pulses and patterns of neural excitation ripple through our brains like endless waves on a pond of a subtle dynamic electric field.

The creation process of frequency binaural beat is very simple to explain. First, we create two audio tones with two frequencies slightly different (i.e. 100 Hz and 107 Hz). When playing a tone in the ear left and the other tone in his right ear, the brain reacts to the stimulus audio by resonance brain activity to the difference between these two tones. Our brain waves adjust to match this frequency differential. For example, if we play a frequency of 100 Hz in the ear and left 107 Hz in the right ear, our brain tune the 7 Hz differential (107 Hz - 100 Hz = 7 Hz). This frequency tracking response makes our brain to resonate at 7 Hz frequencies and this falls within the range of theta brainwaves. This psychoacoustics state can create phenomenal results.

The electrical activity of neurons is changing patterns of electrical potential through all cell membranes. Each cell generates in the membrane potential that can be detected in about one micrometer of the cell and in large sets of brain cells that can work in harmony to generate potential of few micro volts, this can be detected through the skull and scalp by using electrodes. The variation of the electrical potential around the scalp is the basis of operation of the electroencephalogram (EEG). This method of recording the electrical activity of the brain, digitized maps produces the electrical activity of brain. The state in which the two hemispheres are synchronized by showing similar activity in both hemispheres, is sometimes known as “whole brain” and occurs randomly for short periods. Stimulation through the differential tone makes it possible to sustain this state for longer periods.

The Hemi-Sync process has already been tested and implemented in many ways for:

- Sleep better
- Reduce tension or stress
- Control pain
- Accelerate learning
- Study and concentration
- Enhance creativity
- Find solutions to problems

The Induction and Measurement of Altered States of Consciousness by Using Neurotechnology in Transpersonal Psychotherapy

The most frequently heard of studies of altered states of consciousness criticism is that they are hoaxes, some form of mental delusion. A good example is the case of Eastern yogis who for years claimed to be able to control parts of the nervous system and the body such as heart rate, blood pressure, hormone secretion, etc.

Western scientists considered these claims impossible whose theories and personal experience denied this possibility.

Biofeedback research shows that many of the claims made by physicists yogis, changing the sound pattern proved to be true can change particularly the state of consciousness at will. EEG measurements have been based on the research and theories developed from the early work of Adrian and Matthews (1934) that discovered that the brain could go to certain frequencies with electronic brain stimulation, this work led to the discovery that various frequencies were linked to certain psychological states (Kamiya, 1968), and ultimately the work of Green et al. (1977) demonstrated the ability to control these states and frequencies. You could say that these tests were the first to show how the brain can boot, such as a computer with the right input frequency.

What exactly happens neurologically when we walked into alternate states of consciousness is still far from being understood. This gap in our knowledge of these kingdoms is largely due to deficiencies in both research tools and philosophies employed by scientific research, and our general reluctance of society to accept such states as real. Within the traditional scientific practice is important to understand how our brains create the bridge to stimulate altered states of consciousness, but understanding it tells us little or nothing about the correlation with psychological phenomena with which we are able to interpret altered states of consciousness. It is this inner cosmological view or its representation of our quantum reality.

Once we accept this premise as our fundamental metaphor for altered states of consciousness, then it is possible to postulate that our brainwave frequencies are measurement indicators of our psychological states and correspond to the various ways in which we produce. That is, these frequencies are the units of our quantum reality. This is how we create, outside the sphere of influence of the Heisenberg principle that says that our fields are a unified experience. Cade et al (1979) conducted EEG tests in 70 subjects and measure the ESR (electrical resistance of the skin) and with the application of its results to the work of Lesh (1970) was able to build in the table below that represents the objective and subjective correlates of these states.

One of the determinants of the results of the induction of altered states of consciousness in psychotherapy comes from Penfield and Perot (1963) who developed a study where a series of what was called in those days outside the body psychic visions were caused a that emerged not only for his epileptic patients but also in patients who had at the operating table for which they stimulated the surface of their brain. In one case study, one of his epileptic patients actually had visions of God descending from heaven.

An important factor in the development of Neurotechnology step was carried out by Persinger (1983). Persinger is the director of the neuroscience program at Laurentian University. Persinger (1983) is able to induce visions of God and other

Table 2. states of consciousness and frequency measurements

Consciousness	Measured Frequency	Types of Waves
Just he is beginning to relax with difficulty quieting the mind.	25-20	alpha and beta
Not very clear conscience or sense of anesthesia	20-16	Guests beta alpha continuous
Calm and relaxed with memories	16-13	Alpha continues without beta theta intermittent
State definite feeling of floating with increased imagination and more concentration sustained	13-10	Alfa falling Continuous theta
Living consciousness the body modification between awareness internal and external	10-8	alpha continuous theta falling Frequency
Awareness with satisfaction and deep intense alertness and calmness and detachment	8-5	Theta continuous alpha close to theta
New way of feeling by intuitive vision synthesis of opposites in a higher unity	below 4	Delta occasionally

religious and mystical experiences in the laboratory by using a computer and what he calls the koran helmet was also given the nickname God helmet. His most important contribution to the induction of altered states of consciousness came when he had a vision as to the origins of spirituality in human evolution. He found that the temporal lobes of the brain are the source of most spiritual and mystical experiences= of the scientific literature.

The God helmet is a device used to induce altered states of consciousness using weak magnetic signals to direct brain activity. This can induce spiritual experiences and helps auto wing transpersonal exploration and transformation of many people. Persinger (1983) investigated some common perceptions of the inner mind by taking electromagnetic brain patterns seen in people who have near-death experiences. Persinger (1983) found that it can simulate that by applying complex significant magnetic fields in the brain that can also induce altered state of consciousness such as near-death experiences. Persinger et al (2000) conducted an experiment that tested the idea that mystical perception and stimulating the nerve activity in the brain can trigger paranormal experiences. In the experiment, volunteers were blindfolded in a soundproof chamber, this sensory deprivation allowed the mind to concentrate on electromagnetic patterns sent through the brain via a modified helmet. In the experiment, they were able to simulate the exact brain patterns that occur in near-death experiences.

Dr. Persinger (2000) suggests that his research will benefit psychotherapy by producing altered states of consciousness including near death experience, hearing voices and the sense of a presence as patients will able to deal with things like psychological depression by experiencing these altered states. Persinger (2000) suggests that these experiences are so strong that they are completely real to the person who has them. As a tool of science, the God helmet technology can bring us valuable new insight into the dark depths of the human mind. Persinger (1983) conducted experiments of the type of stimulation of the low level temporal lobes of the brain, in order to induce altered states in the subject in the experiment. After an initial feeling of floating in the air, the individual was feeling 'out of body'. Then the experiments used different subjects but whose constant is to describe their feelings with cosmic and spiritual meanings. Persinger mentions "Often intense listening experiences in which the person feels that some messages are communicated to him occurs". This transmission is perceived by the individual through a kind of feeling of "knowing what happens" without being able to necessarily say that hears a voice ". Persinger suggests that people with epilepsy, (temporal lobe dysfunction), are more likely to experiment altered states.

With the aid of Neurotechnology, people can discover hidden deep subconscious events as well as conflicts of personality offering the opportunity to research our personality and discover the depths of our psychology. Green, et al. (1970) mentioned, "every change in mental-emotional state, conscious or unconscious, is accompanied by an appropriate change in the physiological state." Our travels along with the continuous-consciousness is manifested by a wide range of psychological and physiological changes, inducing altered states of consciousness take our mental functions to places normally out of reach of our everyday consciousness, these areas are usually reserved for religion, mysticism and ingestion of psychoactive substances. The experiences one is on a journey through the fall of consciousness into the realm of psychological experience known as the transpersonal, these transpersonal experiences are such that exceed normal limits of our existence and leave the empirical way of knowing, initiating human consciousness in a meeting with those areas of consciousness that are, in normal conditions, being largely inaccessible to us. This process of leaving the empirical normal physical limits of our existence seems to serve as further proof of what was described in this chapter before that religious, mystical and philosophical thought are related to quantum physics.

When individuals use Neurotechnology using the phenomenon of entrainment in the brain for days or weeks in a row, the out of body experience seems to be more the rule than the exception. Normally these experiences manifest as spontaneous feelings flying above a landscape. It is nothing strange that the same feeling out of the body that occurs in many different practices aimed access to altered states of consciousness as well as show as the main subject of near-death experiences. The timing and the subsequent stimulation of the two hemispheres of the brain entrainment can result with the use of Neurotechnology as Fischer and d'Aquili (1986) suggest. Much of what appears to take place within the transcendental experience of parapsychology seems to be what many of us commonly called the synchronicity. The synchronicity can be defined as a causal connecting principle of coincidence of events in space / time. Carl Jung, who is the first to describe the concept of synchronicity, saw that this state could be related to many transcendental experiences. These synchronistic events can be linked dreams, visions, meditative states and other inner experiences with tangible events in the life of the subject.

A growing number of professional researchers postulated that ESP could be linked to the alpha state (Lawrence, 1972). Dr. Edward Bokert of the American Society for Psychical Research analyzed mental states and has concluded that they are, at least in its early stages, "characterized by a highly aroused autonomic nervous system" (Lawrence, 1972) precisely what one finds in the ergotropic excitement associated with the brain and the use of neuro technologies. Dr. Charles Honorton of the Maimonides Medical Center has also found that the ESP seems to be associated with "relaxation, mild dissociation, passivity, and reduced visual imagery" (Honorton, 1970), which is commonly found when waves alpha occur with brain entrainment technologies. Indeed, Honorton found that the higher alpha production, the higher the score obtained in the individual tests ESP. It seems as if many of the psychic states that identified Grof as part of the "Experiential Extension Beyond the consensus reality and space-time" may be associated with changes in one level of consciousness to another.

Proposed Cyber-Psychotherapy System with the Use of Neurotechnology

The state of consciousness of someone can be measured by using physiological changes. Some physiological changes are typically associated with altered state of consciousness so measuring these physiological changes may provide evidence to more accurately determine the state of consciousness someone is in. Cade and Coxhead (1979) was able to map altered state of consciousness with alpha brain waves between 10 to 8 cycles.

The proposed Cyber-psychotherapy system uses EEG to show the ephemeral patterns of the electrical signals from the two hemispheres of the cortex as they are happening (Cade & Coxhead 1979). The EEG captures the users' brainwave signals. After being converted to digital form, the brainwaves are processed, and the results are wirelessly transmitted to the USB receiver. A brain mapping software interprets these signals to displays mental activity in real time. The software displays brain activity in four significant brainwave frequency bands (Delta, Theta, Alpha, Beta) and uses the headset to read data.

An application of quantum physics (Neurotechnology) in the altered states of consciousness was carried out by Persinger (1983). Persinger (1983) was able to induce visions of God and other religious and mystical experiences in the laboratory by using a computer and with what he called the Koran helmet that has also the nickname of the God helmet. He found that the temporal lobes of the brain are the source of the most spiritual experiences and other alternate state of consciousness.

This God helmet is a device to induce altered states of consciousness using weak magnetic signals to direct brain activity that can induce spiritual experiences that helps with transpersonal exploration and transformation of many people that is able to heal because of these transpersonal experiences (Persinger, 2000). It is suggested that altered states of consciousness such as sensed presence and out-of-body experience whether they are produced by magnetic, electric or other stimulations or circumstances can be most effectively explained as the changes of the relative contents and/or intensities of the test subjects' neural quantum entanglement with their surroundings including possibly spiritual environments or information (Hu & Wu, 2012).

The proposed Cyber-psychotherapy system uses the Koran helmet of Persinger (1983). The koran helmet software produces EEG signals. These are applied to the brain using modified commonly available magnetic coils. The magnetic signals are applied to the head at very low strength. The signals are short bursts, followed by intervals of silence. Each signal speaks a language that only one brain structure understands and responds. The brain has two hippocampus and two amygdalas, one on each side. When these structures respond, they can put the person in a positive altered state of consciousness.

The proposed architecture of the Cyber-psychotherapy is depicted in Figure 1. The therapist computer has installed Brain activity map software and Skype. Skype is a telecommunications software that allows verbal and text communications with the patient, the Brain activity map software allows the therapist to visualize the states of consciousness of the patient by detecting the frequency band with the highest level of activity. The therapist is able to access the EEG signals collected by the EEG headset wore by the patient. These digital signals are transmitted over the internet by using a cloud based hub such as Flexihub software (Flexihub 2016), FlexiHub is a USB over IP software solution, it enables sharing access to USB devices over Internet. The EEG headset is connected to the USB of the patient's computer via a USB wireless adaptor. The koran helmet is wore by the patient and is meant to induce altered states of consciousness by receiving modulated signals to both temporal lobes from a signal generator installed in the patient's computer.

Figure 1. Proposed cyber-psychotherapy system

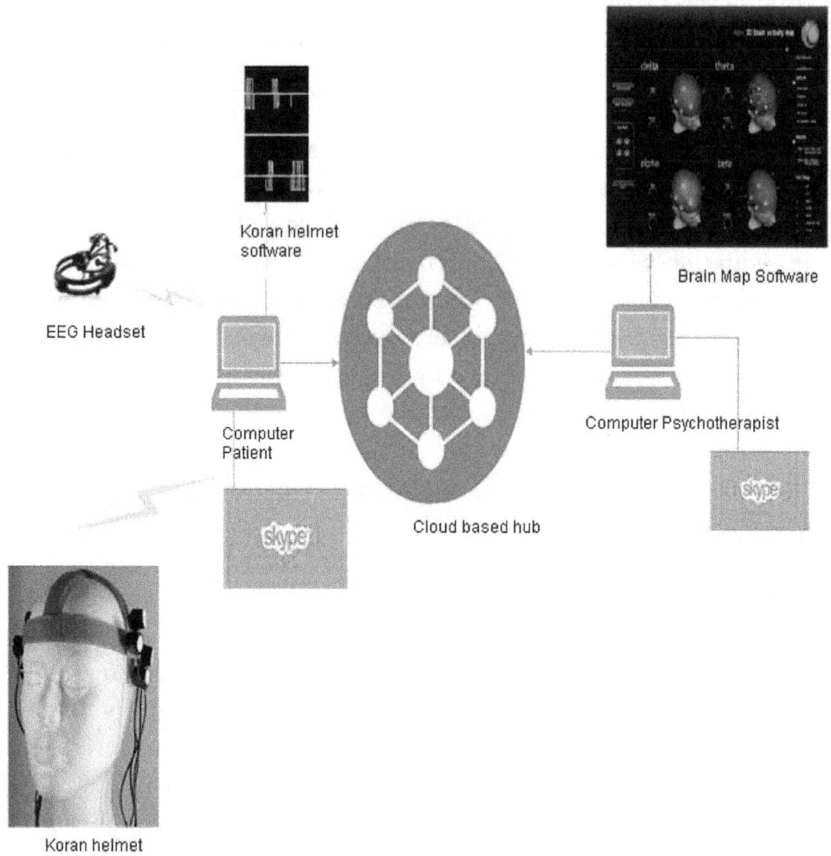

CONCLUSION

Our present understanding of "brain entrainment technology" is still in its infancy, however, this chapter intends to open the eyes of the reader that this technology has great potential particularly for transpersonal therapies.

This chapter introduced Neurotechnology based technologies including quantum biofeedback; the latter has proven curative value for particular diseases that seem to be psychosomatic and also has been proven to help to measure state of consciousness of individuals. Transpersonal psychology was presented as a paradigm that recognizes the immortality of consciousness and relies on spiritual concepts that have roots in mystic religions as reincarnation and survival of consciousness after the brain death. The immortality of consciousness is based largely on the quantum theory explaining the origin of consciousness and its connection to the universe.

Neurotechnology explores the use of technologies of sound, light and radiofrequency to control the frequency of brain waves with the reason to induce altered states of consciousness. Altered states of consciousness have been proposed as therapies for healing in transpersonal psychology, these therapies recognize the spiritual essence of the individual and are based on the concept that psychological illnesses are rooted in the spirit and not in the brain. Once the patient knows the root of his or her problems, seems to find the answer to his or her anxieties and can self heal with these transpersonal experiences.

Inducing altered states of consciousness with Neurotechnology is a relatively new concept and although there are serious studies, they are not incorporated into traditional medicine more than anything by a lack of understanding of this technology in traditional medicine. The aim of this chapter is to open the eyes of the therapists about the potential of these technologies in the use of transpersonal therapies.

In this chapter a Cyber-psychotherapy system is proposed to support transpersonal psychotherapy. The system can be used to induce non-ordinary state of consciousness that can be used by transpersonal psychologists as a healing tool to cure his patients with psychological problems such as psychosis at a distance location with the help of Internet technologies. The proposed cyber psychotherapy system uses quantum signal generator for the induction of altered states of consciousness and has integrated an EEG that serves as a biofeedback device in order to assess if the patient has reached the desired level of consciousness and can be used it to adjust the frequencies of the signal generator in order to improve the psychotherapy experience of the patient if necessary.

REFERENCES

Adrian, E. D., & Matthews, B. H. C. (1934). The Berger Rhythm; potential Changes from the occipital lobes in man. *Brain*, *57*(4), 355–384. doi:10.1093/brain/57.4.355

Becker, R. O., & Selden, G. (1985). *The Body Electric: Electromagnetism and the foundation of life (pp 364-p.)*. New York: Quill.

Botella, C., Garcia-Palacios, A., Banos, R. M., & Quero, S. (2009). Cybertherapy: Advantages, Limitations and Ethical issues. *PsychNology Journal*, *7*(1), 77–100.

Cade, C. Maxwell, and Nona Coxhead. 1979. The Awakened Mind: Biofeedback and the Development of Higher States of Awareness. New York: Delacorte Press.

d'Aquili, E. (1983). The Myth-Ritual Complex: A Biogenetic Structural Analysis. Zygon, 18. doi:10.1111/j.1467-9744.1983.tb00513.x d'Aquili, E. (1986). Myth, Ritual, and the Archetypal Hypothesis. *Zygon*, *21*(2).

Doblin, R. (1991). Pahnke's "Good Friday experiment": A long-term follow-up and methodological critique. *Journal of Transpersonal Psychology*, *23*, 1–28.

Edelman, G. M., & Tononi, G. (2000). *A Universe of Consciousness: How Matter Becomes Imagination*. Basic books.

Ferrer, J. N. (2002). *Revisioning transpersonal theory: A participatory vision of Human spirituality*. Albany, NY: State University of New York Press.

Flexihub. (2016). Flexihub software. Retrieved from http://www.flexihub.com/

Goleman, D., & Davidson, R. J. (1979). *Consciousness: Brain, states of consciousness, and mysticism*. New York: Harper.

Green, E., & Alyce M. (1977). *Beyond Biofeedback*. New York: Delta Books.

Green, E. E., Green, A. M., & Walters, E. D. (1970). Voluntary Control of Internal States: Psychological and Physiological. Journal of Transpersonal Psychology, 2, 1-26.

Greyson, B. (2000). Dissociation in People Who Have near-death experiences: Their bodies out of or out of Their minds? *Lancet*, *355*(9202), 460–463. doi:10.1016/S0140-6736(00)82013-9 PMID:10841127

Greyson, B. (2010). Implications of near-death experiences for a postmaterialist psychology. *Psychology of Religion and Spirituality*, *2*(1), 37–45. doi:10.1037/a0018548

Grinspoon, R. L., & Bakalar, J. (1997). Psychedelic drugs reconsidered (2nd ed.). New York: Lindesmith Center.

Grof, S. (1988). *The Adventure of Self-Discovery*. New York: State University of New York Press.

Grof, S. (2000). *Psychology of the Future: Lessons from modern consciousness research*. Albany, NY: State University of New York Press.

Hall, C. S., & Nordly, V. J. (1973). *A Primer of Jungian Psychology*. New York: Mentor Books.

Hawnser, P. E. (1997). *The Answer*. Mexico: Editorial Diana.

Health and Public Policy Committee, American College of Physicians. (1985). Biofeedback for Hypertension. *Annals of Internal Medicine*, *102*(5), 709–715. doi:10.7326/0003-4819-102-5-709 PMID:3885819

Honorton, C. (1970). Tracing ESP through altered states of consciousness. Psychic Magazine, 2, 18.

Hu, H., & Wu, M. (2012). Scientific GOD: Michael Persinger & the GOD Experiments. *Scientific GOD Journal, 3*(10).

Hutchison, M. (1986). *Megabrain: New tools and techniques for brain growth and mind expansion*. New York: Beech Tree Books.

Jonas, W. B., & Levin, J. S. (Eds.). (1999). *Essentials of complementary and alternative medicine*. Philadelphia, Pa, USA: Lippincott Williams & Wilkins.

Jung, C. G. (1981). *The archetypes and the collective unconscious (No. 20)*. Princeton University Press.

Kamiya, J. (1969). Operant monitoring of the EEG alpha rhythm and some of Its Reported effects on consciousness. In C. Tart (Ed.), *Altered States of Consciousness*. New York: John Wiley and Sons, Inc.

Lawrence, J. (1972). *Alpha Brain Waves*. Los Angeles: Nash Publishing.

Lesh, T. V. (1970). Meditators Zen and the Development of Empathy in Counselors. Aldine Annual.

Liboff, A. R. (1985). Geomagnetic cyclotron resonance in living cells. *Journal of Biological Physics, 13*(4), 99–102. doi:10.1007/BF01878387

Lorber, J. (1978, January). Is Your Brain Really Necessary. Disease in Childhood, 53(10), 834-834.

Ludwig, A. (1972). Altered states of consciousness. In C. T. Tart (Ed.), *Altered states of consciousness* (pp. 11–24). New York: Doubleday.

Magnus, O., & Van der Holst, M. (1987). Zeta waves: A special type of slow delta waves. *Electroencephalography and Clinical Neurophysiology, 67*(2), 140–146. doi:10.1016/0013-4694(87)90036-8 PMID:2439290

Masters, R., & Houston, J. (1966). *The Varieties of Psychedelic Experience*. New York: Delta Books.

Miller, N. E. (1978). Biofeedback and visceral learning. *Annual Review of Psychology, 29*(1), 373–404. doi:10.1146/annurev.ps.29.020178.002105 PMID:341785

Monroe, R. (1982). *The Hemi-Sync process. Monroe Institute Bulletin*. VA: Nellysford.

Ornstein, R. E. (1972). *The psychology of consciousness*. New York: WH Freeman.

Penfield, W., & Perot, P. (1963). The brains record of auditory and visual experience a final summary and discussion. *Brain, 86*(4), 595–696. doi:10.1093/brain/86.4.595 PMID:14090522

Persinger, M. A. (1983). Religious and mystical experiences as artifacts of temporal lobe function: General hypothesis. *Perceptual and Motor Skills, 57*(3f), 1255–1262. doi:10.2466/pms.1983.57.3f.1255 PMID:6664802

Persinger, M. A., Tiller, S. G., & Koren, S. A. (2000). Experimental Simulation Of Experience And A Elicitation Haunt Of Activity By Paroxysmal Electroencephalographic Transcerebral Complex Magnetic Fields: Induction Of A Synthetic ghost? *Perceptual and Motor Skills, 90*(2), 659–674. doi:10.2466/pms.2000.90.2.659 PMID:10833767

Russell, R. J., Murphy, N., & Isham, C. J. (1993). Quantum cosmology and the laws of nature: scientific perspectives on divine action.

Singer, J. L., & Streiner, B. F. (1966). Imaginative content in the dreams and fantasy play of blind and sighted children. *Perceptual and Motor Skills, 22*(2), 475–482. doi:10.2466/pms.1966.22.2.475

Smith, H. (1964). Have religious import drugs do? *The Journal of Philosophy, 61*(18), 517–530. doi:10.2307/2023494

Sutich, A. J. (1969). Some Considerations Regarding transpersonal psychology. *Journal of Transpersonal Psychology, 1*, 11–20.

Tart, C. T. (1971). Scientific foundations for the study of altered states of consciousness. *Journal of Transpersonal Psychology, 3*, 93–124.

Tart, C. T. (1976). The basic nature of altered states of consciousness: A systems approach. *Journal of Transpersonal Psychology, 8*, 45–64.

Tart, C. T. (1983). *States of consciousness*. El Cerrito, CA: Psychological Processes.

Tart, C. T. (1992). Science, states of consciousness, and spiritual experiences: The need for state-specific sciences. In C. T. Tart (Ed.), *Transpersonal psychologies* (pp. 9–58). New York: Harper.

Tornell H. (2001), the quantum man.

Valverde, R. (2011). *Principles of Human Computer Interaction Design*. Lambert Academic Publishing.

Valverde, R. (2015). Channeling as an Altered State of Consciousness in Transpersonal Psychology Therapy. *Journal of Consciousness Exploration & Research*, *6*(7).

Valverde, R. (2016). Possible Role of Quantum Physics in Transpersonal & Metaphysical Psychology. *Journal of Consciousness Exploration & Research*, *7*(4), 303–309.

Wallace, B., & Fisher, L. E. (1991). Consciousness and behavior (3rd ed.). Boston: Allyn & Bacon.

Walter, W. G. (1964). Slow potential waves in the human brain Associated With expectancy, attention and decision. *European Archives of Psychiatry and Clinical Neuroscience*, *206*(3), 309–322. PMID:14345314

Watson, J. B. (1916). The place of the conditioned reflex in psychology. *Psychological Review*, *23*(2), 89–116. doi:10.1037/h0070003

Wilber, K. (1980). Psychologia Perennis: The Spectrum of Consciousness. Walsh and Vaughan.

Chapter 8
The Development of Ethical Guidelines for Online Counselling and Psychotherapy

Stephen Goss
Metanoia Institute, UK

Kate Elizabeth Anthony
Online Therapy Institute, UK

ABSTRACT

The history and development of guidelines on the ethics of providing online counselling and guidance are considered. Some issues the authors have found to be of particular importance are highlighted with reference to particular publications as exemplars of the ongoing development of ethical practice in this field. Changes in ethical guidelines produced by the British Association for Counselling and Psychotherapy (BACP) are examined to elucidate the evolution in ethical thinking and practice that has been necessitated by the continual rapid development of technological applications relevant to mental health care that have typified the field and led to the current approach which defines competencies required. The article ends with a look to the advent of web 2.0 philosophies and the need for practitioners to remain constantly vigilant with regard to their work.

DOI: 10.4018/978-1-5225-3241-5.ch008

INTRODUCTION

As the field of online therapy has developed rapidly in various parts of the world since the mid 1990s many distinct issues have arisen in practising counselling ethically over the Internet that differ from face to face practice. This article will explore some of the ways in which ethical practice has had to change in response to the emerging use of new technologies in psychotherapy.

This article will trace the development of ethical guidance for online counselling, psychotherapy and guidance. It will examine developments in ethical thinking regarding the use of technology from the initial reluctant scepticism to the now growing acceptance of online practice, based on increasingly supportive evidence and robust rules for those offering guidance, counselling or psychotherapy through technological means. It will consider developments in the requirements for doing so in ways that provide adequate, effective services and sufficiently safe practice to protect clients – and practitioners – from the pitfalls that await the unwary when entering this area of work. Throughout this chapter, the ethical matters and guidelines under consideration are especially applicable to the use of email and Internet relay chat (IRC or 'chat'). However, it should be noted that many of the same issues apply to other technologies such as use of video links, text messaging, stand-alone software or virtual reality environments or even more familiar means of communication such as the telephone.

We trace the development of guidelines for online work from around the English-speaking world with particular reference to major developments in ethical thinking regarding online counselling practice. The development of the guidelines and competencies provided by the British Association for Counselling and Psychotherapy (BACP) are considered in more detail as an exemplar of the ways in which ethical practice, and guides for practitioners, have had to be continually evolved merely to keep up with changes in this fast developing field. While written initially for application in the United Kingdom, all the ethical principles and the practices that are recommended in these guidelines apply anywhere in the world, with appropriate adaptation for differing cultural perspectives.

While we provide examples of ethical thinking and guidance this should not be taken as a replacement for reference to the various guidelines available for practitioners themselves. We end by looking at the future impact of 'Web 2.0' developments for counselling and psychotherapy provision over the Internet and the need to pay attention to the shift in power it implies from the practitioner as 'skilled, knowledgeable expert', who dispenses interventions to their clientele towards a more shared knowledge and power over the direction and mechanisms for change.

REACTIONS TO TECHNOLOGY IN COUNSELLING, PSYCHOTHERAPY, AND GUIDANCE

Placing any form of technology between the practitioner and client appears to be met with strong and yet highly polarised responses. As early as the 1940s, Carl Rogers was writing enthusiastically about the advantages of using tape recordings of counselling sessions to improve client care and enhance practitioner training and supervision (Rogers, 1942). Even before that, using the available communication 'technology' of his time, Sigmund Freud carried out his analysis of 'Little Hans' by letter (cited Rothschild, 1997) and self-analysis through correspondence with Fliess (cited Kaplan, 1997). Computers and other forms of technology such as live video links have been used in several kinds of guidance, counselling and mental health care, including psychiatry, since at least the mid 1960s (e.g. Cogswell, 1967; Cogswell & Estavan, 1965; Weizenbaum, 1966,) with encouraging research emerging then and in the 1970s (e.g. Bennet et al 1978; Del Vecchio et al., 1970; Dwyer, 1973; Solow et al., 1971;) right through to the current century. Despite this extensive history, reactions to the idea do not appear to have changed substantially. It is often still treated as if it were something new, unexpected and perhaps even out of place in a profession that is based entirely on the quality of a human-human relationship.

When first coming across the idea, many practitioners, steeped in their experience of nurturing a human bond across a distance of no more than a few feet in their consulting room, are wary or even hostile to the idea of allowing technology to assist them in extending their ability to reach out, (Reynolds & Morris, 2002). Others have been more willing to embrace the idea, some with an enthusiasm that has led them to leap into action ahead of testing whether what they wanted to do was effective, or even safe, for their clients. That pitfalls exist for the unwary or those who do not undertake appropriate training is undoubtedly the case and not only is specialist training now widely available (see for example, www.onlinetherapyinstitute.com) but there is a rapidly expanding literature on the subject (e.g. Anthony and Nagel, 2010; Anthony, Nagel and Goss, 2010; Goss and Anthony, 2003; Kraus et al., 2004; Anthony and Nagel, 2010; Anthony, Nagel and Goss, 2016).

To cite a basic example of just one of the pitfalls to which many untrained practitioners are prone, communicating with clients without encryption (that is, systems that encode content so that it cannot be read by anyone without the required 'key' to decode it) still sometimes occurs even though it is rather like embarking on a counselling session while sitting in a busy room. Should anyone care to overhear, they can and are likely to be able to eavesdrop without either the practitioner or client being aware of it. For example, Internet Service Providers (ISPs) and many email facilities automatically scan the contents of email exchanges for key words either to target advertising (mention 'holiday' and you may see adverts for holiday companies at the side of your screen with some email systems or on your social media profiles) or for the entirely legitimate purpose of preventing criminal activities, such as the distribution of extreme forms of pornography. Nonetheless, there are still examples of counselling and guidance services using insufficiently encrypted services, placing their clients at risk of unwanted disclosure not only of the nature of their problems but of the entire transcript of their therapy in a form that can then easily be distributed far and wide. Untrained practitioners can thus also create risks for themselves in that they risk exposure as insufficiently competent, at best.

Caution is undoubtedly appropriate in any innovative area of care provision. It is a basic principle of any evidence-based activity that we must progress *with* the evidence base, not ahead of it. Consequently, it is right to await thorough testing and research. However, to reject the use of technology simply because it is unfamiliar would be to deny access to services for clients who cannot, or who prefer not to, access face to face services and there is reason to seek to make progress as rapidly as safety and our expanding knowledge base will allow.

It should not, perhaps, be entirely surprising that reactions to the idea of using technology to reach out to clients should be as polarised as they continue to be, however. Every major new development in communications technology seems to have been met with similarly contradictory responses. The invention of printing was initially seen as a threat by the established church in Europe, who sought to control it as a serious threat (see for example, http://homeenglish.ru/refbooks.htm) but also welcomed as "a divinely inspired invention" helpful as a way of spreading its doctrines (Rosenthal, 1998). The telephone was seen as a technology that would undermine society by removing the need to see a person to speak to them but, contradictorily, also as a means by which it would be possible to extend our ability to communicate across large distances. Official reactions to the Internet now vary widely around the world from fearful censorship to deliberate policies of widening access as rapidly as possible. Technologies must be sufficiently developed, and their use sufficiently sophisticated and thoroughly understood for it to be appropriate for our wariness or enthusiasm to settle into a more everyday attitude and it may be that we simply need to follow this process through to a point where the use of technology in mental health care is no longer remarkable. Douglas Adams noted in 1999 that,

Another problem with the net is that it's still 'technology', and 'technology', as the computer scientist Brian Ferren memorably defined it, as 'stuff that doesn't work yet.' We no longer think of chairs as technology, we just think of them as chairs. (Adams, 1999: 1)

When our understanding of, and familiarity with, the communication possibilities of the Internet and computers is as well developed as it is with regards to what we sit on, perhaps we will be better able to make full, and appropriate, use of them. Knowledge about how to make that use safe and productive would then be so widespread as to need no comment. To arrive at that point, however, requires that we consider carefully what can and cannot be done and, vitally, *how* it should be done to be considered ethical. That guidance is needed in what is still often considered a new field more than 50 years after it began to develop is demonstrated by the wariness among practitioners unfamiliar with the possibilities and confirmed by the existence of poor use of technologies, such as those alluded to above.

The rest of this article considers a selection of the ethical guidelines that have been developed in various parts of the world and offers examples of their development and the increasing breadth of the topics with which they have dealt.

THE DEVELOPMENT OF ETHICAL GUIDELINES FOR COUNSELLING AND PSYCHOTHERAPY

This section can offer only a sampling of the work carried out over the years on the ethics of technologically mediated communication in the provision of counselling and guidance. The authors focus on a few exemplars of work that have marked particular milestones or that serve to underline points that the authors have found to be of particular importance for practitioners. We focus on both trends such as the shift from use of technology being seen as a specialist area to a mainstream one, and particularly the work of the American Psychological Association (APA) and BACP to explore work that has been reflected among other professional bodies as well.

While guidance had been available for some time for practitioners interested in the use of some more established technologies, such as the telephone, as early 1997 the APA had published a statement on the use of technologies that included the Internet. However, at this early stage it was tentative "until such time as a more definitive judgment is available" (APA, 1997, p. 1) and primarily comprised emphasising the applicability of certain sections of their existing code of ethics, such as confidentiality, fee structures, the use of research or the standard '1.04c' regarding boundaries of competence:

In those emerging areas in which generally recognized standards for preparatory training do not yet exist, psychologists nevertheless take reasonable steps to ensure the competence of their work and to protect patients, clients, students, research participants, and others from harm. (APA, 1997: 1)

Specialist 'preparatory training' did emerge soon afterwards (cf. Steele, 2002 for an account of two of the earliest examples) rendering even this cautious statement already out of date. The rapidity with which any but the most general ethical guidance for online counselling and guidance practitioners becomes outdated is a notable feature in this field, reflecting the pace of developments in technologically mediated communication. However, it is worthy of note that this early statement already implied that specialist training might be important for those wanting to practice online, now increasingly accepted as a basic element for ethical practice of counselling and guidance online (e.g. Anthony and Goss, 2009; Nagel and Anthony, 2009). Subsequent to these Guidelines from BACP were the introduction of "competences required to deliver psychological therapies 'at a distance" (Hill & Roth, (2014), created by a large group of specialist experts in the field, including the co-author of this article.

In 2002, the APA incorporated reference to the Internet and electronic communication of any kind into their main statement of ethical principles, becoming effective in 2003 (APA, 2002). While this move gave *de facto* recognition to the use of technologically delivered services, and emphasised that general ethical considerations apply to this specialist field, it fell well short of providing detailed insight into how practitioners should handle the particular concerns that arise, for example regarding the greater complexity of ensuring adequate confidentiality for the online practitioner. Indeed, in many ways it progressed only a little way beyond the opinion of the American Psychiatric Association expressed in 1996 that the detail of such questions remained largely unanswered, although it did alter the opinion expressed at that point of a preference for 'traditional' face to face contact (American Psychiatric Association, 1996).

In 1999, the American National Association of Social Workers (NASW) had already inserted reference to use of electronic communication, computers and other technologies into their main ethical guidelines, as did the American Association of Marriage and Family Therapists two years later (AAMFT, 2001) along with other organisations in the field. Such moves have become increasingly common in the following decade, emphasising the steady progress online provision has made from the fringes of the counselling and guidance world to its mainstream. The APA took this approach in its revised main ethical code in 2002 (APA, 2002), which is explicitly applicable to electronic communications and contains a small number of statements directly relating to technologically delivered interventions such as "psychologists who offer services, products, or information via electronic transmission inform clients/patients of the risks to privacy and limits of confidentiality" (APA, 2002). The main ethical framework produced by the British Association for Counselling and Psychotherapy (BACP) explicitly recognised the trend, for example (BACP, 2010), a move which has been seen in the UK as confirming that technologically delivered therapies had become, by 2010, firmly part of mainstream practice. Those who offer such services are, by the time of writing, clearly no longer thought to be outside the norm but more and more to be doing something that is part of the everyday experience of the millions who live at least part of their lives online. Nonetheless, despite the value of overarching statements that general ethical rules apply when working online, none give sufficiently detailed guidance on the use of technologies to give much help to practitioners wanting to avoid the pitfalls. Specialist guidelines to address the ethical concerns of counsellors remain vital.

The last year of the 20th Century also saw activity focussed on online work with the publication of two more focussed attempts to provide more detailed guidance. Ethicscode.com, led by Ron Kraus, published guidance aimed specifically at "professionals who provide clinical services online" (Ethicscode, 1999, p. 1). Comprising 10 relatively brief points, this 'code' covers items such as 'mastery of the modality', supervision, emergency contact and professional standards. However, much of this publication is brief and offers little in the way of concrete guidance on how to proceed, with statements being restricted to, for example, under the heading of privacy, "Online clinicians provide care only through "secure" web sites, using current protective procedures" (Ethicscode, 1999, p. 1) without an indication of what level of protection such 'procedures' should attain to be considered sufficient.

Another American organisation, the National Board for Certified Counselors (NBCC), created a slightly more extensive document entitled 'Standards for the Ethical Practice of Web Counseling' (NBCC, 1999). This document defines face-to-face and online counselling and offers 14 points to which practitioners should adhere, covering the therapeutic relationship, confidentiality, licensure and legal considerations. These standards stress, among other items, the need to identify the client, and for clients to be able to verify the practitioner's credentials, the need for offline emergency support provision in the client's locality, identified in collaboration with the client, technological failure and access.

Encryption is recommended in the NBCC document, but is explicitly not mandatory stating only that it should be used 'whenever possible' (NBCC, 1999, p. 5), which is at sharp variance with more recent work and current opinion and best practice in the field. Interestingly, the document recognises the pace of change in technologically delivered interventions, noting that 'cases should be reviewed in light of delivery systems existing at the moment rather than at the time the standards were adopted' (NBCC, 1999: 4).

In January 2000, the International Society for Mental Health Online (ISMHO) published its 'suggested principles' for counselling online (ISMHO, 2000). These cover informed consent – especially regarding what can and cannot be achieved - but also including response times, standard operating procedures and emergencies. Many would perhaps now consider the stated principles as being useful but limited in their scope and level of detail. Under the heading of standard operating procedures, the principles include notes on the importance of appropriate boundary keeping but these state only that counsellors should not attempt to address issues for which they would consider themselves competent when working face to face, rather than the special competence boundaries for working online. The principles imply that they should be treated as subordinate to the ethical requirements of their main professional association but give no indication of areas where they might be expected to mesh with those. Helpfully, the principles do point out the need for those working online to ensure that access to local services to back up the online work should be arranged in case the client reaches a crisis stage requiring a more immediate response than that offered by their routine contact with their counsellor.

In 2001, BACP published the first edition of their guidelines for online counselling and psychotherapy, which are discussed in more detail below. At the time of their publication, these set out to be the most comprehensive guidelines in existence and have remained among the most detailed on offer. Their contents have been reflected in guidance produced elsewhere in the world, suggestive of a degree of universality in the application of ethics helpful in an environment that inherently erodes national governmental or regulatory boundaries to accessing services. While most guidelines will need some adaptation to allow for differing cultural contexts, it has been our experience that the ethical principles and much of their content can remain unchanged. Practice across international boundaries is more a challenge for those who must enforce practice standards than it is one for ethicists or the ethical practitioner *per se*. Works on the topic on online counselling and guidance appear readily applicable in more than just the country for which they were initially intended (e.g. Goss and Anthony, 2008)

The American Counseling Association (ACA) incorporated a section devoted to the application of technology in their 2005 revision of their main ethical code, updating a 1999 statement on web counselling. A-typically for such guidelines, these are intended to apply to all forms of technology in any kind of counselling intervention, whether it be telephones, computers or any other technology. The guidance includes requirements for practitioners to ensure that clients are able to make good use of the technology concerned, to consider providing the same service face to face in some circumstances and considers matters related to informed consent, such as the duration of data storage, the need to pay attention to the niceties of inter-state provision, technological breakdown and emergency procedures. It also refers to web sites held by counsellors, regardless of whether they offer services online or not.

The increasing spread of the acceptance of technologically mediated counselling and guidance is further evidenced by the numbers of ethical codes that include their use around the world. The New Zealand Association of Counsellors (NZAC), for example, addresses their use (see http://www.nzac.org.nz/ethics/13.html). Of particular value is the ethical framework produced by the Online Therapy Institute (Nagel and Anthony, 2009). These detailed and highly specific guidelines comprise a series of statements to which an ethical practitioner should adhere. This framework is especially useful because of its applicability to *any* form of technologically mediated mental health intervention. They can be reviewed at http://www.onlinetherapyinstitute.com/id43.html.

Other Publications of Relevance

A number of other publications of some relevance to the provision of online counselling and guidance are available. Of particular note is that provided by the non-governmental Health on the Net Foundation, known as the 'HONcode', possibly the most widely accepted reference for online health and medical publishers, who provide certification of trustworthy health related websites to address the serious problem of misinformation being available on the Internet. Based on their own guidelines, the 'HONcode' is not only a route to identifying which sites should be trusted, but also offers practitioners a form of validation based on basic principles such as clear identification of the authors and their credentials, differentiation of advertising and editorial content and other matters (Health on the Net, 2008). More recently, and more appropriate for online guidance and counselling, the Online Therapy Institute introduced its own specialist validation scheme to approve services that meet the standards laid out in their framework. Such marks of approval can be invaluable in assisting clients in identifying practitioners who meet minimum standards and are likely to become essential for services wishing to demonstrate their adherence to adequate ethical safeguards in coming years.

There is now a burgeoning literature on technologically delivered mental health care. Readers are advised to obtain not only a good grounding in the range of technologies available, which is far wider than many imagine. The breadth of options now available runs from email and Internet chat through virtual reality and Computerised Cognitive Behavioural Therapy (CCBT) to the use of film and television, all of which are covered in *The Use of Technology in Mental Health Care: Applications, Ethics and Practice* with the important inclusion not only of explicitly discussion of the ethical implications of each technology but examples of their use in practice, providing a vivid link to actual work grounded in real experience (Anthony, Nagel and Goss, 2010; 2016). Shorter guides are also increasingly available from professional associations and individual authors around the world, some intended for specific audiences. An example is *Launching Into Cyberspace*, produced in 2005 by the MindMatters Plus project and published more recently by the Australian Guidance and Counselling Association (Campbell and Glasheen, 2007), supplemented with video material. This brief introductory text notes several essential items designed primarily for use in school guidance services but with wider applicability as well. Readers should take note of the general caution that no single text – even those far more extensive that this example - can stand as a replacement for the specialist training required before delivering technologically mediated services.

Readers in the United States should be familiar with the implications of the Health Insurance Portability and Accountability Act (HIPAA), which lays down responsibilities for protecting and sharing sensitive information about clients. Most countries have some kind of legislation governing such matters. In the UK, for example, applicable law includes the UK Data Protection Act– see http://www.ico.gov.uk - the Consumer Protection (distance selling) Regulations, 2000 and the Electronic Communications Act, 2000. All practitioners offering services online need to be aware of their implications in their own locale.

The Development of Guidelines for the British Association for Counselling and Psychotherapy: A Case Study in the Development of Ethical Practice

First Studies, Research, and Reports

The British Association for Counselling and Psychotherapy (BACP) was one of the earlier professional bodies to recognise the issue of technologically delivered services and to attempt to offer detailed guidance for practitioners. The development of policy and practice in BACP is used here as an exemplar of what can be achieved and some of the stumbling blocks that can be encountered.

The first publication giving the point of view of the organisation appeared in 1999 following the creation of a special working group by one of its Divisions, the Association for University and College Counsellors (AUCC), in 1997 (Lago et al., 1999). Called *Counselling Online*, comprising 43 pages and 9 chapters, this special report was intended primarily for purchasers and providers of counselling services and was produced precisely because of the recognition that online counselling was beginning to happen anyway and the profession was already in a position of having to respond.

The report considered two questions to be paramount: was online counselling effective and was it safe for clients? The report noted reasons for optimism, such as the long history of counselling and guidance offered via correspondence and what was then growing but still primarily anecdotal evidence. It was noted that the involvement of a practitioner was itself not necessarily a requirement, given that anxiety reduction had been demonstrated from creating soliloquies with a computer

(Slack et al., 1990) while psychiatric patients had been shown to prefer computerised interviews to live therapists, disclosing more to the machines than to their human interviewers (Greist et al., 1973). Process and outcome research available at the time also seemed to indicate equivalence of technologically mediated and face-to-face interventions, including in reductions in anxiety and the degree of self-revelation achieved (Slack and Slack, 1977; Cohen, 1998).

However, difficulties were also foreseen. Even this early report noted that 'therapists may need to acquire a different and broader range of literary skills to compensate' (Lago et al., 1999: 18) for the lack of face-to-face presence but noted only that 'what these skills might consists of remains to be clarified' (Ibid.). The report noted later that

...even if a counsellor is adequately qualified and experienced in face-to-face work, their competency in an e-mail environment may be untested and/or lacking. Not all therapists may have the aptitude for e-mail counselling, and many believe that they do not have this ability...this new and emergent mode of therapy lacks an experienced cohort of practitioners to give training and supervision (Lago et al., 1999, p. 25).

At that point, these statements were correct and the emergence of specialist training in the following years addressed this fundamental issue.

In addressing its two key questions, the report was careful to strike an at least moderately cautious note. It cited much encouraging anecdotal evidence and reports from service providers and, perhaps most notably, clients. Overall, however, it suggested that on the one hand 'substantial and complex relationships can be established, developed and maintained remotely' (Sanders, 1998 cited in Lago et al., 1999: 21) while, on the other hand, noting the opinion of other authors that 'the creation of the relationship that is necessary in client-centred counselling could not be facilitated in its wholeness through computer communication' (Robson and Robson, 1998: 40). The report also noted that safety concerns had not been properly explored (Lago et al., 1999, p. 24). Closer examination, however, reveals that some of the safety concerns revolved around the provision of forms of service so highly limited that they would almost certainly not be considered to constitute counselling or therapy at all, such as the fear that interaction might be reduced to a single question and answer exchange without assessment or knowledge of the client's wider medical history. Such concerns led directly to their being addressed in the BACP ethical guidelines that were to follow. The issues around adequate training and supervision already noted were more serious and, with the absence of definitive comparative outcomes research, largely accounted for the tentative stance taken at this early stage.

The relatively high demands placed on therapists in terms of the care taken to ensure that proper assessment procedures were in place, boundaries and contracting issues were addressed and their own preparation for the work was sufficient were stressed. It was noted, via the experience of the UK Samaritans (perhaps the best known support service in Europe for those at risk of suicide) that working through email had different requirements. In particular, it was emphasised that 'training is essential in the use of language in showing empathy and in exploring feelings. Since people will often feel safe enough to express strong feelings via e-mail, those running such a service need to be prepared for the level of despair that may emerge' (Lago et al., 1999, p. 38).

Quality controls – such as how a client could be sure of the identity and qualifications of any given practitioner – were also raised. The report noted that 'much discussion is undertaken …of the inappropriateness of existing legal and ethical provisions for online therapy' (Lago et al., 1999, p. 26).

Recognising the Need for Guidance

The absence of adequate legal and ethical guidance was, perhaps, the main message of the working party in this case. It was clear that additional guidance was required, not least because those practitioners who were inclined towards incorporating technology into their practice were already taking clients and, furthermore, it was the experience of the working group that clients could not be prevented from making use of the means of communication most comfortable for them – including email. People were doing it and were clearly going to run into difficulties before very long. These concerns and the additional pitfalls, such as the difficulties of legal jurisdiction across national boundaries that the report also highlighted without being able to offer any clear resolutions, served to confirm the already growing view that specialist guidance was indeed required.

Issues that needed to be addressed, many of which are still pertinent today, included the question of their scope. Should they aim to be applicable nationally or internationally, given that Internet based services have a potential global reach? Should we seek to create an internationally acceptable and applicable code? It is the position of the authors that this would indeed be desirable, requiring the co-operation of numerous professional associations in different parts of the world to apply them to their own memberships. Gaining such international co-operation in practice appears to be the major stumbling block along with another issue of concern at the firsts writing of the guidelines, that of differing national legal status of online counselling activities. Some countries have little or no legal regulation of either counselling or psychotherapy while others offer a quite different environment for practitioners. Austria, for example, does not sanction online counselling or psychotherapy while some American States, such as California, definitely prohibit the provision of psychological care across the State boundary. Any practitioner should be aware of these restrictions before accepting clients from outside their own region or professional jurisdiction.

Questions relating to international law also still include which country's legal system would be deemed to control the contract for services between the practitioner and client and thus any liability should things go wrong. Even within the UK, for example, contract law differs for example between Scotland and England, let alone when contracting with clients further afield. Professional bodies, practitioners and clients also need to be concerned about who has jurisdiction, for example in the case of a complaint against a practitioner – could a client in, say, Malawi or Botswana, raise a complaint against a practitioner based in, say New Jersey, Australia or the UK? The position developed in response to this question by the BACP was that any client of a member could indeed raise a complaint against that member regardless of the location of either, thus claiming a world wide jurisdiction limited by membership rather than geography. Not all associations have developed such a position, however.

The extended geographical reach of services also sharpens issues related to cultural sensitivity and awareness. The very meaning of key terms, such as 'counselling', can differ widely in different parts of the world and clients may have very different expectations to those of practitioners steeped in their own culture, training and professional milieu. A useful position was suggested in the original *Counselling Online* document (Lago et al., 1999, p. 20), which emphasised that all relationships are, in any case, 'partial' and incomplete with the development of mutual understanding being a key task of any practitioner with every client. Even if working face to face with a client from the next town, their familial and cultural experiences will be different than those of the practitioner who must use their clinical skills to be able to enter into their client's frame of reference. Thus, the extended cross-cultural possibilities of online work 'merely heighten the problems involved in trying to develop helpful relationships with any other person' (Ibid.). Checking out the expectations of clients, and thus carrying out thorough assessment, became a key component of online work as reflected in the BACP guidelines, significantly adding to the need for clarity in contracting prior to commencing therapy.

It was also a concern that guidance should be applicable to different levels of support with as little translation or adaptation as possible. Those working under the title of 'befriender', 'social worker', 'crisis support worker', 'counsellor', 'psychotherapist' or even 'psychiatrist' – indeed 'e-mental-health' in general –

should, insofar as possible, be able to make use of guidelines that were consistent in laying down what should and should not be done in order for their work to be considered ethical. Thus, while the guidelines were written with counsellors from the UK as their primary audience, the authors were aware from the outset that they would have far wider applicability.

It was also a requirement that the guidelines be applicable to different theoretical orientations. Psychodynamic counsellors often perceive themselves to work in ways different than those from, say a cognitive behavioural therapy or person-centred tradition. The *Counselling Online* document had noted particular questions for person-centred counsellors and questioned whether it would be possible to achieve the first and sixth of Carl Rogers' 'necessary and sufficient conditions' for effective therapy, that 'two persons are in psychological contact' and 'the communication to the client of the therapist's empathic understanding and unconditional positive regard is to a minimal degree achieved' respectively (Rogers, 1957, pp. 95 – 103). That strong, empathetic and highly emotional bonds can be achieved is now confirmed by the literature on online counselling but the essential point for the guidelines was to consider how all the elements considered necessary by each of the major theoretical orientations could be covered. Thus, it was absolutely necessary to adopt a 'pluralist' approach to the work (Goss and Mearns, 1997; Goss, 2000) and to consider all the different pitfalls that might arise from the different orientations.

The authors also considered the question of to which technologies, platforms and means of communication the guidelines should be applicable. While it was tempting to make them as broad as the range of technologies available, even as the first edition of the ethical guidance was being written in 2000, the difference in requirements for the ethical use of, say, CCBT, as compared to, say, email and Internet chat, were so great that it was decided to focus on the latter. However, it was recognised even at this early stage that many of the issues were likely to transfer to other technologies. Later guidance, notably that produced by the Online Therapy Institute, has been framed in terms that are far more widely applicable.

The First Edition

The first edition of the guidelines was written in the absence of definitive research findings regarding email and Internet chat therapy. The authors were also aware that as they were written, the situation was already changing. The first edition appeared in 2001, written by a team of 4 authors (Goss et al., 2001) including experts in ethics as well as specialists in online counselling. It was necessary also to include a much wider team of experts in international ethics of health care and the early drafts were circulated widely to obtain the maximal range of feedback and input possible.

Subsidiarity to Over Arching Ethical Codes and Principles

It was clear from the outset that any guidance for online work was to be considered as subsidiary to the primary ethical codes under which the practitioner worked. Thus, importantly, general principles of non-maleficence (doing no harm), beneficence (seeking to help), trustworthiness, justice and seeking to promote the autonomy of clients, and the practical expression of these values, still applied to all online work. Personal moral qualities required of practitioners also applied in just the same way, such as the ability to empathise, sincerity, integrity and maintaining a level of personal resilience sufficient to carry out the work in a competent manner. Overarching ethical requirements also include awareness of the limitations of competence and training and a commitment to ensuring adequate standards of care, such that clients' needs are met by practitioners who are themselves accountable for the quality of the care they provide. It was notable, however, that these general ethical requirements were frequently phrased in terms that required greater specificity when applied to work online, such as those regarding protecting confidentiality and privacy or regarding training and technical, let alone technological, competence. The more precise statements in the guidelines for online provision were, however, explicitly noted to be supplementary to the more general statements.

Exemplar Features of the First Edition

The first edition of the guidelines was cautiously framed. In the absence of definitive research on the comparable outcomes achieved through email or Internet chat, it was not possible at that stage to state whether the necessary conditions for effective therapy could be created online, despite the existence of anecdotal and supportive research evidence available at the time. Furthermore, it was unclear as to whether online work was best seen as an adjunct to face-to-face methods, as some authors had recommended (e.g. Childress, 1999). Thus, this edition recommended that 'practitioners should consider carefully whether to engage in therapeutic relationships exclusively online or whether their work requires a number of face to face sessions at the outset and at regular intervals thereafter' (Goss et al., 2001, p. 2). It is notable that in the intervening years, evidence to support the equivalence of online therapy has become increasingly available (e.g. Barak, 2008; Hanley, 2010) and the cautiousness of the approach taken in the first edition has been steadily reduced in the light of emerging evidence.

The first edition guidelines also noted that 'competence as a therapist in one medium does not necessarily translate into another medium ... Very few practitioners will be able to engage in online therapy without additional skills, training and experience' (Goss et al., 2001, p. 2) implying that specialist training was necessary. It was also noted that 'practitioners should consider both the limitations and complexities of offering their services online ... [and] should also consider the shift skills and practices required for online work and the effect on the likely experience and outcomes for clients in relation to both their theoretical orientation and personal skills' (Ibid.). With little such training available at this time, however, stronger wording could not achieve consensus, especially given that most practitioners at this time were entering into online work in an exploratory fashion. It is notable that each subsequent edition of the guidelines have strengthened their wording regarding training requirements and that it is the view of the authors that this trend is likely to continue with specialist training probably becoming absolutely required.

The specialist content of training was also briefly indicated, including items such as consideration of the shift from verbal to written communication skills, the importance, and difficulties of building and maintaining adequate therapeutic relationships online, the importance of greater clarification to reduce the risks of misunderstandings, online assessment issues, appropriate administrative procedures (such as legal obligations, data storage, etc.) and adequate knowledge of technical questions relating to security, privacy and so on.

The guidelines also stressed that 'online provision is a specialist area, requiring a level of competence at *least* as high as that for face-to-face work ... Online therapy is NOT appropriate for novice or inexperienced practitioners' (Goss et al., 2001, p. 2, emphasis in the original). It had been the experience of the authors that some novice practitioners saw online work as a way of 'easing themselves in' to the profession, seeing the distance between them and their clients as a kind of emotional safety barrier for themselves. While clients frequently report greater emotional safety thanks to the presences of a computer between themselves and the practitioner, it is a myth to think that adequate safety can be provided by any practitioner who seeks emotional safety in this way.

It was also stressed that clients should be able to verify the identity and credentials of their practitioner and also that how to do so should be made clear in pre-contracting information.

The guidelines also attempted to consider for whom online counselling might be considered appropriate. At that time, little research gave strong indications regarding the suitability of particular client groups and there was a noted lack of consensus. For example, young people were thought by some to be inappropriate for distance provision due to issues of informed consent; others saw young people as especially appropriate on the grounds that they were likely to be more comfortable with Internet communication than their elders. Clients in crisis, such as those who were suicidal, were similarly seen as inappropriate for online work given the possible need for local emergency intervention and yet seen as particularly appropriate by others who saw the Internet as a means of reaching clients who would not otherwise access services at all. The latter position was explicitly that of the Samaritans in the UK who already ran one of the most extensive email services available at the time. This edition of the guidelines was, again, cautious but stressed that it was

… especially important that therapists have in place robust procedures, such as pre-therapy assessment, to identify clients who are unlikely to benefit from their online services, who may at additional risk or with whom they are not competent to work online. (Goss et al., 2001, p. 3)

Brief case studies were provided in appendices to explore and exemplify some of the issues that online work could provide, the development of which are discussed later in the chapter.

Cultural issues were also addressed, as noted above. It was noted that 'competence to practice in one cultural environment does not necessarily imply competence to work in another' (Goss et al., 2001, p. 3) regardless of whether cultural differences arose as a result of working internationally or not. The guidelines noted, however, some positive advantages from online work in reducing the impact of gender, race or disability and the possibility of reducing inequalities on these grounds. It also noted, however, that 'paradoxically online therapy may deny others groups access. For example, it may not be accessible to some people with learning disabilities or those who are unable to read' (Goss et al., 2001, p. 3).

Issues related to age and informed consent were also addressed, emphasising that the definition of a 'minor' who was deemed unable to give informed consent to treatment vary widely around the world.

The increased need for clarity in the contracting process between practitioner and client was already apparent during the drafting of the first edition of the guidelines. It was stressed that 'all information, especially pre-therapy information and contractual issues, should be communicated directly to prospective clients in the body of a message … Practitioners should not assume that their clients will have read information on their website in detail' (Goss et al., 2001, p. 4). Very few people actually read the 'terms and conditions' sections of websites to which they subscribe so this safeguard to ensure that clients were aware of contractual and boundary issues was already seen as absolutely required. Included in the contractual information were issues of time boundaries – how long a client could expect a practitioner to spend reading and responding to an email, for example – response times (how long it would take for messages to be responded to), fees, applicable law and terms of contract to be taken to govern the work, applicable professional bodies, regulatory issues and complaints procedures, the procedures, processes or techniques that the practitioner would offer along with their limitations, contra-indications, likely outcomes and limitations, and responsibility for accuracy, such as ensuring that outgoing emails were correctly addressed. Other contractual issues included the use of attached files, virus checking, how to proceed in the event of technical failure, the extent of confidentiality that could be offered and its limitations and emergency procedures should the client require immediate intervention. Even this fairly long list was not intended to be exhaustive and it was noted that it was especially important in online work for practitioners to ensure adequate arrangements for care of their clients should they die or fall ill to save their clients being left without an indication of the reason for sudden non-response from a person on whom they are likely to have come to rely, at least to a degree, and to ensure adequate onward referral.

The question of complaints and jurisdiction of professional codes and laws received special attention in this first version of the guidelines, as they have in all subsequent editions. The first principle was clearly that any practitioner should conform to '*at least* the standards of practice required by their own professional organisation' (Goss et al., 2001, p. 5, emphasis in the original). However, the authors were aware that practice across international boundaries could readily create conflicts between different legal and professional requirements in different parts of the world. Following extensive consultation it was decided to develop an entirely new position for what was hitherto an association that worked purely within its national boundaries:

...where differences in professional standards exist (e.g. required qualifications, requirements for accreditation/licensure, and models of best practice) practitioners should generally assume that both sets of standards will apply (Goss et al., 2001, p. 5)

This position has held through later editions of the guidelines and implies that any practitioner will uphold whichever is the higher standard. The position taken here suggests that any practitioner should familiarise themselves with the rules and regulations governing their activities in the region to which a prospective client belongs *before* accepting them. Caution again ruled in this draft of the guidelines, which noted that 'therapists ... may prefer to restrict their practice to work clients subject to legal systems [and by implication professional regulations] with which they (or their advisors) are familiar' (Goss et al., 2001: 6). This position has disappointed some practitioners who saw their practice as being able to leap instantly to a global level by transferring to online work. In practice, doing so is far more complicated unless one is to risk falling foul of regulations in countries about which one is insufficiently educated. The guidelines recommended that because 'this is an evolving area of law ... proper advice should be obtained to ensure that online services conform to current legal and professional requirements' (Goss et al., 2001, p. 6).

Onward referral, for example for clients deemed unsuitable for online work with that practitioner or who required emergency interventions, were also seen as having the potential to restrict the ethical provision of care across regional or national boundaries. 'Referral practices may vary widely between countries, and practitioners should bear in mind that making referrals across international boundaries may be difficult ... [to the extent that such difficulties might] preclude working with some clients' in other parts of the world (Goss et al., 2001, p. 6). However, where local referral information (such as the contact details of the client's doctor, physician or psychiatric services) could be obtained from the client, this was not seen as an insurmountable barrier.

On technological competence, the first edition of the guidelines noted that practitioners should ensure that a secondary means of contact (such as a telephone number) was available for use in case of technological breakdown in addition to taking all reasonable steps to minimise the risk of such things occurring. It was also noted that practitioners should ensure that their systems and hardware were as up to date as possible, that they ran with optimal stability, were compatible with those of their intended clients, and that they took steps to prevent transmission of viruses or other malware.

Confidentiality and data storage were also addressed. Interestingly, at the time of their preparation, these guidelines were not able to be worded as strongly as subsequent editions noting that 'it is strongly recommended that message are encoded to restrict access to them' (Goss et al., 2001: 7) whereas later editions have noted encryption as an absolute requirement, thanks not least to the ready availability of free software that makes it widely available through services such as Hushmail and the dedicated online therapy platform PlusGuidance. The guidelines also noted the still existing problem of third party access to messages. Internet Service Providers, for example, may routinely monitor the content of email messages as has already been noted above. Large institutions may also give access to emails for their technical staff as a matter of routine, rendering such systems inadequate for the purposes of any confidential transmission of sensitive information. Furthermore, most breaches of security are low-tech ones such as leaving an email message on a screen or due to the use of computers in environments that do not offer sufficient privacy, such as an Internet café or public library. Practitioners were required to inform their clients of these kinds of issues. Subsequent editions strengthened this position to make it the practitioner's responsibility to ensure that their clients become adequately educated about the risks to security (including the fact that deleted messages may remain recoverable) and strategies for 'covering their tracks' should it be required.

Practitioners were also urged to ensure that their professional insurance cover extended to online work. As the first guidelines were being prepared this was a new issue for most insurers and few had definitive answers to the question. This is a situation that has changed in subsequent years but it is worth noting that not all professional insurance covers work via the Internet and it is still the case that practitioners should take care to ensure that they are adequately covered, not least because the level of liability can be considerably higher in some countries, such as the United States.

The concluding section of the guidelines reflected the level of caution about online work that prevailed at the time. While it noted that counselling and psychotherapy over the Internet might have 'significant potential for extending, perhaps even enhancing, conventional means of service delivery' it also noted that 'there are many areas of uncertainty and there also exists the potential for harm both to clients and to practitioners' (Goss et al., 2001, p. 8).

The Second Edition

It has been the experience of BACP and the authors of this chapter that new editions of ethical guidelines are required approximately every 4 or 5 years, at least. Indeed, it has often seemed that the need to adapt them in the light of emerging new technologies or new uses of existing ones arises before each edition appears in print. This may give reason to doubt the applicability, and in some cases even the validity, of guidance that remains unchanged for a longer period. In the case of the BACP guidelines, work on new editions has been unceasing with notes and contributions being collected from the time of the creation of the first AUCC working party that led to the 1999 *Counselling Online* report (Lago et al., 1999) onwards.

The essential changes to the guidelines for their second edition in 2005 (Anthony and Jamieson, 2005) comprised a restructuring of the document to improve clarity; a positive shift in attitude towards therapeutic work being conducted online; more accessible appendices in light of Internet access to resources; and a significant extension by the addition of guidelines for online supervision.

The restructuring of the document meant that the paragraphs within the original document that had been superseded by technological or legal developments and so needed to be spelled out in less detail could be consumed within other sections. Conversely, those sections that had been alluded to but not fully explicated in light of lack of empirical evidence could be expanded to their own sections to give more concrete guidance. Thus, clinical issues regarding client safety in crisis was given its own section, whereas practical considerations such as rules governing intellectual property rights were condensed. Ease of reference was therefore much improved, specifically in relation to the guidelines being used as part of professional conduct or complaints procedures. This was particularly relevant at the time as a complaint had already gone through BACP previously in relation to practitioners' use of unencrypted and unsecure forums for peer supervision, and so the 2nd edition was extended to mention forums as part of "text-based communication" alongside email and IRC.

In light of the growth of empirical evidence since the first publication, the 2nd edition also allowed for a more positive, although still rightly cautious, attitude to working online. For example, where the first edition stated that it was 'not possible to assert that written communication over the Internet should, or should not, be considered as an adequate replacement for, or equivalent to, face-to-face provision', the second edition stated that it was 'unwise to definitively claim' that position. The statement that BACP was optimistic about the role of technology was explicitly included. However, much more definitive statements about the complexity of online work were also added, and appropriate caution with proceeding remained the theme. This caution was evident by stronger, more definitive statements regarding items such as the use of tools such as encryption and password protection being essential rather than merely recommended.

Case studies in the second edition remained the same brief indicative outlines as in the first due to budget restrictions, which made them technologically insufficient in light of developments with encryption and other suitable software applications, although robust as realistic scenarios to give stimulus for consideration and debate. However, the authors made a decision that – apart from textbooks that were by then available – all appendices would be accessible via the Internet rather than only as printed resources, which would become quickly out-of-date and difficult to access.

The addition of the guidelines for online supervision in 2005 within the profession was a major milestone, as they remain the only such specific ones worldwide. So as not to simply replicate the main guidelines (and there were many overlaps), they concentrated on four major themes: authentication of the other party; legal and professional regulatory constraints; contracting protocol (in particular); security and confidentiality (also at length); and a statement on the importance of research and development in such a new and evolving domain.

The Third Edition

The third edition of the BACP guidelines in 2009 (Anthony and Goss, 2009) reviewed current guidance of all kinds throughout the field, worldwide. Five sources were particularly highlighted either due to their content or the influence they or the organisation behind them has had in the field. These were previous editions of the BACP guidelines, the ethical notes produced by the American Counseling Association, the 13 item code produced by the National Board for Certified Counselors in the USA, the EthicsCode, noted above, and the far more detailed ethical guidance that had more recently become available from the Online Therapy Institute (OTI). It is the view of the current authors that the guidance produced by BACP and OTI are by far the most comprehensive and practically applicable of the guidance available at the time of writing (April, 2010).

There were two major additions to the third edition. The first was a specific section on maintaining a responsible online presence in light of social and professional networking over the Internet – the first such guidelines worldwide. The rise of social networking has already raised increasingly complex boundary issues for practitioners. For example, a practitioner who maintains an online presence through a service such as Facebook will need to be aware not only that their colleagues may be able to see information and photographs of them posted by family and friends – possibly from many years previously and possibly not showing them in the most professional of circumstances – but that clients and potential clients may also make seeking out their profiles and consequently will need to take steps to protect their privacy and professional image.

The second was the rewrite of the case studies into that of a single full-length scenario with one client - that of 'Johanna'. The authors set out to include as many "perils" of online work as possible, including technological breakdown; the client blogging her opinion of the therapy; keystroke recording by employers; and the use of mobile SMS, chat and encrypted email.

The Transition to Competencies

Although plans for a fourth edition of the Guidelines were planned, it was decided that a new approach (not least away from paper publication) was needed to fit with overall future planning of Guidance by the organisation towards developing competencies for different areas of the profession. Therefore, an expert group of BACP staff and members was put together to create a set of competencies for the budding distance counsellor. The uptake and application of these competencies by practitioners is unknown, but they should have a firm place on the timeline of ethical developments in the field (and within training and CPD courses).

Extending Ethical Guidance to Other Kinds of Intervention

The Online Therapy Institute's Ethical Framework (Nagel & Anthony, 2009; Anthony & Nagel, 2010) offers the basics of the originally developed codes and guidelines of BACP, ACA, NBCC, ISMHO and EthicsCode, incorporating additions that appear in the revised ACA Code of Ethics and the 2nd and 3rd editions of the BACP guidelines. What is interesting about the framework is its ability to be applicable to other areas of mental health, such as career and school guidance (Schmelter-Davis, Anthony & Nagel, 2009a; 2009b). With minimal adaptation, they are designed to be extended to other kinds of intervention within the mental health arena. The authors welcome collaboration with other bodies around the world to continue their development and to consider new areas – geographical or professional – to which they might be applied.

CONCLUSION: WEB 2.0 AND THE NEW BALANCE OF POWER

The term 'web 2.0' is used to refer to what has been called the second incarnation of the World Wide Web. It is particularly used to indicate the shift away from static web pages towards interactive sites and applications that facilitate reactive information sharing, collaborative social and professional networking based on communities comprising groups of people with a common interest. It does not so much denote a new form of technology as a change in the uses to which the Internet can be put. Communities from Facebook and Twitter to Linkedln are examples of Web 2.0 in action.

By promoting connections between people, the advent of Web 2.0 thinking has the potential to create a further egalitarian shift in power from experts dispensing their knowledge and skills towards a more balanced sharing of information. It will be increasingly the case that clients approach services with as much information on their issues as that held by the professional to whom they turn for help. In some cases, help seeking has been shown to develop quite naturally into help providing within Internet communities (e.g. Greidanus and Everall, 2010).

Rather than practitioners retaining their expert 'intellectual capital', Web 2.0 is characterised by the pooling of that capital to create situations in which those seeking help can readily equip themselves with knowledge and can choose to contact a vast range of professional and non-professional or peer resources for help, advice and guidance. This probably irreversible trend means that clients of services have more control over the kinds of interventions they receive and how those services are delivered.

Practitioners in any form of human helping, perhaps especially counselling and guidance, must respond positively to this new situation and be willing to share at least part of what was previously a privileged position with their clientele or face being increasingly confronted with clients who are as well informed on their own conditions as the professionals from whom they seek help. The role of the professional itself thus needs to evolve to one of facilitating growth rather than defining and delivering interventions *per se*.

Just as social networking contains the possibility for creating new mutually assistive communities, practitioners also have a great deal to gain from the pooling of knowledge and access to expertise professional networks allow. With continuing development of the evidence base for online counselling and guidance and continued developments in the ways we live with technology we must look forward to further editions not only of the BACP guidelines but possibly also to their extension to a more international acceptance befitting the worldwide nature of the Internet.

REFERENCES

AAMFT. (2001). *AAMFT Code of Ethics*. Retrieved from http://www.aamft.org/resources/lrm_plan/Ethics/ethicscode2001.asp

Adams, D. (1999). *How to Stop Worrying and learn to Love the Internet*. Retrieved from http://www.douglasadams.com/dna/19990901-00-a.html

American Psychiatric Association. (1996). Opinions of the Ethics Committee on The Principles of Medical Ethics. Retrieved from http://onlinetherapy.wikispaces.com/Ethics

Anthony, K., & Goss, S. P. (2009). Guidelines for online counselling and psychotherapy (3rd ed.). Lutterworth: BACP.

Anthony, K., & Jamieson, A. (2005). Guidelines for Online Counselling and Psychotherapy (2nd ed.). BACP: Lutterworth.

Anthony, K., & Nagel, D. M. (2009). Ethical Framework for the Use of Technology in Mental Health. *Online Therapy Institute*. Retrieved from http://www.onlinetherapyinstitute.com/ethical-training/

Anthony, K., & Nagel, D. M. (2010). *Therapy Online: A Practical Guide*. London: Sage.

Anthony, K., Nagel, D. M., & Goss, S. P. (2010). *The Use of Technology in Mental Health Care: Applications, Ethics and Practice*. Springfield, IL: CC Thomas.

APA. (1997). APA Statement on Services by Telephone, Teleconferencing, and Internet. *American Psychological Association*. Retrieved from http://web.archive.org/web/20070929104840/www.apa.org/ethics/stmnt01.html

APA. (2002). Ethical Principles of Psychologists and Code of Conduct. *American Psychological Association*. Retrieved from http://web.archive.org/web/20071009031511/www.apa.org/ethics/code2002.html

BACP. (2010). *Ethical Framework for Good Practice in Counselling and Psychotherapy*. Lutterworth: BACP.

Barak, A., Hen, L., Boniel-Nissim, M., & Shapira, N. (2008). A comprehensive review and meta-analysis of the effectiveness of Internet based psychotherapeutic interventions. *Technology in Human Services*, *26*(2-4), 109–160. doi:10.1080/15228830802094429

Bennett, A. M., Rappaport, W. H., & Skinner, F. L. (1978). Telehealth Handbook: A Guide to Telecommunications Technology for Rural health Care. Hyattsville, MD: NCHSR Publications and Information Branch.

Campbell, M., & Glasheen, K. (2007). Launching Into Cyberspace A Short Guide for Providing Online Support for Students. Queensland: Australian Guidance and Counselling Association. Retrieved from http://mhws.agca.com.au/onlcoun_home.php

Childress, C. (1999, July 23). E-mail communication to the ISMHO mailing list.

Cogswell, J. F. (1967). *Exploratory Study of Information-processing Procedures and Computer-based Technology in Vocational Counseling, Final Report*. Santa Monica, CA: System Development Corp.

Cogswell, J. F., & Estavan, D. P. (1965). *Explorations in Computer Assisted Counselling*. Santa Monica, CA: System Development Corp.

Cohen, G., & Kerr, B. A. (1998). Computer mediated counseling: An empirical view of a new mental health treatment. *Computers in Human Services*, *15*(4), 13–26. doi:10.1300/J407v15n04_02

Del Vecchio, R., & Dundas, E. (1970). Telecommunications for mental health: prospects for the seventies and eighties. In M.M. Berger (Ed.), Videotape Techniques in Psychiatric Training and Treatment (pp. 251-257). New York: Brunner/Mazel.

Dwyer, T. F. (1973). Telepsychiatry: Psychiatric Consultation by Interactive Television. *The American Journal of Psychiatry*, *1308*(August), 865–869. doi:10.1176/ajp.130.8.865 PMID:4716685

Ethicscode. (1999). Guidelines for Mental Health and Healthcare Practice Online. EthicsCode. Retrieved from http://web.archive.org/web/20070809083408/www.ethicscode.com/pages/698182/index.htm

Goss, S., Anthony, K. & Nagel, D.M. (2016). *Technology in Mental Health: Applications in practice, supervision and training (2nd ed.)*. Springfield: CCThomas Publishing.

Goss, S. P. (2000) *An exploratory study in aspects of the philosophy, method and application of pluralist evaluation of counselling*. Unpublished Ph.D. thesis, Strathclyde University Counselling Unit, Glasgow.

Goss, S. P., & Anthony, K. (2003). *Technology in Counselling and psychotherapy: A Practitioner's Guide*. Basingstoke, UK: Palgrave MacMillan. doi:10.1007/978-0-230-50015-0

Goss, S. P., & Anthony, K. (2008). *Uudet Teknologiat Terapiassa*. Helsinki: Edita Publishing Oy.

Goss, S. P., Anthony, K., Jamieson, A., & Palmer, S. (2001). *Guidelines for Online Counselling and Psychotherapy*. Rugby: BACP.

Goss, S. P., & Mearns, D. (1997). A call for a pluralist epistemological understanding in the assessment and evaluation of counselling. *British Journal of Guidance & Counselling*, *25*(2), 189–198. doi:10.1080/03069889708253801

Greidanus, E., & Everall, R. D. (2010). Helper therapy in an online suicide prevention community. *British Journal of Guidance & Counselling*, *38*(2), 191–204. doi:10.1080/03069881003600991

Greist, J., Gustafson, D. H., Stauss, F., Rowse, M. S., Laughren, T. P., & Chiles, J. A. (1973). A computer interview for suicide-high risk prediction. *The American Journal of Psychiatry*, *130*(12), 12. doi:10.1176/ajp.130.12.1327 PMID:4585280

Hanley, T. (2010, March). Does online counselling work? Reviewing the research into outcomes and alliances. Proceedings of the OCTIA 2010 conference, Manchester, UK.

Health on the Net. (1995, updated 2008) The HONcode in brief. Retrieved from http://www.hon.ch/HONcode/Pro/Conduct.html

Hill, A., & Roth, A. (2014). The competences required to deliver psychological therapies 'at a distance'. Lutterworth: BACP.

International Society for Mental Health Online (ISMHO). (2000). *Suggested Principles for the Online Provision of Mental Health Services*. Retrieved from https://www.ismho.org/suggestions.asp

Kaplan, E. H. (1997). Telepsychotherapy. Psychotherapy by telephone, videotelephone, and computer videoconferencing. *The Journal of Psychotherapy Practice and Research*, *6*, 227–237. PMID:9185068

Kraus, R., Zack, J., & Stricker, G. (2004). *Online Counseling A Handbook for Mental health professionals*. San Diego, CA: Elsevier.

Lago, C., Baughan, R., Copinger Binns, P., Brice, A., Caleb, R., Goss, S., & Lindeman, P. (1999). *Counselling Online...A BAC Special Report for Purchasers and Providers*. Rugby: BAC.

Nagel, D. M., & Anthony, K. (2009). *Ethical Framework for the Use of Technology in Mental Health*. Retrieved from http://www.onlinetherapyinstitute.com/id43.html

NBCC. (1999). Standards for the Ethical Practice of Web Counseling. Retrieved from http://www.nbcc.org/AssetManagerFiles/ethics/internetCounseling.pdf

Reynolds, P., & Morris, T. (2002). Intimacy as we know it? *Counselling and Psychotherapy Journal, 13*(3), 11.

Robson, D., & Robson, M. (1998). Intimacy and computer communication. *British Journal of Guidance & Counselling, 26*(1), 33–41. doi:10.1080/03069889808253836

Rogers, C. (1942). The use of electronically recorded interviews in improving psychotherapeutic techniques. *The American Journal of Orthopsychiatry, 12*(12), 429–434. doi:10.1111/j.1939-0025.1942.tb05930.x

Rosenthal, M. (1998). Elaborations and Digressions on Histories of the Book. Retrieved from http://www.mtbs.com/bkhist1.html

Rothschild, E. (1997). E-mail therapy [letter]. *The American Journal of Psychiatry, 154*(10), 1476–1477. doi:10.1176/ajp.154.10.1476b PMID:9326843

Sanders, P. (1998). *Paper presented at the British Association for the Person Centred Approach Annual Conference.*

Schmelter-Davis, H., Anthony, K., & Nagel, D. M. (2009a). Ethical Framework for the Use of Technology in Career and School Guidance. Retrieved from http://www.onlinetherapyinstitute.com/id51.html

Schmelter-Davis, H., Anthony, K. & Nagel, D.M. (2009b). Using technology to deliver career and School Guidance services: Establishing a global and inclusive ethical framework. *Student Assistance Journal,* Winter.

Slack, W. V., Porter, D., Balkin, P., Kowaloff, H. B., & Slack, C. W. (1990). Computer assisted soliloquy as an approach to psychotherapy. *M.D. Computing, 7*, 37–42. PMID:2308504

Slack, W. V., & Slack, C. W. (1977). Talking to a computer about emotional problems; a comparative study. *Psychotherapy (Chicago, Ill.), 14*(2), 156–164. doi:10.1037/h0086523

Solow. C., Weiss, R.J., Bergen, B., & Sanborn, C.J. (1971). 24-hour psychiatric consultation via TV. *American Journal of Psychiatry, 127*(12), 1684-1687.

Steele, P. (2002). Online Counselling Training. *Counselling and Psychotherapy Journal, 13*(3), 36–37.

Weizenbaum, J. (1966). ELIZA – A computer program for the study of natural language communication between man and machine. *Proceedings of Conference of Association for Computer Machinery,* New York. doi:10.1145/365153.365168

ADDITIONAL READING

Alcañiz, M., Botella, C., Baños, R. M., Zaragoza, I., & Guixeres, J. (2009). The Intelligent e-Therapy system: A new paradigm for telepsychology and cybertherapy. *British Journal of Guidance & Counselling*, *37*(3), 287–296. doi:10.1080/03069880902957015

Baños, R. M., Botella, C., Guillen, V., García-Palacios, A., Quero, S., Bretón-López, J., & Alcañiz, M. (2009). An adaptive display to treat stress-related disorders: EMMAs World. *British Journal of Guidance & Counselling*, *37*(3), 347–356. doi:10.1080/03069880902957064

Bauer, S., Moessner, M., Wolf, M., Haug, S., & Kordy, H. (2009). ES[S]PRIT – an Internet-based programme for the prevention and early intervention of eating disorders in college students. *British Journal of Guidance & Counselling*, *37*(3), 327–336. doi:10.1080/03069880902957049

Botella, C., Gallego, M. J., Garcia-Palacios, A., Baños, R. M., Quero, S., & Alcañiz, M. (2009). The acceptability of an Internet-based self-help treatment for fear of public speaking. *British Journal of Guidance & Counselling*, *37*(3), 297–311. doi:10.1080/03069880902957023

Efstathiou, G. (2009). Students psychological web consulting: Function and outcome evaluation. *British Journal of Guidance & Counselling*, *37*(3), 243–255. doi:10.1080/03069880902956983

Fink, J. (1999). *How to use Computers and Cyberspace in the Clinical Practice of Psychotherapy*. London: Aronson.

Goss, S., & Anthony, K. (2009). Developments in the use of technology in counselling and psychotherapy. *British Journal of Guidance & Counselling*, *37*(3), 223–230. doi:10.1080/03069880902956967

Goss, S. P., & Anthony, K. (2003). *Technology in Counselling and psychotherapy: A Practitioner's Guide*. Basingstoke, UK: Palgrave MacMillan. doi:10.1007/978-0-230-50015-0

Hanley, T. (2009). The working alliance in online therapy with young people: Preliminary findings. *British Journal of Guidance & Counselling*, *37*(3), 257–269. doi:10.1080/03069880902956991

Hsuing, R. C. (2002) e-Therapy Case Studies, Guiding Principles, and the Clinical Potential of the Internet. New York: W.W. Norton.

Jones, G., & Stokes, A. (2009). *Online Counselling A Handbook for Practitioners*. London: Palgrave MacMillan. doi:10.1007/978-0-230-23085-9

Malone, J. F., Miller, R. M., & Walz, G. R. (2007). *Distance Counselling: Expanding the Counselor's Reach and Impact*. Ann Arbor, MI: Counseling Outfitters.

Nagel, D. M., & Anthony, K. (2009). *Ethical Framework for the Use of Technology in Mental Health*. Retrieved from http://www.onlinetherapyinstitute.com/id43.html

Preziosa, A., Grassi, A., Gaggioli, A., & Riva, G. (2009). Therapeutic applications of the mobile phone. *British Journal of Guidance & Counselling, 37*(3), 313–325. doi:10.1080/03069880902957031

Richards, D. (2009). Features and benefits of online counselling: Trinity College online mental health community. *British Journal of Guidance & Counselling, 37*(3), 231–242. doi:10.1080/03069880902956975

Riva, G. (2009). Virtual reality: An experiential tool for clinical psychology. *British Journal of Guidance & Counselling, 37*(3), 337–345. doi:10.1080/03069880902957056

Simpson, S. (2009). Psychotherapy via videoconferencing: A review. *British Journal of Guidance & Counselling, 37*(3), 271–286. doi:10.1080/03069880902957007

Stofle, G. S. (2001). *Choosing and Online Therapist*. Harrisburg, PA: White Hate Communications.

Tyler, J.M. and Sabella, R.A. (2004) *Using Technology to Improve Counselling Practice A Primer for the 21st Century*. Alexandria: ACA.

Chapter 9
Revisiting the Issue of Trust in E-Health

Elizabeth Sillence
Northumbria University, UK

Pam Briggs
Northumbria University, UK

Peter R. Harris
University of Sussex, UK

ABSTRACT

As people continue to go online for their health information needs we revisit the issue of trust in relation to e-health. This chapter begins by briefly presenting an overview of e-health and describing current ways in which people are using the Internet for health advice and information. Models of trust are revisited and we then explore two emerging areas within the e-health field: peer resources and mobile health applications. Finally, we revisit and update our guidelines and point to further sources of information in this field.

INTRODUCTION

Over the past few years the scope of e-health has continued to increase yet the concept remains stubbornly difficult to define. A systematic review of published definitions identified a wide range of themes but no clear consensus about the meaning of the term e-health, other than the presence of two universal themes (health and technology) (Oh et al., 2005). Over the last ten years the term e-health has been used to describe the provision of web-based information, technology delivered behaviour change

DOI: 10.4018/978-1-5225-3241-5.ch009

interventions, the use of social media within a health context (Sadah et al., 2015), and more recently health-related mobile applications (Krebs and Duncan, 2015). This evolving domain is further complicated by the fact that e-health continues to incorporate a range of health services and providers with a shifting and growing pattern of stakeholders.

For many conditions, the Internet provides a major source of health information (Fox, Duggan & Purcell, 2013, Harris, Sillence & Briggs, 2011). Over the last ten years, the number of people using the internet for health information and advice has increased. 72% of adult internet users say they looked online for health information (Fox et al., 2013) and the nature of those health resources has altered. Patients themselves now provide a crucial source of online health material and the number of people accessing patient-authored content, in particular those with chronic conditions, has greatly increased. 16% of people are looking for people that might share the same health concerns (Fox, 2011). A wide range of people are accessing online resources. 84% of teens have gone online for health information and 21% have used mobile apps (Wartella, Rideout, Montague et al., 2016). There has also been a rise in surrogate seekers, people looking online for someone else. Surrogate seekers are more likely to engage with user-generated content online in comparison to those who seek health information for only themselves. This might involve using social networking sites (SNSs) and emailing healthcare providers (Cutrona et al., 2015). Indeed, we know that carers are using the Internet to support their coping role (Fox et al, 2013). People caring for a friend or relative with a serious or long-term chronic condition have been shown to use the internet for information, support and communication (James et al., 2007; Coleman, et al., 2005; White & Dorman, 2000). Finally, there are interesting demographic differences in relation to health-related SNSs with the majority of users being older females (Sadah et al., 2015).

As user profiles become better understood we recognise that the e-health space is becoming more crowded with more providers, authors and more delivery modes. This in turn poses questions for health consumers about which information, providers and technologies to trust. Research over the last 15 -20 years has examined the issue of trust in relation to online services and e-health services in particular. In this chapter, we revisit the issue of trust within the context of e-health. The rest of this chapter is organized as follows. We begin by briefly discuss the role of technology in the context of health information and advice. We then re-examine the context of trust in relation to e-health and in particular online or web-based health advice and information and re-visit our model of trust in e-health. The next section highlights a number of emerging research areas, peer-to-peer resources and mobile health applications. Finally, we discuss guidelines for trust in e-health and point towards future research directions.

THE EVOLVING ROLE OF TECHNOLOGY IN THE CONTEXT OF HEALTH INFORMATION AND ADVICE

Technology continues to play an evolving role within health care. Electronic patient records, online appointment booking systems and internet pharmacy services, technology to log, monitor and share health and wellbeing information to mobile applications that allow you to connect to a family doctor (GP) in real time for an online consultation (see for example: http://www.drnow.com). Online health resources, however, continue to be the most accessible and well used source of advice and information and as people are continually encouraged to take a more pro-active role in their own health (Coulter and Colins, 2011) so these resources become more important. People search online for health information and advice for a number of reasons. Some people want to be better informed, better prepared when meeting the doctor, or are searching for support, alternative answers or reassurance (Rozmovits & Ziebland, 2004, Harris et al., 2011).

One key change over recent years is the increasing importance of user-generated content (Ziebland & Wyke, 2012). User generated health information, created by patients or carers, typically consists of personal experiences of a particular treatment or health condition often in narrative form. In the UK, nearly 25% of people have accessed and shared personal experiences of health online (O'Neill et al, 2014). Such narratives or personal experiences are rapidly becoming a central part of health-related Internet use (Mo & Coulson, 2008; France, Wyke, Ziebland, Entwistle et al., 2011; Hinton, Kurinczuk, & Ziebland, 2010). Patient experiences offer opportunities for social comparison, helping patients understand how well they are coping with a particular illness (Locock & Brown, 2010) or allowing them to understand that they are not alone in their situation and become more optimistic about their own condition (Powell & Clarke, 2006). Access to patients' stories is also associated with a sense of feeling supported, of maintaining relationships with others and for some people an ability to visualize the disease (Ziebland & Wyke, 2012). Finally, people engaged with behavioural and lifestyle changes, for example weight loss and smoking cessation are using online support groups as a way of sharing personal experiences (Brindal, 2012; van Mierlo, 2012). However, given the diverse experiences online it is not surprising that personal narratives can also cause problems. Strong emotional content can be challenging for some individuals whilst others suggest engaging with online personal stories can have an isolating effect with respect to friends and family (Hinton, et al., 2010).

One of the benefits (and the disadvantages) of the Internet is the range of material available regarding health and lifestyle advice. Sites can vary in the type of advice and information they present (see Table 1), and in terms of their scope, health topic, ownership and funding model, country of origin and mode of presentation. To indicate

Table 1. The range of health websites available to consumers

Type of Site	Description of Site
Web providers and portal sites	Information and advice supplied by web provider rather than a physical organisation. Portals act as catalogues of information providing a gateway to many other sites providing information and advice.
Support groups	Often run by individuals or on behalf of support groups. May be local, national or global in scale. Contain forums where consumers can read comments and contribute to discussions.
Charity sites	Registered charity sites provide information and advice on specific health issues and provide a focal point for fund raising activities. Often include personal experiences in written, audio or video format and forum.
Government websites	Provide patient information in the form of news, features and fact sheets. May contain patient testimonials, forum or advice line. Links to additional sources of information.
Pharmaceutical sites	Sponsored by pharmaceutical companies these sites are often biased in favour of their own drug remedies and regimes.
Sales sites	Sales sites promote and sell certain drugs, medical devices or health plans often in addition to some information.
Personal sites	Contains personal experiences of illness and health issues. These may be written or video based.
Social networking sites	Contains profiled members connected via network. Health topic may be focus of network or part of a broader set of topics.
Medical databases	Provide access to research papers on health and illness issues.
Media sites	Extensions of print or television media sites that provide the latest news and commentary on health features.
Clinician sites	Information on specific health issues or specialist clinics run by medical professionals.

the range of different sites available Table 2 provides an overview of three different UK based sites highlighting their main features and the range of services available on each site. Compared with ten years ago, many of these sites have introduced a stronger peer resources element with some including interactive forums and others more curated patient stories.

Given the huge variety of sites and resources available, how are consumers searching for and evaluating the trustworthiness and quality of health information online? A body of literature developed around 15 years ago focussed on the quality of the information available on the Internet (Wyatt, 1997; Jadad & Gagliardi, 1998; Smart & Burling, 2001), embracing diverse topics such as Viagra, rheumatoid arthritis and diabetes. A systematic meta-analysis of health website evaluations noted that the most frequently used quality criteria included accuracy, completeness, readability, and design (Eysenbach et al., 2002). Seventy percent of the studies they reviewed concluded that quality is a problem on the Internet. The issue of information quality remains a problem with recent studies showing poor levels of information completeness in relatively less well-understood conditions (Hardy & Sillence, 2015).

Table 2. Health websites and range of features/services

	Website		
	Netdoctor www.netdoctor.co.uk	**Healthtalkonline www.healthtalkonline.org**	**NHS Choices www.nhschoices.gov.uk**
Domain	General health	High blood pressure	General health
Owner	Web provider	Charity	Government
Type of advice	• Patient fact sheets • Ask the doctor service • News • Discussion boards	• Curated personal accounts in video, audio and written format • Medical information • Frequently Asked Questions • Discussion board	• Health encyclopaedia • Self help guide • Clinical evidence based research reports • Curated patient stories • Links to further information • Contact numbers for national and local information and support
Commercial aspects	Health related advertising	Donations requested	None
Notable features	• SMS alert service e.g. contraceptive pill reminder • Discussion boards	• Video clips • Links to support groups • Quality logo	• Locate nearest NHS services facility • Chat to an advisor • Quality logo

These quality assessments provide a useful starting point but offer little in terms of understanding the patient experience. How do different stakeholders e.g. patients, carers, friends and family access and evaluate the information available online? Studies looking at a range of health issues including HIV/AIDS, cancer and medicine requirements have suggested that patients use online information to help them make treatment decisions, interpret information, find support groups and seek alternative therapies (Mo and Coulson, 2008; Ziebland et al., 2004; Peterson et al., 2003, Entwistle et al., 2011). Other studies have suggested that whilst the Internet can increase patients' knowledge about their health conditions, they can be left feeling too overwhelmed by the information available online to be able to make an informed decision about their own health care (Hart, Henwood &Wyatt, 2004).

TRUST AND MISTRUST IN E-HEALTH

Early studies trying to understand the components of trust in relation to e-health from a consumer perspective often used artificial search tasks (e.g. Eysenbach & Köhler, 2002) and it may be that people in a 'real setting' with a greater stake in the outcome may well pay more attention to the content of the websites, in terms of markers of quality. This failure to engage with real Internet consumers in a realistic setting is a common problem in studies of online trust. Thus, over the last ten years we have engaged in a programme of research aimed at systematically exploring the ways in which people evaluate the trustworthiness of health information and advice online.

The literature suggests that trust is multi-faceted, multi-dimensional, and not easy to tie down in a single space (Marsh & Dibben, 2003). A key point to note is that trust is intimately associated with risk – indeed it is possible to argue that in the absence of risk, trust is meaningless (Brien, 1998). Even within seemingly simple acts of trust complex sets of judgements are invoked and a risk assessment is involved. Indeed, some of the trust models that have been developed in recent years have explicitly included risk (Corritore, Kracher & Wiedenbeck, 2003). In online advice, there is no doubt that people are more willing to trust a site if perceived risk is low. This came out very clearly in a study of over two and a half thousand people who said they had sought advice online (Briggs et al., 2002). Those that sought advice in relatively high-risk domains (e.g. finance) were less likely to trust and subsequently act on the advice than those who sought advice in low risk domains (e.g. entertainment).

Originally, we turned to the e-commerce literature for an understanding of trust in online settings. This provided a useful starting point for exploring the ways in which people evaluate the trustworthiness of health information and advice online (see Beatty et al., 2011 or Grabner-Krauter & Kaluscha, 2003 for reviews. Based on this literature we can assume that various factors are likely to govern the extent to which individuals feel they can trust health advice online. Firstly, they may be influenced by the look and feel of the site – trusting, for example, those sites rated high in visual appeal and mistrusting those sites with poor visual design or with unprofessional errors (Fogg et al., 2002; Stanford et al., 2002, Kim & Moon, 1998, Harris et al., 2009). Secondly, they may be influenced by the branding of the site or by presence of familiar images or trusted logos (Riegelsberger, Sasse & McCarthy, 2003). Thirdly, they may be influenced by the quality of information available on the site, trusting those sites with greater perceived expertise or competence, (Bhattacherjee, 2002; McKnight & Chervany, 2001) and fourthly, they may be influenced by the extent to which the advice is personalised to the individual – i.e. the extent to which the advice appears to come from and be directed to similar individuals (i.e. those with a shared social identity) (Briggs, De Angeli & Simpson, 2004).

We reconciled these different findings by proposing a staged model of trust in which it is possible to distinguish between relatively 'hasty' and more 'considered' processing strategies for the evaluation of trust in high and low risk environments. Chaiken (1980) identified two processing strategies by which an evaluation of trustworthiness may be made: firstly, a heuristic strategy which follows a 'cognitive miser' principle - where people base decisions on only the most obvious or apparent information; and secondly, a systematic strategy that involves the detailed processing of message content. A number of other studies in the persuasion literature support the two-process model, namely that people use cognitively intense analytical processing when the task is an important or particularly engaging one, whereas they use affect or other simple heuristics to guide their decisions when they lack the motivation or capacity to think properly about the issues involved. Such different processing strategies also reflect the distinction between the preliminary stage of (i) intention to trust and the later stage of (ii) trusting activity (McKnight and Chervany, 2001). We went a stage further and suggested that a more realistic assessment of the development of trust should include a third stage in which a trusting relationship develops between the consumer and the website.

In summary, people make a relatively quick assessment based on the look and feel of the site before going on to consider the content in more detail. Over time, a trusting relationship may develop as people integrate the online information with their other information sources and begin to contribute to engage with the site further perhaps generating their own content. This model has been validated through a series of qualitative studies across a number of different health domains (Sillence et al., 2007) most recently in relation to raw milk consumption (Sillence et al., 2016).

The important trust antecedents identified in our qualitative work have been explored in a series of large-scale questionnaire based studies looking at trust in and intention to act on e-health advice (Harris et al., 2011). Here, we took measures of trust antecedents i.e. information quality, impartiality, personalisation and design credibility derived from our qualitative work and earlier work by Briggs et al (2002) and combined them with variables to capture elements of the response to uncongenial, online health-risk information e.g. threat, control and coping. This study demonstrated that adding variables specific to e-health enhanced the ability of a model of trust to predict trust and readiness to act on advice.

THE CHANGING FACE OF TRUST IN E-HEALTH: PEER-TO-PEER RESOURCES AND MOBILE HEALTH APPLICATIONS

Over the past ten years, there has been a marked shift towards the use of peer-to-peer resources in e-health. Personal experiences in e-health have always been important to consumers and were valued in our qualitative studies (Sillence, Briggs & Herxheimer, 2004). The range and availability of personal experiences has grown enormously in recent times as online social networks have become more widespread. Contributing to forums, writing blogs or testimonials have become a regular feature in sites provided by individuals through to charities and governmental organisations. Curated material is also present in sites such as www.healthtalkonline.org. Peer resources once again put the concept of a trusting relationship centre stage. Here the technology, the website itself and the other network participants can all be considered as objects of trust (Grabner-Kräuter, 2010). People involved in these kinds of trusting relationships are typically engaging in identification-based trust emerging from a history of personal interactions with the other (van der Zee et al., 2009). Trust is influenced by joint values, tasks and goals, a sense of collective identity, and emotional closeness (Grabner-Kräuter, 2010). Online support communities have a long history of harnessing the Internet to develop long term supportive relationships, providing empathy and alleviating patients' sense of isolation (Rozmovits & Ziebland, 2004; Ziebland & Wyke, 2012). The role of peer resources in relation to trust and engagement with e-health information and advice is something we have studied both qualitatively and in are ongoing, 5-yearly questionnaire based studies (see for example Sillence, Hardy & Briggs, 2013).

In a series of qualitative studies, looking at how people select and engage with online personal experiences (Sillence, Hardy, Briggs & Harris, 2014) we noted that patients and carers sifted through experiences rejecting those that were dissimilar to themselves and engaging with those that resonated with their own experience, background or values in some way. People with relatively mild asthma, for example, preferred to read experiences from other people with a similar diagnosis or from similarly aged contributors (Sillence, Hardy, Briggs & Harris, 2013). Carers of people with multiple sclerosis wanted to hear from other carers who shared their outlook regarding the caring experience or from those with similar backgrounds and difficulties (Sillence Hardy, Briggs & Harris, 2015). Overall, we found that participants were more willing to trust others like themselves, exhibiting homophily in their preferences for health information and advice (Sillence et al 2014). Homophily addresses the extent to which two or more individuals who interact are similar in certain attributes, beliefs, education, social status, and preferences (Rogers, 2003). Certainly, homophily appears to increase the source credibility of information (Phua, 2014) and this, in turn, can lead to greater acceptance of persuasive messages (Hovland &Weiss, 1951). In our work, we have found that across a range of measures, we found evidence that preference matching (for quitting method) was effective in motivating smokers to engage with the online material. We also found modest support for the role of personal experience resources in reducing message resistance (Sillence, Harris and Briggs, 2015).

Including personal stories and testimonials in a broader range of e-health resources has potential problems. The inclusion of personal narratives within patient decision-making aids has shown that different parts of these personal experiences affect decision making (Bekker et al., 2013). In experimental settings, narratives that convey the outcome of health decisions may impact upon or bias treatment choices whilst those that contain information about the experience of the treatment or the process of decision-making are less likely to have an impact in this way (Shaffer & Zikmund-Fisher, 2013). We also know that whilst people may like sites that contain personal experiences, trust is not necessarily simultaneously conferred. Sillence et al (2013) suggested that the presence of commercial elements on sites containing personal experiences led people to question the credibility of the site and the experiences. This is something we are examining further in our latest five-year follow-up.

Mobile health applications are increasing in popularity. A US based survey found that 58% of smartphone users had downloaded a health app. The majority of those respondents believed that the apps had improved their health, and a majority had a strong degree of faith in health apps' accuracy and effectiveness (Krebs & Duncan, 2015). A small-scale conducted by researchers in our lab examined people's use of health apps and the factors important in assessing the trustworthiness of those applications. Nine participants, (7 females, 2 males) aged 20-21, all undergraduate students, took part in an interview to discuss their use of health apps (see Table 3). The participants were asked about their use of health apps and to describe how they searched for and chose particular apps to download.

Most participants used self-monitoring apps concerned with exercise and sleep. In relation to trust, a number of key themes emerged from the interviews. The main trust issues centred on the decision to download the app. In choosing an app, the key issue was cost with all 9 participants only using free apps despite acknowledging that paid for apps may confer some benefits. Only one participant suggested that they might consider paying for an app. However, most thought that paid for apps might be more reliable and accurate and were likely to be based on a more robust set of

Table 3. Participant information regarding health app use

Participant	Gender	Age	Health Apps Installed on Mobile Device
1	M	20	Fitbit, Strava
2	F	21	My fitness Pal
3	F	20	My fitness Pal
4	F	21	Sleep Cycle, Tabata
5	M	20	IIFYM
6	F	20	My Fitness Pal, Run Watch Lite
7	F	20	My Fitness Pal
8	F	21	Sleep Time
9	F	20	Fitbit

research. After cost, a number of factors played into a trust assessment of the app. These centred on the popularity of the app. Apps with a large number of downloads indicated that other people were using the app satisfactorily and many people reported that they often downloaded one of the top three results from any search.

If it was popular to be honest it would be a really big thing like erm if I can see that its got like hundreds of thousands of downloads then that would make me feel more comfortable than if it had like si, yeah that would make me feel more comfortable cause its like obviously a lot people have kind of put their faith in it and its been fine so that would be a big thing. (Participant 3)

A number of people noted the star rating, avoiding those with low ratings but few made use of the reviews choosing instead to rely upon word of mouth recommendations from known others e.g. friends or family. Participants thought that apps developed by large well-known companies would be more trustworthy than those from smaller developers. However, the majority admitted that they paid little attention to the developer and often replied upon the reputation and integrity of the Apple store.

So I guess I put all my trust in Apple they've allowed it to be on their app store to me it's good enough, its good enough. (Participant 1)

Although a couple of participants thought that data privacy and control were important issues in assessing the trustworthiness of a health app for most people trust related to the idea of confidence in the product. An app must be reliable, easy to use and have the advertised functionality or it was simply deleted. Using the apps was mostly about self-monitoring and few people were keen to share their data with other users.

I wouldn't trust one if it was asking me questions that were non relatable in my opinion err or just like if it didn't seem relevant I probably wouldn't trust it erm I wouldn't trust it if it took my bank details. (Participant 8)

Overall, there was a sense that cost was the main priority with regard to mobile health apps and that given that the perceived risk associated with using mobile health apps was low trust per se was not a priority for many people. Selecting which apps to download was usually driven by simple heuristics although issues around subsequent use, information disclosure and sharing did factor into secondary trust evaluations.

SUMMARY AND GUIDELINES

As the digital space becomes more crowded and people are able to access a greater range and diversity of health resources the issue of trust becomes ever more important. Being able to sift through and select health information and advice or engage with digital resources requires careful trust assessments. Understanding the complex set of factors involved in making these decisions is an ongoing process but some suggestions for guidance and future research directions are given below.

In our previous work, we have attempted to capture our findings in a set of guidelines for developing trustworthy e-health websites. These guidelines have considered how users initially evaluate online resources and recommended using a professional and attractive design, maintaining a consistent look and feel through the site to encourage engagement regardless of the landing page and avoiding mixing advertising and content. In terms of evaluating content, we have suggested: including a mixture of expert and peer expert resources, making clear the motivations of the authors – provide good links to independent websites in the same domain to provide reassurances on bias and ensuring that the website reflects the social identity of the user. Finally, in relation to longer-term engagement we recommend that: content is updated regularly and time stamped, posters are encouraged to develop their own profile and that the website contains clearly stated privacy policies. We have also recently compiled some guidelines specifically related to the development of online personal experiences within e-health materials, these can be found in Ziebland et al, (2016).

FUTURE TRENDS

As we have noted the field of e-health is rapidly evolving. We are witnessing greater use of video resources with more examples of lived-experience expertise (Mazanderani, O'Neill & Powell, 2013). There is also an increasing sense of integration as people use technology to contact healthcare professionals and share information between different sources. The use of social networking sites as a peer health resource raises further questions about the layered nature of trusting relationships, who or what is it that we are trusting?

The demand for increasingly personalised e-health services also raises issues of trust privacy and self-disclosure. Our ongoing qualitative work with websites and health apps indicates that people desire personalised health services, in fact, that is one of the key drivers for mobile health app use. Despite this, they are often reluctant to register all their information and are wary of sharing more than they have to. The increase in personalisation coupled with increasing 'public technologies' raises a number of important points regarding privacy and security. Burgoon (1982) described two kinds of privacy; informational privacy and physical privacy both of which will have to be addressed in future work on e-health.

We are continuing to collect data at 5-yearly intervals on e-health and trust. These data provide a useful snapshot of how the landscape is changing. To understand how people come to develop trusting relationships with e-health resources in relation to different health conditions will demand a more longitudinal approach in which we can follow people along their health and wellbeing journeys. This in turn poses a number of methodological problems. Whilst our qualitative paradigm has allowed people to behave naturally during their search and evaluation of websites there is often some reluctance to engage with more interactive content e.g. clicking on videos or registering and posting messages. Participants tell us that they would do that 'at home' but not here in the lab. Capturing that natural data, actual posts and web histories proves ethically and practically challenging. Again, in terms of a natural understanding of trust practises that exist this becomes more complicated as social networks develop. Many health organisations, charities and individuals now have multiple platforms providing information and connectivity with people using some, part or all of the available platforms. Trying to understand the different trust issues here in relation to personal preference, disclosure and identity will be interesting. Finally, a big challenge is to improve the integration of e-health with offline resources as it is interesting to note that people still trust their healthcare professionals and see them as a key source of information.

REFERENCES

Beatty, P., Reay, I., Dick, S., & Miller, J. (2011). Consumer trust in e-commerce web sites: A meta-study. [CSUR]. *ACM Computing Surveys, 43*(3), 14. doi:10.1145/1922649.1922651

Bekker, H. L., Winterbottom, A. E., Butow, P., Dillard, A. J., Feldman-Stewart, D., Fowler, F. J., & Volk, R. J. et al. (2013). Do personal stories make patient decision aids more effective? A critical review of theory and evidence. *BMC Medical Informatics and Decision Making, 13*(Suppl. 2), S9. doi:10.1186/1472-6947-13-S2-S9 PMID:24625283

Bhattacherjee, A. (2002). Individual trust in online firms: Scale development and initial test. *Journal of management Information Systems*, *19*(1), 211-241.

Brien, A. (1998). Professional ethics and the culture of trust. *Journal of Business Ethics*, *17*(4), 391–409. doi:10.1023/A:1005766631092

Briggs, P., Burford, B., De Angeli, A., & Lynch, P. (2002). Trust in Online advice. *Social Science Computer Review*, *20*(3), 321–332. doi:10.1177/089443930202000309

Briggs, P., de Angeli, A., & Simpson, B. (2004). Personalisation and Trust: A Reciprocal Relationship? In M. C. Karat, J. Blom, & J. Karat (Eds.), *Designing Personalized User Experiences for ECommerce*. Kluwer. doi:10.1007/1-4020-2148-8_4

Brindal, E., Freyne, J., Saunders, I., Berkovsky, S., Smith, G., & Noakes, M. (2012). Features predicting weight loss in overweight or obese participants in a web-based intervention: randomized trial. *Journal of Medical Internet Research*, *14*(6). doi:10.2196/jmir.2156

Burgoon, J. K. (1982). Privacy & Communication. *Communication yearbook*, *6*, 206-249.

Chaiken, S. (1980). Heuristic versus systematic information processing and the use of source versus message cues in persuasion. *Journal of Personality and Social Psychology*, *39*(5), 752–766. doi:10.1037/0022-3514.39.5.752

Coleman, J., Olsen, S., Sauter, P., Baker, D., Hodgin, M. B., Stanfield, C., & Nolan, M. T. et al. (2005). The effect of a frequently asked questions module on a pancreatic web site patient/family chat room. *Cancer Nursing*, *28*(6), 460–468. doi:10.1097/00002820-200511000-00009 PMID:16330968

Corritore, C. C. L. L., Kracher, B., & Wiedenbeck, S. (2003). On-line trust: Concepts, evolving themes, a model. *International Journal of Human-Computer Studies*, *58*(6), 737–758. doi:10.1016/S1071-5819(03)00041-7

Coulter, A., & Collins, A. (2011). Making shared decision-making a reality: no decision about me, without me. *Proceedings of King's Fund '11*.

Cutrona, S. L., Mazor, K. M., Vieux, S. N., Luger, T. M., Volkman, J. E., & Finney Rutten, L. J. (2015). Health Information-Seeking on Behalf of Others: Characteristics of Surrogate Seekers. *Journal of Cancer Education*, *30*(1), 12–19. doi:10.1007/s13187-014-0701-3 PMID:24989816

Entwistle, V. A., France, E. F., Wyke, S., Jepson, R., Hunt, K., Ziebland, S., & Thompson, A. (2011). How information about other people's personal experiences can help with healthcare decision-making: A qualitative study. *Patient Education and Counseling*, *85*(3), 291–298. doi:10.1016/j.pec.2011.05.014 PMID:21652162

Eysenbach, G. Powell, J., Kuss, O., & Sa, E.R. (2002). Empirical studies assessing the quality of health information for consumers on the world wide web, a systematic review. *Journal of the American Medical Association*, *287*(20), 2691-2700.

Eysenbach, G., & Köhler, C. (2002). How do consumers search for and appraise health information on the world wide web? Qualitative study using focus groups, usability tests and in-depth interviews. *BMJ (Clinical Research Ed.)*, *324*(7337), 573–577. doi:10.1136/bmj.324.7337.573 PMID:11884321

Fogg, B. J., Kameda, T., Boyd, J., Marchall, J., Sethi, R., Sockol, M., & Trowbridge, T. (2002). Stanford-Makovsky Web Credibiltiy Study 2002: Investigating what makes Web sites credible today, A research report by the Stanford Persuasive Technology Lab & Makovsky & Company, Stanford University. Retrieved from http://www.webcredibility.org

Fox, S. (2011). The social life of health information, 2011. Pew Research Centre. Retrieved from http://pewinternet.org/~/media/Files/Reports/2011/PIP_Social_Life_of_Health_Info.pdf

Fox, S., Duggan, M., & Purcell, K. (2013). Family Caregivers are Wired for Health. Pew Internet Report. Retrieved from http://www.pewinternet.org/2013/06/20/family-caregivers-are-wired-for-health

France, E. F., Wyke, S., Ziebland, S., Entwistle, V. A., & Hunt, K. (2011). How personal experiences feature in women's accounts of use of information for decisions about antenatal diagnostic testing for foetal abnormality. *Social Science & Medicine*, *72*(5), 755–762. doi:10.1016/j.socscimed.2010.11.031 PMID:21257248

Grabner-Kräuter, S. (2010). Toward A Better Understanding of Trust in WEB 2.0 Social Networks. *Marketing Theory and Applications*, *313*.

Grabner-Krauter, S., & Kaluscha, E. A. (2003). Empirical research in online-trust: A review and critical assessment. *International Journal of Human-Computer Studies*, *58*(6), 783–812. doi:10.1016/S1071-5819(03)00043-0

Hardy, C., & Sillence, E. (2015). What are women being exposed to? A review of the quality, content and ownership of websites on premenstrual dysphoric disorder (PMDD). *Women's Health Issues*. PMID:26747724

Harris, P. R., Sillence, E., & Briggs, P. (2009). The effect of trust-related design cues on responses to a Web-based message about the breast cancer risks from alcohol. *J. Med. Internet Res.* doi:10.2196/jmir.1097

Harris, P.R., Sillence, E., & Briggs, P. (2011). Perceived Threat and Corroboration: Key Factors That Improve a Predictive Model of Trust in Internet-based Health Information and Advice. *J. Med. Internet Res.*, *13*(3). doi:10.2196/jmir.1821

Hart, A., Henwood, F., & Wyatt, S. (2004). The role of the Internet in patient practitioner relationships: Findings from a qualitative research study. *Journal of Medical Internet Research*, *6*(3), e36. doi:10.2196/jmir.6.3.e36 PMID:15471762

Hinton, L., Kurinczuk, J. J., & Ziebland, S. (2010, December). Infertility; isolation and the Internet: A qualitative interview study. *Patient Education and Counseling*, *81*(3), 436–441. doi:10.1016/j.pec.2010.09.023 PMID:21036506

Hovland, C. I., & Weiss, W. (1951). The influence of source credibility on communication effectiveness. *Public Opinion Quarterly*, *15*(4), 635–650. doi:10.1086/266350

Jadad, A. R. & Gagliardi A. (1998). Rating health information on the Internet: navigating to knowledge or to Babel? *Journal of the American Medical Association*, *279*(8), 611-614.

James, N., Daniels, H., Rahman, R., McConkey, C., Derry, J., & Young, A. (2007). A study of information seeking by cancer patients and their carers. *Clinical Oncology*, *19*(5), 356–362. doi:10.1016/j.clon.2007.02.005 PMID:17399963

Kim, J., & Moon, J. (1998). Designing towards emotional usability in customer interfaces: Trustworthiness of cyber-banking system interfaces. *Interacting with Computers*, *10*(1), 1–29. doi:10.1016/S0953-5438(97)00037-4

Klein, J. D., & Wilson, K. M. (2003). Delivering quality care: Adolescents discussion of health risks with their providers. *The Journal of Adolescent Health*, *30*(3), 190–195. doi:10.1016/S1054-139X(01)00342-1 PMID:11869926

Krebs, P., & Duncan, D. T. (2015). Health App Use Among US Mobile Phone Owners: A National Survey. *JMIR mHealth uHealth*, 3(4). doi: http://www.ehealthnews.eu/research/4601-national-survey-of-americans-health-app-use-shows-technology-s-promise-and-weakness10.2196/mhealth.4924 Retrieved from

Locock, L., & Brown, J. B. (2010, October). All in the same boat? Patient and carer attitudes to peer support and social comparison in Motor Neurone Disease (MND). *Social Science & Medicine*, *71*(8), 1498–1505. doi:10.1016/j.socscimed.2010.06.043 PMID:20719422

Marsh, S., & Dibben, M. (2003). The role of trust in information science and technology. In B. Cronin (Ed.), *Annual Review of Information Science and Technology*, *37* (pp. 465–498). Medford, NJ: Learned Information. doi:10.1002/aris.1440370111

Mazanderani, F., ONeill, B., & Powell, J. (2013). People power or pester power? YouTube as a forum for the generation of evidence and patient advocacy. *Patient Education and Counseling*, *93*(3), 420–425. doi:10.1016/j.pec.2013.06.006 PMID:23830239

McKnight, D. H., & Chervany, N. L. (2001). Trust and Distrust Definitions: One Bite at a Time. In R. Falcone, M. Singh, & Y.-H. Tan (Eds.), *Trust in Cybersocieties Berlin*. Springer-Verlag.

Mo, P. K. H., & Coulson, N. S. (2008). Exploring the communication of social support within virtual communities: A content analysis of messages posted to an online HIV/AIDS support group. *Cyberpsychology & Behavior*, *11*(3), 371–374. doi:10.1089/cpb.2007.0118 PMID:18537512

Oh, H., Rizo, C., Enkin, M., Jadad, A., Powell, J., & Pagliari, C. (2005). What Is eHealth (3): A Systematic Review of Published Definitions. *Journal of Medical Internet Research*, *7*(1), e1. doi:10.2196/jmir.7.1.e1 PMID:15829471

ONeill, B., Ziebland, S., Valderas, J., & Lupiáñez-Villanueva, F. (2014). User-Generated Online Health Content: A Survey of Internet Users in the United Kingdom J Med. *Internet Research*, *16*(4), e118. doi:10.2196/jmir.3187 PMID:24784798

Peterson, G., Aslani, P., & Williams, K. A. (2003). How do Consumers Search for and Appraise Information on Medicines On the Internet? A Qualitative Study Using Focus Groups. *Journal of Medical Internet Research*, *5*(4), e33. doi:10.2196/jmir.5.4.e33 PMID:14713661

Phua, J. (2014). The effects of similarity, parasocial identification, and source credibility in obesity public service announcements on diet and exercise self-efficacy. *J. Health Psych.*

Powell, J., & Clarke, A. (2006, September). Internet information-seeking in mental health. *The British Journal of Psychiatry*, *189*(3), 273–277. doi:10.1192/bjp.bp.105.017319 PMID:16946364

Riegelsberger, J., Sasse, M. A., & McCarthy, J. (2003). Shiny happy people building trust? Photos on e-commerce websites and consumer trust. *Proceedings CHI '03*. ACM Press.

Rogers, E. M. (2003). *Diffusion of innovations*. New York: Free Press.

Rozmovits, L., & Ziebland, S. (2004). What do patients with prostate or breast cancer want from an internet site? A qualitative study of information needs. *Patient Education and Counseling*, *53*(1), 57–64. doi:10.1016/S0738-3991(03)00116-2 PMID:15062905

Sadah, S. A., Shahbazi, M., Wiley, M. T., & Hristidis, V. (2015). A Study of the Demographics of Web-Based Health-Related Social Media Users. *Journal of Medical Internet Research*, *17*(8), e194. doi:10.2196/jmir.4308 PMID:26250986

Shaffer, V. A., & Zikmund-Fisher, B. J. (2013). All Stories Are Not Alike A Purpose-, Content-, and Valence-Based Taxonomy of Patient Narratives in Decision Aids. *Medical Decision Making*, *33*(1), 4–13. doi:10.1177/0272989X12463266 PMID:23065418

Sillence, E., Briggs, P., Harris, P. R., & Fishwick, L. (2007). How do patients evaluate and make use of online health information? *Social Science & Medicine*, *64*(9), 1853–1862. doi:10.1016/j.socscimed.2007.01.012 PMID:17328998

Sillence, E., Briggs, P. Herxheimer, A. (2004). Personal experiences matter: What patients think about hypertension information online. *He@lth Information on the Internet*, *42*, 3-5.

Sillence, E., Hardy, C., & Briggs, P. (2013, May 2-5). Why don't we trust health websites that help us help each other? *Proceedings of ACM Web Science '13*, Paris. doi:10.1145/2464464.2464488

Sillence, E., Hardy, C., Briggs, P., & Harris, P. R. (2013). How do people with asthma use Internet sites containing patient experiences? *Patient Education and Counseling*, *93*(3), 439–443. doi:10.1016/j.pec.2013.01.009 PMID:23415631

Sillence, E., Hardy, C., Briggs, P., & Harris, P. R. (2015). How do carers of people with multiple sclerosis engage with websites containing the personal experiences of other carers and patients? *Health Informatics Journal*. PMID:26460102

Sillence, E., Hardy, C., Harris, P. R., & Briggs, P. (2014). Modelling Patient Engagement in Peer-to-Peer Healthcare. *Proceedings of WWW'14 Proceedings of the companion publication of the 23rd international conference on World wide web companion* (pp. 481-486). doi:10.1145/2567948.2576937

Sillence, E., Hardy, C., Medeiros, L. C., & LeJeune, J. T. (2016). Examining trust factors in online food risk information: The case of unpasteurized or raw milk. *Appetite*, *99*, 200–210. doi:10.1016/j.appet.2016.01.010 PMID:26792772

Sillence, E., Harris, P. R., & Briggs, P. (2015, May). Assessing Patient Experience and Patient Preference when Designing Web Support for Smoking Cessation. *Proceedings of the 5th International Conference on Digital Health 2015* (pp. 25-26). ACM. doi:10.1145/2750511.2750516

Smart, J. M., & Burling, D. (2001). Radiology and the Internet: A systematic review of patient information resources. *Clinical Radiology*, *56*(11), 867–870. doi:10.1053/crad.2001.0738 PMID:11603887

Stanford, J., Tauber, E., Fogg, B. J., & Marable, L. (2002). Experts vs. Online Consumers: A Comparative Credibility Study of Health and Finance Web Sites. Consumer Web Watch Research Report. Retrieved from http://www.consumerwebwatch.org/news/report3_credibility research/slicebread_abstract.htm

Van der Zee, K., Vos, M., & Luijters, K. (2009). Social identity patterns and trust in demographically diverse work teams. *Social Sciences Information. Information Sur les Sciences Sociales*, *48*(2), 175–198. doi:10.1177/0539018409102406

Van Mierlo, T., Voci, S., Lee, S., Fournier, R., & Selby, P. (2012). Superusers in Social Networks for Smoking Cessation: Analysis of Demographic Characteristics and Posting Behavior From the Canadian Cancer Societys Smokers Helpline Online and StopSmokingCenter.net. *Journal of Medical Internet Research*, *14*(3), e66. doi:10.2196/jmir.1854 PMID:22732103

Wartella, E., Rideout, V., Montague, H., Beaudoin-Ryan, L., & Lauricella, A. (2016). Teens, health and technology: A national survey. *Media and Communication*, *4*(3).

White, M. H., & Dorman, S. M. (2000). Online support for caregivers. Analysis of an Internet Alzheimer mailgroup. *Computers in Nursing*, *18*, 168–176. PMID:10939186

Wyatt, J. C. (1997). Measuring quality and impact of the World Wide Web. *British Medical Journal*, *314*(7098), 1879–1881. doi:10.1136/bmj.314.7098.1879 PMID:9224133

Ziebland, S., Chapple, A., Dumelow, C., Evans, J., Prinjha, S., & Rozmovits, L. (2004). How the internet affects patients experience of cancer: A qualitative study. *British Medical Journal*, *328*(7439), 564. doi:10.1136/bmj.328.7439.564 PMID:15001506

Ziebland S, Powell J, Briggs P, Jenkinson C, Wyke S, Sillence E, et al. (2016). Examining the role of patient's experiences as a resource for choice and decision-making in health care: a creative, interdisciplinary mixed-method study in digital health. *Programme Grants Appl. Res.*, *4*(17).

Ziebland, S., & Wyke, S. (2012). Health and illness in a connected world: How might sharing experiences on the Internet affect people's health? *The Milbank Quarterly*, *90*(2), 219–249. doi:10.1111/j.1468-0009.2012.00662.x PMID:22709387

Compilation of References

AAMFT. (2001). *AAMFT Code of Ethics*. Retrieved from http://www.aamft.org/resources/lrm_plan/Ethics/ethicscode2001.asp

Abramowitz, J. S., Taylor, S., & McKay, D. (2009). Obsessive-compulsive disorder. *Lancet*, *374*(9688), 491–499. doi:10.1016/S0140-6736(09)60240-3 PMID:19665647

Adams, D. (1999). *How to Stop Worrying and learn to Love the Internet*. Retrieved from http://www.douglasadams.com/dna/19990901-00-a.html

Adrian, E. D., & Matthews, B. H. C. (1934). The Berger Rhythm; potential Changes from the occipital lobes in man. *Brain*, *57*(4), 355–384. doi:10.1093/brain/57.4.355

Albaina, I. M., Visser, T., van der Mast, C. A., & Vastenburg, M. H. (2009, April). Flowie: A persuasive virtual coach to motivate elderly individuals to walk. *Proceedings of the 3rd International Conference on Pervasive Computing Technologies for Healthcare Pervasive Health '09* (pp. 1-7). IEEE. doi:10.4108/ICST.PERVASIVEHEALTH2009.5949

Albritton, T., Angley, M., Gibson, C., Sipsma, H., & Kershaw, T. (2015). Mental health utilization among diverse parenting young couples. *American Journal of Community Psychology*, *56*(1/2), 89–100. doi:10.1007/s10464-015-9738-7 PMID:26163272

Alhola, P., & Polo-Kantola, P. (2007). Sleep deprivation: Impact on cognitive performance. *Neuropsychiatric Disease and Treatment*, *3*(5), 553. PMID:19300585

Allen, M. D., & Green, B. L. (2012). A multilevel analysis of consultant attributes that contribute to effective mental health consultation services. *Infant Mental Health Journal*, *33*(3), 234–245. doi:10.1002/imhj.21333

American Psychiatric Association. (1996). Opinions of the Ethics Committee on The Principles of Medical Ethics. Retrieved from http://onlinetherapy.wikispaces.com/Ethics

Amstadter, A. B., Broman-Fulks, J., Zinzow, H., Ruggiero, K. J., & Cercone, J. (2009). Internet-based interventions for traumatic stress-related mental health problems: A review and suggestion for future research. *Clinical Psychology Review*, *29*(5), 410–420. doi:10.1016/j.cpr.2009.04.001 PMID:19403215

Andersson, J., & Kjerrman, V. (2013). Patient Empowerment and User Experience in eHealth Services: A Design-Oriented Study of eHealth Services in Uppsala County Council.

Andersson, G., & Cuijpers, P. (2009, December). Internet-based and other computerized psychological treatments for adult depression: A Meta-analysis. *Cognitive Behaviour Therapy*, *38*(4), 196–205. doi:10.1080/16506070903318960 PMID:20183695

Andersson, G., Cuijpers, P., Carlbring, P., Riper, H., & Hedman, E. (2014). Guided Internet-based vs. face-to-face cognitive behavior therapy for psychiatric and somatic disorders: A systematic review and meta-analysis. *World Psychiatry; Official Journal of the World Psychiatric Association (WPA)*, *13*(3), 288–295. doi:10.1002/wps.20151 PMID:25273302

Andersson, G., Paxling, B., Wiwe, M., Vernmark, K., Felix, C. B., Lundborg, L., & Carlbring, P. et al. (2012). Therapeutic alliance in guided internet-delivered cognitive behavioural treatment of depression, generalized anxiety disorder and social anxiety disorder. *Behaviour Research and Therapy*, *50*(9), 544–550. doi:10.1016/j.brat.2012.05.003 PMID:22728647

Andersson, G., & Titov, N. (2014). Advantages and limitations of Internet-based interventions for common mental disorders. *World Psychiatry; Official Journal of the World Psychiatric Association (WPA)*, *13*(1), 4–11. doi:10.1002/wps.20083 PMID:24497236

Andrews, G., Henderson, S., & Hall, W. (2002). Prevalence, comorbidity, disability and service utilisation: Overview of the Australian National Mental Health Survey. *Yearbook of Psychiatry and Applied Mental Health*, *2002*(1), 230-231.

Andrews, G., Cuijpers, P., Craske, M. G., McEvoy, P., & Titov, N. (2010). Computer therapy for the anxiety and depressive disorders is effective, acceptable and practical health care: A meta-analysis. *PLoS ONE*, *5*(10), e13196. doi:10.1371/journal.pone.0013196 PMID:20967242

Andrews, G., & Williams, A. D. (2015). Up-scaling clinician assisted internet cognitive behavioural therapy (iCBT) for depression: A model for dissemination into primary care. *Clinical Psychology Review*, *41*, 40–48. doi:10.1016/j.cpr.2014.05.006 PMID:25043445

Anthony, K., & Goss, S. P. (2009). Guidelines for online counselling and psychotherapy (3rd ed.). Lutterworth: BACP.

Anthony, K., & Jamieson, A. (2005). Guidelines for Online Counselling and Psychotherapy (2nd ed.). BACP: Lutterworth.

Anthony, K., & Nagel, D. M. (2009). Ethical Framework for the Use of Technology in Mental Health. *Online Therapy Institute*. Retrieved from http://www.onlinetherapyinstitute.com/ethical-training/

Anthony, K., & Nagel, D. M. (2010). *Therapy Online: A Practical Guide*. London: Sage.

Anthony, K., Nagel, D. M., & Goss, S. P. (2010). *The Use of Technology in Mental Health Care: Applications, Ethics and Practice*. Springfield, IL: CC Thomas.

APA. (1997). APA Statement on Services by Telephone, Teleconferencing, and Internet. *American Psychological Association*. Retrieved from http://web.archive.org/web/20070929104840/www.apa.org/ethics/stmnt01.html

APA. (2002). Ethical Principles of Psychologists and Code of Conduct. *American Psychological Association*. Retrieved from http://web.archive.org/web/20071009031511/www.apa.org/ethics/code2002.html

Aromaa, E., Tolvanen, A., Tuulari, J., & Wahlbeck, K. (2011). Personal stigma and use of mental health services among people with depression in a general population in Finland. *BMC Psychiatry*, *11*(1), 52. doi:10.1186/1471-244X-11-52 PMID:21453504

Aronson, J. K. (2007). Compliance, concordance, adherence. *British Journal of Clinical Pharmacology*, *63*(4), 383–384. doi:10.1111/j.1365-2125.2007.02893.x PMID:17378797

Austin, J., Williams, W., Ross, L., & Hutchison, S. (2008). Five-year follow-up findings from a randomized controlled trial of cardiac rehabilitation for heart failure. *European Journal of Cardiovascular Prevention and Rehabilitation*, *15*(2), 162–167. doi:10.1097/HJR.0b013e3282f10e87 PMID:18391642

Australian Psychological Society. (2011). *Guidelines for providing psychological services and products using the internet and telecommunications technologies*. Melbourne, Australia: Australian Psychological Society.

BACP. (2010). *Ethical Framework for Good Practice in Counselling and Psychotherapy*. Lutterworth: BACP.

Bagozzi, R. P., Bergami, M., & Leone, L. (2003). Hierarchical representation of motives in goal setting. *The Journal of Applied Psychology*, *88*(5), 915–943. doi:10.1037/0021-9010.88.5.915 PMID:14516253

Bandura, A. (1986). *Social foundations of thought and action* (pp. 5–107). Englewood Cliffs, NJ: Prentice Hall.

Banti, S., Mauri, M., Oppo, A., Borri, C., Rambelli, C., Ramacciotti, D., & Cassano, G. B. et al. (2011). From the third month of pregnancy to 1 year postpartum. Prevalence, incidence, recurrence, and new onset of depression. Results from the Perinatal Depression-Research & Screening Unit study. *Comprehensive Psychiatry*, *52*(4), 343–351. doi:10.1016/j.comppsych.2010.08.003 PMID:21683171

Barak, A., Hen, L., Boniel-Nissim, M., & Shapira, N. (2008). A comprehensive review and meta-analysis of the effectiveness of Internet based psychotherapeutic interventions. *Technology in Human Services*, *26*(2-4), 109–160. doi:10.1080/15228830802094429

Barak, A., Klein, B., & Proudfoot, J. G. (2009). Defining Internet-supported therapeutic interventions. *Annals of Behavioral Medicine*, *38*(1), 4–17. doi:10.1007/s12160-009-9130-7 PMID:19787305

Barnoski, T., & Aos, S. (2004). *Outcome evaluation of Washington State's research-based programs for juvenile offenders*. Washington, DC: Washington State Institute for Public Policy.

Bathory, D. S. (2015). Behavioral health and relational dynamics. *International Journal of Applied Behavioral Economics*, *4*(2), 36–52. doi:10.4018/ijabe.2015040103

Bauer, A., Parsonage, M., Knapp, M., Iemmi, V., & Adelaja, B. (2014). *The costs of perinatal mental health problems*. London, UK: London School of Economics & Centre for Mental Health.

Baumel, A., Faber, K., Mathur, N., Kane, J. M., & Muench, F. (2017). Enlight: A Comprehensive Quality and Therapeutic Potential Evaluation Tool for Mobile and Web-Based eHealth Interventions. *Journal of Medical Internet Research*, *19*(3), e82. doi:10.2196/jmir.7270 PMID:28325712

Beattie, A., Shaw, A., Kaur, S., & Kessler, D. (2009). Primary-care patients expectations and experiences of online cognitive behavioural therapy for depression: A qualitative study. *Health Expectations*, *12*(1), 45–59. doi:10.1111/j.1369-7625.2008.00531.x PMID:19250152

Beatty, P., Reay, I., Dick, S., & Miller, J. (2011). Consumer trust in e-commerce web sites: A meta-study. [CSUR]. *ACM Computing Surveys*, *43*(3), 14. doi:10.1145/1922649.1922651

Beck, A. T., Ward, C., & Mendelson, M. (1961). Beck depression inventory (BDI). *Archives of General Psychiatry*, *4*(6), 561–571. doi:10.1001/archpsyc.1961.01710120031004 PMID:13688369

Becker, R. O., & Selden, G. (1985). *The Body Electric: Electromagnetism and the foundation of life (pp 364-p.)*. New York: Quill.

Bekker, H. L., Winterbottom, A. E., Butow, P., Dillard, A. J., Feldman-Stewart, D., Fowler, F. J., & Volk, R. J. et al. (2013). Do personal stories make patient decision aids more effective? A critical review of theory and evidence. *BMC Medical Informatics and Decision Making*, *13*(Suppl. 2), S9. doi:10.1186/1472-6947-13-S2-S9 PMID:24625283

Benbasat, I. (2010). HCI research: Future challenges and directions. *AIS Transactions on Human-Computer Interaction*, *2*(2), 1.

Benca, R. M., & Peterson, M. J. (2008). Insomnia and depression. *Sleep Medicine*, *9*, S3–S9. doi:10.1016/S1389-9457(08)70010-8 PMID:18929317

Bendelin, N., Hesser, H., Dahl, J., Carlbring, P., Nelson, K. Z., & Andersson, G. (2011). Experiences of guided Internet-based cognitive-behavioural treatment for depression: A qualitative study. *BMC Psychiatry*, *11*(1), 107. doi:10.1186/1471-244X-11-107 PMID:21718523

Bennett, A. M., Rappaport, W. H., & Skinner, F. L. (1978). Telehealth Handbook: A Guide to Telecommunications Technology for Rural health Care. Hyattsville, MD: NCHSR Publications and Information Branch.

Bergner, R. M. (1995). Promoting Constructive Modes of Self-Criticism. In Pathological Self-Criticism (pp. 107-129). Springer US. doi:10.1007/978-1-4757-2410-3_7

Bhattacherjee, A. (2002). Individual trust in online firms: Scale development and initial test. *Journal of management Information Systems*, *19*(1), 211-241.

Bickmore, T. W., & Gruber, A. (2010). Relational agents in clinical psychiatry. *Harvard Review of Psychiatry*, *18*(2), 119–130. doi:10.3109/10673221003707538 PMID:20235777

Billett, S. (2010). *The practices of learning through occupations* (pp. 59–81). Springer Netherlands. doi:10.1007/978-90-481-3939-2_4

Blase, K. A., & Fixsen, D. L. (2013). *Core intervention components: Identifying and operationalizing what makes programs work*. Washington, DC: US Department of Health and Human Services.

Bohnenkamp, J. H., Stephan, S. H., & Bobo, N. (2015). Supporting student mental health: The role of the school nurse in coordinated school mental health care. *Psychology in the Schools*, *52*(7), 714–727. doi:10.1002/pits.21851

Bonny, H. L. (1975). Music and consciousness. *Journal of Music Therapy*, *12*(3), 121–135. doi:10.1093/jmt/12.3.121

Botella, A. M., Banos, C., Zaragoza, R. M., & Guixeres, J. (2009). The Intelligent e-Therapy system: A new paradigm for telepsychology and cybertherapy. *British Journal of Guidance & Counselling*, *37*(3), 287–296. doi:10.1080/03069880902957015

Botella, C., Garcia-Palacios, A., Banos, R. M., & Quero, S. (2009). Cybertherapy: Advantages, Limitations and Ethical issues. *PsychNology Journal*, *7*(1), 77–100.

Braun, V., & Clarke, V. (2006). Using thematic analysis in psychology. *Qualitative Research in Psychology*, *3*(2), 77–101. doi:10.1191/1478088706qp063oa

Brewer, J., & Hunter, A. (1989). *Multimethod research: A synthesis of styles*. Sage Publications, Inc.

Brien, A. (1998). Professional ethics and the culture of trust. *Journal of Business Ethics*, *17*(4), 391–409. doi:10.1023/A:1005766631092

Briggs, P., Burford, B., De Angeli, A., & Lynch, P. (2002). Trust in Online advice. *Social Science Computer Review*, *20*(3), 321–332. doi:10.1177/089443930202000309

Briggs, P., de Angeli, A., & Simpson, B. (2004). Personalisation and Trust: A Reciprocal Relationship? In M. C. Karat, J. Blom, & J. Karat (Eds.), *Designing Personalized User Experiences for ECommerce*. Kluwer. doi:10.1007/1-4020-2148-8_4

Brindal, E., Freyne, J., Saunders, I., Berkovsky, S., Smith, G., & Noakes, M. (2012). Features predicting weight loss in overweight or obese participants in a web-based intervention: randomized trial. *Journal of Medical Internet Research*, *14*(6). doi:10.2196/jmir.2156

Briñol, P., & Petty, R. E. (2009). Persuasion: Insights from the self-validation hypothesis. *Advances in Experimental Social Psychology*, *41*, 69–118.

Brown, D., & Engler, J. (1980). The stages of meditation: A validation study. *Journal of Transpersonal Psychology*, *12*, 143–192.

Brudal, L. H. (2014). *Empatisk kommunikasjon: Et verktøy for menneskemøter* [Empathic communication: The missing link]. Oslo: Gyldendal Akademisk.

Brunero, S., Jeon, Y. H., & Foster, K. (2012). Mental health education programmes for generalist health professionals: An integrative review. *International Journal of Mental Health Nursing, 21*(5), 428–444. doi:10.1111/j.1447-0349.2011.00802.x PMID:22500589

Burgoon, J. K. (1982). Privacy & Communication. *Communication yearbook, 6*, 206-249.

Burke, R., Jones, J., Ho, P., & Bekelman, D. (2014). Caregivers' perceived roles in caring for patients with heart failure: What do clinicians need to know? *Journal of Cardiac Failure, 20*(10), 731–738. doi:10.1016/j.cardfail.2014.07.011 PMID:25084216

Burns, J., Blanchard, M., & Metcalf, A. (2013). Bridging the digital divide in Australia: The potential implications for the mental health of young people experiencing marginalisation. In *Digital literacy: Concepts, methodologies, tools, and applications* (pp. 772–793). Hershey, PA: IGI Global. doi:10.4018/978-1-4666-1852-7.ch040

Buysse, D. J. (2013). Insomnia. *Journal of the American Medical Association, 309*(7), 706–716. doi:10.1001/jama.2013.193 PMID:23423416

Byrne, L., Happell, B., Welch, T., & Moxham, L. J. (2013). "Things you can't learn from books": Teaching recovery from a lived experience perspective. *International Journal of Mental Health Nursing, 22*(3), 195–204. doi:10.1111/j.1447-0349.2012.00875.x PMID:23020070

Cabana, M. D., Rand, C. S., Powe, N. R., Wu, A. W., Wilson, M. H., Abboud, P.-A. C., & Rubin, H. R. (1999). Why dont physicians follow clinical practice guidelines? A framework for improvement. *Journal of the American Medical Association, 282*(15), 1458–1465. doi:10.1001/jama.282.15.1458 PMID:10535437

Cade, C. Maxwell, and Nona Coxhead. 1979. The Awakened Mind: Biofeedback and the Development of Higher States of Awareness. New York: Delacorte Press.

Cade, C. M., & Coxhead, N. (1979). *The Awakened Mind: Biofeedback and the Development of Higher States of Awareness*. New York: Delacorte Press.

Cajanding, R. J. M. (2016). The effectiveness of a nurse-led cognitive–behavioral therapy on the quality of life, self-esteem and mood among Filipino patients living with heart failure: A randomized controlled trial. *Applied Nursing Research, 31*, 86–93. doi:10.1016/j.apnr.2016.01.002 PMID:27397824

Calvo, R. A., Hussain, M. S., Milne, D., Nordbo, K., Hickie, I., & Danckwerts, P. (2016). Augmenting online mental health support services. In D. Villani, P. Cipresso, A. Gaggioli, & G. Riva (Eds.), *Integrating technology in positive psychology practice* (pp. 82–103). Hershey, PA: IGI Global. doi:10.4018/978-1-4666-9986-1.ch004

Cameron, P. S. (2014). Learning with a curve: Young women's "depression" as transformative learning. In V. Wang (Ed.), *Handbook of research on adult and community health education: Tools, trends, and methodologies* (pp. 100–122). Hershey, PA: IGI Global. doi:10.4018/978-1-4666-6260-5.ch007

Campbell, M., & Glasheen, K. (2007). Launching Into Cyberspace A Short Guide for Providing Online Support for Students. Queensland: Australian Guidance and Counselling Association. Retrieved from http://mhws.agca.com.au/onlcoun_home.php

Carels, R., Musher-Eizenman, D., Cacciapaglia, H., Pérez-Benítez, C., Christie, S., & O'Brien, W. (2004). Psychosocial functioning and physical symptoms in heart failure patients: A within-individual approach. *Journal of Psychosomatic Research*, *56*(1), 95–101. doi:10.1016/S0022-3999(03)00041-2 PMID:14987970

Cassin, S. E., Sockalingam, S., Du, C., Wnuk, S., Hawa, R., & Parikh, S. V. (2016). A pilot randomized controlled trial of telephone-based cognitive behavioural therapy for preoperative bariatric surgery patients. *Behaviour Research and Therapy*, *80*, 17–22. doi:10.1016/j.brat.2016.03.001 PMID:26990279

Chaiken, S. (1980). Heuristic versus systematic information processing and the use of source versus message cues in persuasion. *Journal of Personality and Social Psychology*, *39*(5), 752–766. doi:10.1037/0022-3514.39.5.752

Childress, C. (1999, July 23). E-mail communication to the ISMHO mailing list.

Choe, E. K., Consolvo, S., Watson, N. F., & Kientz, J. A. (2011, May). Opportunities for computing technologies to support healthy sleep behaviors. *Proceedings of the SIGCHI Conference on Human Factors in Computing Systems* (pp. 3053-3062). ACM. doi:10.1145/1978942.1979395

Christensen, H., & Griffiths, K. (2007). Reaching standards for dissemination: A case study. *Studies in Health Technology and Informatics*, *129*(Pt 1), 459–463. PMID:17911759

Cinquin, O., & Demongeot, J. (2002). Positive and negative feedback: Striking a balance between necessary antagonists. *Journal of Theoretical Biology*, *216*(2), 229–241. doi:10.1006/jtbi.2002.2544 PMID:12079373

Cogswell, J. F. (1967). *Exploratory Study of Information-processing Procedures and Computer-based Technology in Vocational Counseling, Final Report*. Santa Monica, CA: System Development Corp.

Cogswell, J. F., & Estavan, D. P. (1965). *Explorations in Computer Assisted Counselling*. Santa Monica, CA: System Development Corp.

Cohen, G., & Kerr, B. A. (1998). Computer mediated counseling: An empirical view of a new mental health treatment. *Computers in Human Services*, *15*(4), 13–26. doi:10.1300/J407v15n04_02

Coleman, J., Olsen, S., Sauter, P., Baker, D., Hodgin, M. B., Stanfield, C., & Nolan, M. T. et al. (2005). The effect of a frequently asked questions module on a pancreatic web site patient/family chat room. *Cancer Nursing*, *28*(6), 460–468. doi:10.1097/00002820-200511000-00009 PMID:16330968

Collins, E., Tranter, S., & Irvine, F. (2012). The physical health of the seriously mentally ill: An overview of the literature. *Journal of Psychiatric and Mental Health Nursing*, *19*(7), 638–646. doi:10.1111/j.1365-2850.2011.01831.x PMID:22070657

Consolvo, S., McDonald, D. W., & Landay, J. A. (2009, April). Theory-driven design strategies for technologies that support behavior change in everyday life. *Proceedings of the SIGCHI Conference on Human Factors in Computing Systems* (pp. 405-414). ACM. doi:10.1145/1518701.1518766

Cooper, G. J. (2010). Mental health management in New Zealand: The pathways model for client-based treatment. In W. Pease, M. Cooper, & R. Gururajan (Eds.), *Biomedical knowledge management: Infrastructures and processes for e-health systems* (pp. 253–266). Hershey, PA: IGI Global. doi:10.4018/978-1-60566-266-4.ch018

Corritore, C. C. L. L., Kracher, B., & Wiedenbeck, S. (2003). On-line trust: Concepts, evolving themes, a model. *International Journal of Human-Computer Studies*, *58*(6), 737–758. doi:10.1016/S1071-5819(03)00041-7

Coulter, A., & Collins, A. (2011). Making shared decision-making a reality: no decision about me, without me. *Proceedings of King's Fund '11.*

Cox, J. L., Holden, J. M., & Sagovsky, R. (1987). Detection of postnatal depression. Development of the 10-item Edinburgh Postnatal Depression Scale. *The British Journal of Psychiatry*, *150*(6), 782–786. doi:10.1192/bjp.150.6.782 PMID:3651732

Crutzen, R., Cyr, D., & de Vries, N. K. (2012). The role of user control in adherence to and knowledge gained from a website: Randomized comparison between a tunneled version and a freedom-of-choice version. *Journal of Medical Internet Research*, *14*(2), e45. doi:10.2196/jmir.1922 PMID:22532074

Cuijpers, P. (1997, June). Bibliotherapy in unipolar depression: A meta-analysis. *Journal of Behavior Therapy and Experimental Psychiatry*, *28*(2), 139–147. doi:10.1016/S0005-7916(97)00005-0 PMID:9194011

Cuijpers, P., Donker, T., Johansson, R., Mohr, D. C., van Straten, A., & Andersson, G. (2011). Self-guided psychological treatment for depressive symptoms: A meta-analysis. *PLoS ONE*, *6*(6), e21274. doi:10.1371/journal.pone.0021274 PMID:21712998

Cuijpers, P., Donker, T., van Straten, A., Li, J., & Andersson, G. (2010). Is guided self-help as effective as face-to-face psychotherapy for depression and anxiety disorders? A systematic review and meta-analysis of comparative outcome studies. *Psychological Medicine*, *40*(12), 1943–1957. doi:10.1017/S0033291710000772 PMID:20406528

Cunningham, N. R., Jagpal, A., Tran, S. T., Kashikar-Zuck, S., Goldschneider, K. R., Coghill, R. C., & Lynch-Jordan, A. M. (2016). Anxiety adversely impacts response to cognitive behavioral therapy in children with chronic pain. *The Journal of Pediatrics*, *171*, 227–233. doi:10.1016/j.jpeds.2016.01.018 PMID:26879812

Cutrona, S. L., Mazor, K. M., Vieux, S. N., Luger, T. M., Volkman, J. E., & Finney Rutten, L. J. (2015). Health Information-Seeking on Behalf of Others: Characteristics of Surrogate Seekers. *Journal of Cancer Education*, *30*(1), 12–19. doi:10.1007/s13187-014-0701-3 PMID:24989816

d'Aquili, E. (1983). The Myth-Ritual Complex: A Biogenetic Structural Analysis. Zygon, 18. doi:10.1111/j.1467-9744.1983.tb00513.x

d'Aquili, E. (1986). Myth, Ritual, and the Archetypal Hypothesis. *Zygon*, *21*(2).

Dardas, L. A., & Simmons, L. A. (2015). The stigma of mental illness in Arab families: A concept analysis. *Journal of Psychiatric and Mental Health Nursing*, *22*(9), 668–679. doi:10.1111/jpm.12237 PMID:26118332

Davis, F. D., & Yi, M. Y. (2004). Improving Computer Skill Training: Behavior Modeling, Symbolic Mental Rehearsal, and the Role of Knowledge Structures. *The Journal of Applied Psychology*, *89*(3), 509–523. doi:10.1037/0021-9010.89.3.509 PMID:15161409

de Shazer, S., & Dolan, Y. (2007). *More than miracles: The state of the art of solution-focused brief therapy*. New York, NY: Routledge.

Deacon, B., Fawzy, T., Lickel, J., & Wolitzky-Taylor, K. (2011). Cognitive defusion versus cognitive restructuring in the treatment of negative self-referential thoughts: An investigation of process and outcome. *Journal of Cognitive Psychotherapy*, *25*(3), 218–232. doi:10.1891/0889-8391.25.3.218

Del Vecchio, R., & Dundas, E. (1970). Telecommunications for mental health: prospects for the seventies and eighties. In M.M. Berger (Ed.), Videotape Techniques in Psychiatric Training and Treatment (pp. 251-257). New York: Brunner/Mazel.

DeNatale, L. M. (2013). Intersubjective experience of the infant and early childhood mental health consultant–program administrator consultee relationship. *Infant Mental Health Journal*, *34*(5), 470–482. doi:10.1002/imhj.21403

Dennis, C. L., & Chung-Lee, L. (2006). Postpartum depression help-seeking barriers and maternal treatment preferences: A qualitative systematic review. *Birth*, *33*(4), 323–331. doi:10.1111/j.1523-536X.2006.00130.x PMID:17150072

Dey, A. K. (2001). Understanding and using Context. *Pers. Ubiquit. Comput.* 5, 1, 4–7.

Diener, E., Emmons, R. A., Larsen, R. J., & Griffin, S. (1985). The satisfaction with life scale. *Journal of Personality Assessment*, *49*(1), 71–75. doi:10.1207/s15327752jpa4901_13 PMID:16367493

Dimidjian, S., & Davis, K. (2009). Newer variations of cognitive-behavioral therapy: Behavioral activation and mindfulness-based cognitive therapy. *Current Psychiatry Reports*, *11*(6), 453–458. doi:10.1007/s11920-009-0069-y PMID:19909667

Doblin, R. (1991). Pahnke's "Good Friday experiment": A long-term follow-up and methodological critique. *Journal of Transpersonal Psychology*, *23*, 1–28.

Donkin, L., & Glozier, N. (2012). Motivators and motivations to persist with online psychological interventions: A qualitative study of treatment completers. *Journal of Medical Internet Research*, *14*(3), e91. doi:10.2196/jmir.2100 PMID:22743581

Dowling, N., Thomas, N., Blair-West, S., Bousman, C., Yap, K., Smith, D. J., & Ng, C. H. (2016). Intensive residential treatment for obsessive-compulsive disorder: Outcomes and predictors of patient adherence to cognitive-behavioural therapy. *Journal of Obsessive-Compulsive and Related Disorders*, *9*, 82–89. doi:10.1016/j.jocrd.2016.04.006

Drozd, F. (2013). A web-based program for depressive symptoms and life satisfaction during pregnancy and after childbirth. Retrieved June 24, 2015, from http://www.webcitation.org/6ZWKG3j4P

Drozd, F., Lehto, T., & Oinas-Kukkonen, H. (2012). Exploring perceived persuasiveness of a behavior change support system: A structural model. In M. Bång & E. Ragnmalm (Eds.), *The 7th Conference on Persuasive Technology* (pp. 157–168). Linköping, Sweden: Springer-Verlag. doi:10.1007/978-3-642-31037-9_14

Drozd, F., Andersen, C. A., Haga, S. M., Slinning, K., & Bjørkli, C. A. (2017). User experiences and perceptions of internet interventions for depression. In S. U. Langrial & A. Sharieh (Eds.), *Web-based behavioral therapies for mental disorders* (pp. xx–xx). Hershey, PA: IGI Global.

Drozd, F., Haga, S. M., Brendryen, H., & Slinning, K. (2015). An Internet-based intervention (Mamma Mia) for postpartum depression: Mapping the development from theory to practice. *JMIR Research Protocols*, *4*(4), e120. doi:10.2196/resprot.4858 PMID:26476481

Drozd, F., Vaskinn, L., Bergsund, H. B., Haga, S. M., Slinning, K., & Bjørkli, C. A. (2016). The implementation of internet interventions for depression: A scoping review. *Journal of Medical Internet Research*, *18*(9), e236. doi:10.2196/jmir.5670 PMID:27608548

Dumit, J. (1995). Brain-mind machines and American technological dream marketing: towards an ethnography of cyborg envy. In *The cyborg handbook* (pp. 347-362).

Dwyer, T. F. (1973). Telepsychiatry: Psychiatric Consultation by Interactive Television. *The American Journal of Psychiatry*, *1308*(August), 865–869. doi:10.1176/ajp.130.8.865 PMID:4716685

Eapen, V., & Walter, A. (2016). Mind the gap: Developmental vulnerability and mental health. In R. Gopalan (Ed.), *Handbook of research on diagnosing, treating, and managing intellectual disabilities* (pp. 11–32). Hershey, PA: IGI Global. doi:10.4018/978-1-5225-0089-6.ch002

Edelman, G. M., & Tononi, G. (2000). *A Universe of Consciousness: How Matter Becomes Imagination*. Basic books.

Emotiv. (2016). 3D-Brain. Retrieved from https://emotiv.com/store/product_74.html

Entwistle, V. A., France, E. F., Wyke, S., Jepson, R., Hunt, K., Ziebland, S., & Thompson, A. (2011). How information about other people's personal experiences can help with healthcare decision-making: A qualitative study. *Patient Education and Counseling*, *85*(3), 291–298. doi:10.1016/j.pec.2011.05.014 PMID:21652162

Espie, C. A., Barrie, L. M., & Forgan, G. S. (2012). Comparative investigation of the psychophysiologic and idiopathic insomnia disorder phenotypes: Psychologic characteristics, patients' perspectives, and implications for clinical management. *Sleep*, *35*(3), 385–393. PMID:22379245

Espie, C. A., Kyle, S. D., Williams, C., Ong, J. C., Douglas, N. J., Hames, P., & Brown, J. S. (2012). A randomized, placebo-controlled trial of online cognitive behavioral therapy for chronic insomnia disorder delivered via an automated media-rich web application. *Sleep*, *35*(6), 769–781. doi:10.5665/sleep.1872 PMID:22654196

Ethicscode. (1999). Guidelines for Mental Health and Healthcare Practice Online. EthicsCode. Retrieved from http://web.archive.org/web/20070809083408/www.ethicscode.com/pages/698182/index.htm

Evans, E., Howlett, S., Kremser, T., Simpson, J., Kayess, R., & Trollor, J. (2012). Service development for intellectual disability mental health: A human rights approach. *Journal of Intellectual Disability Research*, *56*(11), 1098–1109. doi:10.1111/j.1365-2788.2012.01636.x PMID:23106753

Eysenbach, G. Powell, J., Kuss, O., & Sa, E.R. (2002). Empirical studies assessing the quality of health information for consumers on the world wide web, a systematic review. *Journal of the American Medical Association*, *287*(20), 2691-2700.

Eysenbach, G. (2000). Recent advances: Consumer health informatics. *BMJ: British Medical Journal*, *320*(7251), 1713–1716. doi:10.1136/bmj.320.7251.1713 PMID:10864552

Eysenbach, G. (2005). The law of attrition. *Journal of Medical Internet Research*, *7*(1), e11. doi:10.2196/jmir.7.1.e11 PMID:15829473

Eysenbach, G., & Köhler, C. (2002). How do consumers search for and appraise health information on the world wide web? Qualitative study using focus groups, usability tests and in-depth interviews. *BMJ (Clinical Research Ed.)*, *324*(7337), 573–577. doi:10.1136/bmj.324.7337.573 PMID:11884321

Farrell, N. R., Deacon, B. J., Dixon, L. J., & Lickel, J. J. (2013). Theory-based training strategies for modifying practitioner concerns about exposure therapy. *Journal of Anxiety Disorders*, *27*(8), 781–787. doi:10.1016/j.janxdis.2013.09.003 PMID:24210013

Farzanfar, R., Frishkopf, S., Friedman, R., & Ludena, K. (2007). Evaluating an automated mental health care system: Making meaning of human-computer interaction. *Computers in Human Behavior*, *23*(3), 1167–1182. doi:10.1016/j.chb.2004.11.015

Faubel, R., Lopez-Garcia, E., Guallar-Castillón, P., Balboa-Castillo, T., Gutiérrez-Fisac, J. L., Banegas, J. R., & Rodríguez-Artalejo, F. (2009). Sleep duration and health-related quality of life among older adults: A population-based cohort in Spain. *Sleep*, *32*(8), 1059. PMID:19725257

Fereday, J., & Muir-Cochrane, E. (2008). Demonstrating rigor using thematic analysis: A hybrid approach of inductive and deductive coding and theme development. *International Journal of Qualitative Methods*, *5*(1), 80–92.

Ferrer, J. N. (2002). *Revisioning transpersonal theory: A participatory vision of Human spirituality*. Albany, NY: State University of New York Press.

Ferrer, J. N. (2002). *Revisioning transpersonal theory: A participatory vision of human spirituality*. Suny Press.

Fetterman, D. M. (2001). Foundations of empowerment evaluation. *Sage (Atlanta, Ga.)*.

Fixsen, D. L., Naoom, S. F., Blase, K. A., Friedman, R. M., & Wallace, F. (2005). *Implementation research: A synthesis of the literature*. Tampa, FL: National Implementation Research Network, University of Florida.

Fleury, M. J., Bamvita, J. M., Farand, L., Aubé, D., Fournier, L., & Lesage, A. (2012). GP group profiles and involvement in mental health care. *Journal of Evaluation in Clinical Practice*, *18*(2), 396–403. doi:10.1111/j.1365-2753.2010.01597.x PMID:21114798

Flexihub. (2016). Flexihub software. Retrieved from http://www.flexihub.com/

Flynn, H. A., Blow, F. C., & Marcus, S. M. (2006). Rates and predictors of depression treatment among pregnant women in hospital-affiliated obstetrics practices. *General Hospital Psychiatry*, *28*(4), 289–295. doi:10.1016/j.genhosppsych.2006.04.002 PMID:16814627

Foa, E. B., Liebowitz, M. R., Kozak, M. J., Davies, S., Campeas, R., Franklin, M. E., & Tu, X. (2005). Randomized, placebo-controlled trial of exposure and ritual prevention, clomipramine, and their combination in the treatment of obsessive-compulsive disorder. *The American Journal of Psychiatry*, *162*(1), 151–161. doi:10.1176/appi.ajp.162.1.151 PMID:15625214

Fogg, B. J. (2009, April 26 - 29). A behaviour model for persuasive design. In *Proceedings of the 4th International Conference on Persuasive Technology Persuasive '09*, Claremont, CA. . ACM, New York, NY. doi:10.1145/1541948.1541999

Fogg, B. J., Kameda, T., Boyd, J., Marchall, J., Sethi, R., Sockol, M., & Trowbridge, T. (2002). Stanford-Makovsky Web Credibiltiy Study 2002: Investigating what makes Web sites credible today, A research report by the Stanford Persuasive Technology Lab & Makovsky & Company, Stanford University. Retrieved from http://www.webcredibility.org

Fogg, B. J. (2002). Persuasive technology: Using computers to change what we think and do. *Ubiquity*, *2002*(December), 5. doi:10.1145/764008.763957

Forman, E. M., Herbert, J. D., Moitra, E., Yeomans, P. D., & Geller, P. A. (2007). A randomized controlled effectiveness trial of acceptance and commitment therapy and cognitive therapy for anxiety and depression. *Behavior Modification*, *31*(6), 772–799. doi:10.1177/0145445507302202 PMID:17932235

Fox, S. (2011). The social life of health information, 2011. Pew Research Centre. Retrieved from http://pewinternet.org/~/media/Files/Reports/2011/PIP_Social_Life_of_Health_Info.pdf

Fox, S., Duggan, M., & Purcell, K. (2013). Family Caregivers are Wired for Health. Pew Internet Report. Retrieved from http://www.pewinternet.org/2013/06/20/family-caregivers-are-wired-for-health

France, E. F., Wyke, S., Ziebland, S., Entwistle, V. A., & Hunt, K. (2011). How personal experiences feature in women's accounts of use of information for decisions about antenatal diagnostic testing for foetal abnormality. *Social Science & Medicine*, *72*(5), 755–762. doi:10.1016/j.socscimed.2010.11.031 PMID:21257248

Freedland, K. E., Carney, R. M., Rich, M. W., Steinmeyer, B. C., & Rubin, E. H. (2015). Cognitive behavior therapy for depression and self-care in heart failure patients: A randomized clinical trial. *JAMA Internal Medicine*, *175*(11), 1773–1782. doi:10.1001/jamainternmed.2015.5220 PMID:26414759

Frenda, S. J., & Fenn, K. M. (2016). Sleep Less, Think Worse: The Effect of Sleep Deprivation on Working Memory. *Journal of Applied Research in Memory and Cognition*, *5*(4), 463–469. doi:10.1016/j.jarmac.2016.10.001

Fry, J. P., & Neff, R. A. (2009, April-June). Periodic Prompts and Reminders in Health Promotion and Health Behavior Interventions: Systematic Review. *Journal of Medical Internet Research*, *11*(2), e16. doi:10.2196/jmir.1138 PMID:19632970

Galatzer-Levy, I. R., & Bonanno, G. A. (2014). Optimism and death predicting the course and consequences of depression trajectories in response to heart attack. *Psychological Science*. PMID:25298294

Gaudiano, B. A., & Herbert, J. D. (2006). Acute treatment of inpatients with psychotic symptoms using Acceptance and Commitment Therapy: Pilot results. *Behaviour Research and Therapy*, *44*(3), 415–437. doi:10.1016/j.brat.2005.02.007 PMID:15893293

Gavin, N., Gaynes, B. N., Lohr, K., Meltzer-Brody, S., Gartlehner, G., & Swinson, T. (2005). Perinatal depression: A systematic review of prevalence and incidence. *Obstetrics and Gynecology*, *106*(5), 1071–1083. doi:10.1097/01.AOG.0000183597.31630.db PMID:16260528

Gefen, D., & Straub, D. (2000). The relative importance of perceived ease of use in IS adoption: A study of e-commerce adoption. *Journal of the Association for Information Systems, 1*(1). Retrieved from http://aisel.aisnet.org/jais/vol1/iss1/8

Gega, L., Smith, J., & Reynolds, S. (2013). Cognitive behaviour therapy (CBT) for depression by computer vs. therapist: Patient experiences and therapeutic processes. *Psychotherapy Research*, *23*(2), 218–231. doi:10.1080/10503307.2013.766941 PMID:23390994

Georgakopoulos, P., Chatzidimitriou, M., & Tsolaki, M. (2015). A review of interventions with assistive technologies for patients with cognitive impairment. In P. Bamidis, I. Tarnanas, L. Hadjileontiadis, & M. Tsolaki (Eds.), *Handbook of research on innovations in the diagnosis and treatment of dementia* (pp. 118–129). Hershey, PA: IGI Global. doi:10.4018/978-1-4666-8234-4.ch006

Gerhards, S. A. H., Abma, T. A., Arntz, A., de Graaf, L. E., Evers, S. M. A. A., Huibers, M. J. H., & Widdershoven, G. A. M. (2011). Improving adherence and effectiveness of computerised cognitive behavioural therapy without support for depression: A qualitative study on patient experiences. *Journal of Affective Disorders*, *129*(1-3), 117–125. doi:10.1016/j.jad.2010.09.012 PMID:20889214

Gillin, J. C. (1998). Are sleep disturbances risk factors for anxiety, depressive and addictive disorders? *Acta Psychiatrica Scandinavica*, *98*(s393), 39–43. doi:10.1111/j.1600-0447.1998.tb05965.x PMID:9777046

Gilula, M. F., & Kirsch, D. L. (2005). Cranial electrotherapy stimulation review: A safer alternative to psychopharmaceuticals in the treatment of depression. *Journal of Neurotherapy*, *9*(2), 7–26. doi:10.1300/J184v09n02_02

Goel, N., Rao, H., Durmer, J. S., & Dinges, D. F. (2009, September). Neurocognitive consequences of sleep deprivation. [). NIH Public Access.]. *Seminars in Neurology*, *29*(4), 320–339. doi:10.1055/s-0029-1237117 PMID:19742409

Goldberg, D. P., Krueger, R. F., Andrews, G., & Hobbs, M. J. (2009). Emotional disorders: Cluster 4 of the proposed meta-structure for DSM-V and ICD-11. *Psychological Medicine*, *39*(12), 2043–2059. doi:10.1017/S0033291709990298 PMID:19796429

Goleman, D., & Davidson, R. J. (1979). *Consciousness: Brain, states of consciousness, and mysticism*. New York: Harper.

Gomez, B., Grønlie, A. A., Kristiansen, D. E., & Richardsen, K. (2014). *Implementering av Tidlig innsats for barn i risiko (TIBIR): Fra teori til praksis* [Implementation of Early Initative for Children at Risk: From theory to practice]. Oslo: The Norwegian Center for Child Behavioral Development.

González-Prendes, A., & Resko, S. (2012). Cognitive-behavioral theory. In S. Ringel & J. Brandell (Eds.), *Trauma: Contemporary directions in theory, practice, and research* (pp. 14–40). Thousand Oaks, CA: Sage Publications. doi:10.4135/9781452230597.n2

Goodman, J. H. (2009). Womens attitudes, preferences, and perceived barriers to treatment for perinatal depression. *Birth*, *36*(March), 60–69. doi:10.1111/j.1523-536X.2008.00296.x PMID:19278385

Goss, S. P. (2000) *An exploratory study in aspects of the philosophy, method and application of pluralist evaluation of counselling*. Unpublished Ph.D. thesis, Strathclyde University Counselling Unit, Glasgow.

Goss, S., Anthony, K. & Nagel, D.M. (2016). *Technology in Mental Health: Applications in practice, supervision and training (2nd ed.)*. Springfield: CCThomas Publishing.

Goss, S. P., & Anthony, K. (2003). *Technology in Counselling and psychotherapy: A Practitioner's Guide*. Basingstoke, UK: Palgrave MacMillan. doi:10.1007/978-0-230-50015-0

Goss, S. P., & Anthony, K. (2008). *Uudet Teknologiat Terapiassa*. Helsinki: Edita Publishing Oy.

Goss, S. P., Anthony, K., Jamieson, A., & Palmer, S. (2001). *Guidelines for Online Counselling and Psychotherapy*. Rugby: BACP.

Goss, S. P., & Mearns, D. (1997). A call for a pluralist epistemological understanding in the assessment and evaluation of counselling. *British Journal of Guidance & Counselling*, *25*(2), 189–198. doi:10.1080/03069889708253801

Grabner-Kräuter, S. (2010). Toward A Better Understanding of Trust in WEB 2.0 Social Networks. *Marketing Theory and Applications*, *313*.

Grabner-Krauter, S., & Kaluscha, E. A. (2003). Empirical research in online-trust: A review and critical assessment. *International Journal of Human-Computer Studies*, *58*(6), 783–812. doi:10.1016/S1071-5819(03)00043-0

Graham, D., Killoran, I., & Parekh, G. (2016). Supporting students' mental health and emotional well-being in inclusive classrooms. In M. Gordon (Ed.), *Challenges surrounding the education of children with chronic diseases* (pp. 86–116). Hershey, PA: IGI Global. doi:10.4018/978-1-4666-9452-1.ch005

Gravel, K., Légaré, F., & Graham, I. D. (2006). Barriers and facilitators to implementing shared decision-making in clinical practice: A systematic review of health professionals perceptions. *Implementation Science; IS*, *1*(1), 16. doi:10.1186/1748-5908-1-16 PMID:16899124

Green, E. E., Green, A. M., & Walters, E. D. (1970). Voluntary Control of Internal States: Psychological and Physiological. Journal of Transpersonal Psychology, 2, 1-26.

Green, E., & Alyce M. (1977). *Beyond Biofeedback*. New York: Delta Books.

Greidanus, E., & Everall, R. D. (2010). Helper therapy in an online suicide prevention community. *British Journal of Guidance & Counselling*, *38*(2), 191–204. doi:10.1080/03069881003600991

Greist, J., Gustafson, D. H., Stauss, F., Rowse, M. S., Laughren, T. P., & Chiles, J. A. (1973). A computer interview for suicide-high risk prediction. *The American Journal of Psychiatry*, *130*(12), 12. doi:10.1176/ajp.130.12.1327 PMID:4585280

Greyson, B. (2000). Dissociation in People Who Have near-death experiences: Their bodies out of or out of Their minds? *Lancet*, *355*(9202), 460–463. doi:10.1016/S0140-6736(00)82013-9 PMID:10841127

Greyson, B. (2010). Implications of near-death experiences for a postmaterialist psychology. *Psychology of Religion and Spirituality*, *2*(1), 37–45. doi:10.1037/a0018548

Grinspoon, R. L., & Bakalar, J. (1997). Psychedelic drugs reconsidered (2nd ed.). New York: Lindesmith Center.

Grof, S. (1988). *The Adventure of Self-Discovery*. New York: State University of New York Press.

Grof, S. (2000). *Psychology of the Future: Lessons from modern consciousness research*. Albany, NY: State University of New York Press.

Gulliksson, M., Burell, G., Vessby, B., Lundin, L., Toss, H., & Svärdsudd, K. (2011). Randomized controlled trial of cognitive behavioral therapy vs. standard treatment to prevent recurrent cardiovascular events in patients with coronary heart disease: Secondary prevention in Uppsala primary health care project (SUPRIM). *Archives of Internal Medicine*, *171*(2), 134–140. doi:10.1001/archinternmed.2010.510 PMID:21263103

Hadjistavropoulos, H. D., Thompson, M., Ivanov, M., Drost, C., Butz, C. J., Klein, B., & Austin, D. W. (2011). Considerations in the development of a therapist-assisted internet cognitive behavior therapy service. *Professional Psychology, Research and Practice*, *42*(6), 463–471. doi:10.1037/a0026176

Hadzic, M., & Dillon, D. S. (2010). Role of multi-agents system in creation of collaborative environments within mental health domain. In R. Paranjape & A. Sadanand (Eds.), *Multi-agent systems for healthcare simulation and modeling: Applications for system improvement* (pp. 196–214). Hershey, PA: IGI Global. doi:10.4018/978-1-60566-772-0.ch011

Haga, S. M., Drozd, F., Brendryen, H., & Slinning, K. (2013). Mamma Mia: A feasibility study of a web-based intervention to reduce the risk of postpartum depression and enhance subjective well-being. *JMIR Research Protocols*, *2*(2), e29. doi:10.2196/resprot.2659 PMID:23939459

Hall, C. S., & Nordly, V. J. (1973). *A Primer of Jungian Psychology*. New York: Mentor Books.

Hall, M., Buysse, D. J., Nowell, P. D., Nofzinger, E. A., Houck, P., Reynolds, C. F. III, & Kupfer, D. J. (2000). Symptoms of stress and depression as correlates of sleep in primary insomnia. *Psychosomatic Medicine*, *62*(2), 227–230. doi:10.1097/00006842-200003000-00014 PMID:10772402

Hamari, J., Koivisto, J., & Pakkanen, T. (2014, May). Do persuasive technologies persuade?-a review of empirical studies. *Proceedings of the International Conference on Persuasive Technology* (pp. 118-136). Springer International Publishing. doi:10.1007/978-3-319-07127-5_11

Hamdan-Mansour, A. M., Al-Gamal, E., Puskar, K., Yacoub, M., & Marini, A. (2011). Mental health nursing in Jordan: An investigation into experience, work stress and organizational support. *International Journal of Mental Health Nursing*, *20*(2), 86–94. doi:10.1111/j.1447-0349.2010.00716.x PMID:21371223

Hameroff, S. R. (1994). Quantum coherence in microtubules: A neural basis for emergent consciousness? *Journal of Consciousness Studies*, *1*(1), 91–118.

Hanley, T. (2010, March). Does online counselling work? Reviewing the research into outcomes and alliances. Proceedings of the OCTIA 2010 conference, Manchester, UK.

Happell, B., Byrne, L., Platania-Phung, C., Harris, S., Bradshaw, J., & Davies, J. (2014). Lived-experience participation in nurse education: Reducing stigma and enhancing popularity. *International Journal of Mental Health Nursing*, *23*(5), 427–434. doi:10.1111/inm.12077 PMID:24898260

Happell, B., & McAllister, M. (2014). Implementing a major stream in mental health nursing: Barriers to effectiveness. *International Journal of Mental Health Nursing*, *23*(5), 435–441. doi:10.1111/inm.12075 PMID:24890753

Happell, B., Palmer, C., & Tennent, R. (2010). Mental health nurse incentive program: Contributing to positive client outcomes. *International Journal of Mental Health Nursing*, *19*(5), 331–339. doi:10.1111/j.1447-0349.2010.00679.x PMID:20887607

Happell, B., & Platania-Phung, C. (2012). Mental health placements in a general health setting: No substitute for the real thing! *Journal of Clinical Nursing*, *21*(13/14), 2026–2033. doi:10.1111/j.1365-2702.2011.04016.x PMID:22564033

Happell, B., Platania-Phung, C., & Scott, D. (2011). Placing physical activity in mental health care: A leadership role for mental health nurses. *International Journal of Mental Health Nursing*, *20*(5), 310–318. doi:10.1111/j.1447-0349.2010.00732.x PMID:21896121

Happell, B., Platania-Phung, C., & Scott, D. (2013). Mental health nurse incentive program: Facilitating physical health care for people with mental illness? *International Journal of Mental Health Nursing*, *22*(5), 399–408. doi:10.1111/inm.12006 PMID:23279365

Happell, B., Scott, D., & Platania-Phung, C. (2013). Nurse views on the cardiometabolic health nurse as an approach to improving the physical health of people with serious mental illness in Australia. *International Journal of Mental Health Nursing*, *22*(5), 418–429. doi:10.1111/j.1447-0349.2012.00892.x PMID:23211091

Hardy, C., & Sillence, E. (2015). What are women being exposed to? A review of the quality, content and ownership of websites on premenstrual dysphoric disorder (PMDD). *Women's Health Issues*. PMID:26747724

Hardy, S., & Thomas, B. (2012). Mental and physical health comordibity: Political imperatives and practice implications. *International Journal of Mental Health Nursing*, *21*(3), 289–298. doi:10.1111/j.1447-0349.2012.00823.x PMID:22533336

Harri, O.-K. (2013, August). A foundation for the study of behavior change support systems. *Personal and Ubiquitous Computing*, *17*(6), 1223–1235. doi:10.1007/s00779-012-0591-5

Harris, P. R., Sillence, E., & Briggs, P. (2009). The effect of trust-related design cues on responses to a Web-based message about the breast cancer risks from alcohol. *J. Med. Internet Res.* doi:10.2196/jmir.1097

Harris, P.R., Sillence, E., & Briggs, P. (2011). Perceived Threat and Corroboration: Key Factors That Improve a Predictive Model of Trust in Internet-based Health Information and Advice. *J. Med. Internet Res.*, *13*(3). doi:10.2196/jmir.1821

Hart, A., Henwood, F., & Wyatt, S. (2004). The role of the Internet in patient practitioner relationships: Findings from a qualitative research study. *Journal of Medical Internet Research*, *6*(3), e36. doi:10.2196/jmir.6.3.e36 PMID:15471762

Hashim, A. H., Kaur, M., Bahar, N., & Ismail, W. S. (2016). Mental health issues among family members of children with mental disability. In R. Gopalan (Ed.), *Handbook of research on diagnosing, treating, and managing intellectual disabilities* (pp. 54–81). Hershey, PA: IGI Global. doi:10.4018/978-1-5225-0089-6.ch004

Hassenzahl, M., & Tractinsky, N. (2006). User experience – a research agenda. *Behaviour & Information Technology*, *25*(2), 91–97. doi:10.1080/01449290500330331

Hatch, G. P., & Stelter, R. E. (2001). Magnetic design considerations for devices and particles used for biological high-gradient magnetic separation (HGMS) systems. *Journal of Magnetism and Magnetic Materials*, *225*(1), 262–276. doi:10.1016/S0304-8853(00)01250-6

Haug, T., Nordgreen, T., Ost, L. G., Tangen, T., Kvale, G., Hovland, O. J., & Havik, O. E. et al. (2016). Working alliance and competence as predictors of outcome in cognitive behavioral therapy for social anxiety and panic disorder in adults. *Behaviour Research and Therapy*, *77*, 40–51. doi:10.1016/j.brat.2015.12.004 PMID:26708332

Hawnser, P. E. (1997). *The Answer*. Mexico: Editorial Diana.

Hayes, S. C., Luoma, J. B., Bond, F. W., Masuda, A., & Lilles, J. (2005). Acceptance and Commitment Therapy: Model, Processes and Outcomes. *Behaviour Research and Therapy*, *44*(1), 1–25. doi:10.1016/j.brat.2005.06.006 PMID:16300724

Hayes, S. C., Strosahl, K. D., & Wilson, K. G. (1999). *Acceptance and commitment therapy: An experiential approach to behavior change*. Guilford Press.

Health and Public Policy Committee, American College of Physicians. (1985). Biofeedback for Hypertension. *Annals of Internal Medicine*, *102*(5), 709–715. doi:10.7326/0003-4819-102-5-709 PMID:3885819

Health on the Net. (1995, updated 2008) The HONcode in brief. Retrieved from http://www.hon.ch/HONcode/Pro/Conduct.html

Heffernan, K. J., Chang, S., Maclean, S. T., Callegari, E. T., Garland, S. M., Reavley, N. J., ... & Wark, J. D. (2016). Guidelines and recommendations for developing interactive eHealth apps for complex messaging in health promotion. *JMIR mHealth and uHealth, 4*(1).

Heller, S. S., Boothe, A., Keyes, A., Nagle, G., Sidell, M., & Rice, J. (2011). Implementation of a mental health consultation model and its impact on early childhood teachers' efficacy and competence. *Infant Mental Health Journal, 32*(2), 143–164. doi:10.1002/imhj.20289

Hemmeter, U. M., Hemmeter-Spernal, J., & Krieg, J. C. (2010). Sleep deprivation in depression. *Expert Review of Neurotherapeutics, 10*(7), 1101–1115. doi:10.1586/ern.10.83 PMID:20586691

Hess, D. J. (1996). Technology and alternative cancer therapies: An analysis of heterodoxy and constructivism. *Medical Anthropology Quarterly, 10*(4), 657–674. doi:10.1525/maq.1996.10.4.02a00140 PMID:8979243

Hill, A., & Roth, A. (2014). The competences required to deliver psychological therapies 'at a distance'. Lutterworth: BACP.

Hinton, L., Kurinczuk, J. J., & Ziebland, S. (2010, December). Infertility; isolation and the Internet: A qualitative interview study. *Patient Education and Counseling, 81*(3), 436–441. doi:10.1016/j.pec.2010.09.023 PMID:21036506

Hoeve, M., Colins, O. F., Mulder, E. A., Loeber, R., Stams, G. J. J. M., & Vermeiren, R. R. J. M. (2015). The association between childhood maltreatment, mental health problems, and aggression in justice-involved boys. *Aggressive Behavior, 41*(5), 488–501. doi:10.1002/ab.21586 PMID:25788428

Ho, F. Y. Y., Chan, C. S., & Tang, K. N. S. (2016). Cognitive-behavioral therapy for sleep disturbances in treating posttraumatic stress disorder symptoms: A meta-analysis of randomized controlled trials. *Clinical Psychology Review, 43*, 90–102. doi:10.1016/j.cpr.2015.09.005 PMID:26439674

Hoff, T., Straumsheim, P., Bjørkli, C. A., & Bjørklund, R. A. (2009). An external validation of two psychosocial work environment surveys - A SWOT approach. *Scandinavian Journal of Organization Psychology, 1*(1), 12–19.

Honorton, C. (1970). Tracing ESP through altered states of consciousness. Psychic Magazine, 2, 18.

Hovland, C. I., & Weiss, W. (1951). The influence of source credibility on communication effectiveness. *Public Opinion Quarterly, 15*(4), 635–650. doi:10.1086/266350

Hsiao, C. Y., Lu, H. L., & Tsai, Y. F. (2015). Factors influencing mental health nurses' attitudes towards people with mental illness. *International Journal of Mental Health Nursing, 24*(3), 272–280. doi:10.1111/inm.12129 PMID:25963120

Hu, H., & Wu, M. (2012). Scientific GOD: Michael Persinger & the GOD Experiments. *Scientific GOD Journal, 3*(10).

Hutchison, M. (1986). *Megabrain: New tools and techniques for brain growth and mind expansion*. William Morrow & Company.

International Society for Mental Health Online (ISMHO). (2000). *Suggested Principles for the Online Provision of Mental Health Services*. Retrieved from https://www.ismho.org/suggestions.asp

Iwashita, N. (2003). Negative feedback and positive evidence in task-based interaction. *Studies in Second Language Acquisition*, *25*(01), 1–36. doi:10.1017/S0272263103000019

Jaafar, W. A., & Nur, S. (2009). Applying Virtual Rehearsal Principle in Developing a Persuasive Multimedia Learning Environment (PMLE). In Visual Informatics: Bridging Research and Practice (pp. 427-435). Springer Berlin Heidelberg.

Jadad, A. R. & Gagliardi A. (1998). Rating health information on the Internet: navigating to knowledge or to Babel? *Journal of the American Medical Association*, *279*(8), 611-614.

James, N., Daniels, H., Rahman, R., McConkey, C., Derry, J., & Young, A. (2007). A study of information seeking by cancer patients and their carers. *Clinical Oncology*, *19*(5), 356–362. doi:10.1016/j.clon.2007.02.005 PMID:17399963

Jimison, H. B., Gorman, P., Woods, S., Nygren, P., Walker, M., Norris, S., & Hersh, W. (2008). *Barriers and drivers of health information technology use for the elderly, chronically ill, and underserved.* Rockville, MD: Agency for Healthcare Research and Quality.

Johansson, R., & Andersson, G. (2012). Internet-based psychological treatments for depression. *Expert Review of Neurotherapeutics*, *12*(7), 861–870. doi:10.1586/ern.12.63 PMID:22853793

Johns, M. W. (1991). A new method for measuring daytime sleepiness: The Epworth sleepiness scale. *Sleep*, *14*(6), 540–545. doi:10.1093/sleep/14.6.540 PMID:1798888

Johns, M. W. (1992). Reliability and factor analysis of the Epworth Sleepiness Scale. *Sleep*, *15*(4), 376–381. PMID:1519015

Jonas, W. B., & Levin, J. S. (Eds.). (1999). *Essentials of complementary and alternative medicine*. Philadelphia, Pa, USA: Lippincott Williams & Wilkins.

Josephson, B. D. (1962). Possible new effects in superconductive tunneling. *Physics Letters*, *1*(7), 251–253. doi:10.1016/0031-9163(62)91369-0

Jung, C. G. (1981). *The archetypes and the collective unconscious (No. 20)*. Princeton University Press.

Kahn-Greene, E. T., Killgore, D. B., Kamimori, G. H., Balkin, T. J., & Killgore, W. D. (2007). The effects of sleep deprivation on symptoms of psychopathology in healthy adults. *Sleep Medicine*, *8*(3), 215–221. doi:10.1016/j.sleep.2006.08.007 PMID:17368979

Kamiya, J. (1969). Operant monitoring of the EEG alpha rhythm and some of Its Reported effects on consciousness. In C. Tart (Ed.), *Altered States of Consciousness*. New York: John Wiley and Sons, Inc.

Kaplan, B., & Duchon, D. (1988). Combining qualitative and quantitative methods in information systems research: A case study. *Management Information Systems Quarterly*, *12*(4), 571–586. doi:10.2307/249133

Kaplan, E. H. (1997). Telepsychotherapy. Psychotherapy by telephone, videotelephone, and computer videoconferencing. *The Journal of Psychotherapy Practice and Research*, *6*, 227–237. PMID:9185068

Karppinen, P., & Oinas-Kukkonen, H. (2013, April). Three approaches to ethical considerations in the design of behavior change support systems. *Proceedings of the International Conference on Persuasive Technology* (pp. 87-98). Springer Berlin Heidelberg. doi:10.1007/978-3-642-37157-8_12

Kasemsap, K. (2017a). Analyzing the role of health information technology in global health care. In N. Wickramasinghe (Ed.), *Handbook of research on healthcare administration and management* (pp. 287–307). Hershey, PA: IGI Global. doi:10.4018/978-1-5225-0920-2.ch017

Kasemsap, K. (2017b). The fundamentals of health literacy. In N. Wickramasinghe (Ed.), *Handbook of research on healthcare administration and management* (pp. 507–527). Hershey, PA: IGI Global. doi:10.4018/978-1-5225-0920-2.ch030

Kasemsap, K. (2017c). Promoting health literacy in global health care. In N. Wickramasinghe (Ed.), *Handbook of research on healthcare administration and management* (pp. 485–506). Hershey, PA: IGI Global. doi:10.4018/978-1-5225-0920-2.ch029

Kasemsap, K. (2017d). Promoting critical thinking in the modern learning environments. In R. Batko & A. Szopa (Eds.), *Strategic imperatives and core competencies in the era of robotics and artificial intelligence* (pp. 50–80). Hershey, PA: IGI Global. doi:10.4018/978-1-5225-1656-9.ch004

Kasemsap, K. (2017e). Advocating problem-based learning and creative problem-solving skills in global education. In C. Zhou (Ed.), *Handbook of research on creative problem-solving skill development in higher education* (pp. 351–377). Hershey, PA: IGI Global. doi:10.4018/978-1-5225-0643-0.ch016

Kasemsap, K. (2017f). Investigating the roles of neuroscience and knowledge management in higher education. In S. Mukerji & P. Tripathi (Eds.), *Handbook of research on administration, policy, and leadership in higher education* (pp. 112–140). Hershey, PA: IGI Global. doi:10.4018/978-1-5225-0672-0.ch006

Kasemsap, K. (2017g). Mastering cognitive neuroscience and social neuroscience perspectives in the information age. In M. Dos Santos (Ed.), *Applying neuroscience to business practice* (pp. 82–113). Hershey, PA: IGI Global. doi:10.4018/978-1-5225-1028-4.ch005

Kashikar-Zuck, S., Ting, T. V., Arnold, L. M., Bean, J., Powers, S. W., Graham, T. B., & Lovell, D. J. et al. (2012). Cognitive behavioral therapy for the treatment of juvenile fibromyalgia: A multisite, single-blind, randomized, controlled clinical trial. *Arthritis and Rheumatism*, *64*(1), 297–305. doi:10.1002/art.30644 PMID:22108765

Kauer, S., & Reid, S. (2015). Mobile tracking for mental health and wellbeing. In Z. Yan (Ed.), *Encyclopedia of mobile phone behavior* (pp. 860–870). Hershey, PA: IGI Global. doi:10.4018/978-1-4666-8239-9.ch071

Kelders, S. M., Van Gemert-Pijnen, J. E., Werkman, A., Nijland, N., & Seydel, E. R. (2011). Effectiveness of a Web-based intervention aimed at healthy dietary and physical activity behavior: a randomized controlled trial about users and usage. *Journal of Medical Internet Research, 13*(2), e32.

Kelders, S. M., Bohlmeijer, E. T., & Van Gemert-Pijnen, J. E. (2013). Participants, usage, and use patterns of a web-based intervention for the prevention of depression within a randomized controlled trial. *Journal of Medical Internet Research, 15*(8), e172. doi:10.2196/jmir.2258 PMID:23963284

Kelders, S. M., Kok, R. N., Ossebaard, H. C., & Van Gemert-Pijnen, J. E. (2012). Persuasive system design does matter: A systematic review of adherence to web-based interventions. *Journal of Medical Internet Research, 14*(6), e152. doi:10.2196/jmir.2104 PMID:23151820

Kidd, S., Kenny, A., & McKinstry, C. (2015). The meaning of recovery in a regional mental health service: An action research study. *Journal of Advanced Nursing, 71*(1), 181–192. doi:10.1111/jan.12472 PMID:25040239

Kilner, W. J. (1965). *The human aura.* Citadel Press.

Kim, D., & Chang, H. (2007). Key functional characteristics in designing and operating health information websites for user satisfaction: An application of the extended technology acceptance model. *International Journal of Medical Informatics, 76*(11), 790–800. doi:10.1016/j.ijmedinf.2006.09.001 PMID:17049917

Kim, J., & Moon, J. (1998). Designing towards emotional usability in customer interfaces: Trustworthiness of cyber-banking system interfaces. *Interacting with Computers, 10*(1), 1–29. doi:10.1016/S0953-5438(97)00037-4

Kirlian, S. D., & Kirlian, V. (1973). *Photography by means of high-frequency currents. Galaxies of life.* New York: Interface.

Kiropoulos, L. A., Klein, B., Austin, D. W., Gilson, K., Pier, C., Mitchell, J., & Ciechomski, L. (2008). Is internet-based CBT for panic disorder and agoraphobia as effective as face-to-face CBT? *Journal of Anxiety Disorders, 22*(8), 1273–1284. doi:10.1016/j.janxdis.2008.01.008 PMID:18289829

Kleine-Budde, K., Müller, R., Kawohl, W., Bramesfeld, A., Moock, J., & Rössler, W. (2013). The cost of depression–a cost analysis from a large database. *Journal of Affective Disorders, 147*(1), 137–143. doi:10.1016/j.jad.2012.10.024 PMID:23164461

Klein, J. D., & Wilson, K. M. (2003). Delivering quality care: Adolescents discussion of health risks with their providers. *The Journal of Adolescent Health, 30*(3), 190–195. doi:10.1016/S1054-139X(01)00342-1 PMID:11869926

Knopp, J., Knowles, S., Bee, P., Lovell, K., & Bower, P. (2013). A systematic review of predictors and moderators of response to psychological therapies in OCD: Do we have enough empirical evidence to target treatment? *Clinical Psychology Review*, *33*(8), 1067–1081. doi:10.1016/j.cpr.2013.08.008 PMID:24077387

Knowles, S. E., Toms, G., Sanders, C., Bee, P., Lovell, K., Rennick-Egglestone, S., & Bower, P. et al. (2014). Qualitative meta-synthesis of user experience of computerised therapy for depression and anxiety. *PLoS ONE*, *9*(1), e84323. doi:10.1371/journal.pone.0084323 PMID:24465404

Knutson, K. L., Spiegel, K., Penev, P., & Van Cauter, E. (2007). The metabolic consequences of sleep deprivation. *Sleep Medicine Reviews*, *11*(3), 163–178. doi:10.1016/j.smrv.2007.01.002 PMID:17442599

Knutson, K. L., & Van Cauter, E. (2008). Associations between sleep loss and increased risk of obesity and diabetes. *Annals of the New York Academy of Sciences*, *1129*(1), 287–304. doi:10.1196/annals.1417.033 PMID:18591489

Kraft, P., & Yardley, L. (2009). Current issues and new directions in Psychology and Health: What is the future of digital interventions for health behaviour change?

Kraft, P., & Yardley, L. (2009). Current issues and new directions in Psychology and Health: What is the future of digital interventions for health behaviour change?.

Kraus, R., Zack, J., & Stricker, G. (2004). *Online Counseling A Handbook for Mental health professionals*. San Diego, CA: Elsevier.

Krebs, P., & Duncan, D. T. (2015). Health App Use Among US Mobile Phone Owners: A National Survey. *JMIR mHealth uHealth*, 3(4). doi: http://www.ehealthnews.eu/research/4601-national-survey-of-americans-health-app-use-shows-technology-s-promise-and-weakness10.2196/mhealth.4924 Retrieved from

Krippner, S. (2000). The epistemology and technologies of shamanic states of consciousness. *Journal of Consciousness Studies*, *7*(11-12), 93–118.

Krolikowski, A. M. (2013). The effectiveness of Internet-based mindfulness interventions for physical and mental illnesses: A narrative review. *International Journal of Cyber Behavior, Psychology and Learning*, *3*(4), 84–96. doi:10.4018/ijcbpl.2013100106

Kuonanoja, L., Langrial, S., Lappalainen, R., Lappalainen, P., & Oinas-Kukkonen, H. (2015). Treating depression with a behavior change support system without face-to-face therapy. *AIS Transactions on Human-Computer Interaction*, *7*(3), 192–210.

Kuyken, W., & Tsivrikos, D. (2009). Therapist competence, comorbidity and cognitive-behavioral therapy for depression. *Psychotherapy and Psychosomatics*, *78*(1), 42–48. doi:10.1159/000172619 PMID:19018156

LaBerge, S., & Rheingold, H. (1990). *Exploring the world of lucid dreaming*. New York: Ballantine Books.

Lago, C., Baughan, R., Copinger Binns, P., Brice, A., Caleb, R., Goss, S., & Lindeman, P. (1999). *Counselling Online...A BAC Special Report for Purchasers and Providers*. Rugby: BAC.

Langrial, S., Lehto, T., Oinas-Kukkonen, H., Harjumaa, M., & Karppinen, P. (2012, July). Native Mobile Applications For Personal Well-Being: A Persuasive Systems Design Evaluation. In PACIS (p. 93).

Langrial, S., Oinas-Kukkonen, H., Lappalainen, P., & Lappalainen, R. (2014, May). Managing depression through a behavior change support system without face-to-face therapy. *Proceedings of the International Conference on Persuasive Technology* (pp. 155-166). Springer International Publishing.

Langrial, S. (2012). From digital interventions to behavior change support systems: Understanding persuasive systems' development and evaluation process. *Proceedings of IRIS*, *2012*, 1–16.

Langrial, S., Oinas-Kukkonen, H., Lappalainen, P., & Lappalainen, R. (2014). *Influence of Persuasive reminders and Virtual Rehearsal on Information Systems for Sleep Deprivation* (p. 228). PACIS.

Langrial, S., Oinas-Kukkonen, H., & Wang, S. (2012). Design of a Web-Based Information System for Sleep Deprivation–A Trial Study. In *Exploring the Abyss of Inequalities* (pp. 41–51). Springer Berlin Heidelberg. doi:10.1007/978-3-642-32850-3_4

Lappalainen, P., Granlund, A., Siltanen, S., Ahonen, S., Vitikainen, M., Tolvanen, A., & Lappalainen, R. (2014). ACT Internet-based vs face-to-face? A randomized controlled trial of two ways to deliver Acceptance and Commitment Therapy for depressive symptoms: An 18-month follow-up. *Behaviour Research and Therapy*, *61*, 43–54. doi:10.1016/j.brat.2014.07.006 PMID:25127179

Lappalainen, P., Langrial, S., Oinas-Kukkonen, H., Tolvanen, A., & Lappalainen, R. (2015). Web-based acceptance and commitment therapy for depressive symptoms with minimal support: A randomized controlled trial. *Behavior Modification*, *39*(6), 805–834. doi:10.1177/0145445515598142 PMID:26253644

Laursen, T. M., Nordentoft, M., & Mortensen, P. B. (2014). Excess early mortality in schizophrenia. *Annual Review of Clinical Psychology*, *10*(1), 425–448. doi:10.1146/annurev-clinpsy-032813-153657 PMID:24313570

Lawrence, J. (1972). *Alpha Brain Waves*. Los Angeles: Nash Publishing.

Ledley, D. R., Marx, B. P., & Heimberg, R. G. (2011). *Making cognitive-behavioral therapy work: Clinical process for new practitioners*. New York, NY: The Guilford Press.

Lee, E.-J. (2009). I like you, but I wont listen to you: Effects of rationality on affective and Behavioral responses to computers that flatter. *International Journal of Human-Computer Studies*, *67*(8), 628–663. doi:10.1016/j.ijhcs.2009.03.003

Lehto, T., & Oinas-Kukkonen, H. (2011). Persuasive features in web-based alcohol and smoking interventions: A systematic review of the literature. *Journal of Medical Internet Research*, *13*(3), e46. doi:10.2196/jmir.1559 PMID:21795238

Lesh, T. V. (1970). Meditators Zen and the Development of Empathy in Counselors. Aldine Annual.

Lesh, T. V. (1970). Meditators Zen and the Development of Empathy in Counselors. *Journal of Humanistic Psychology*, *10*(1), 39–74. doi:10.1177/002216787001000105

Levita, L., Duhne, P. G. S., Girling, C., & Waller, G. (2016). Facets of clinician's anxiety and the delivery of cognitive behavioral therapy. *Behaviour Research and Therapy*, *77*, 157–161. doi:10.1016/j.brat.2015.12.015 PMID:26764585

Liboff, A. R. (1985). Geomagnetic cyclotron resonance in living cells. *Journal of Biological Physics*, *13*(4), 99–102. doi:10.1007/BF01878387

Likert, R. (1932). A technique for the measurement of attitudes. *Archives de Psychologie*.

Lillevoll, K. R., Wilhelmsen, M., Kolstrup, N., Høifødt, R. S., Waterloo, K., Eisemann, M., & Risør, M. B. (2013). Patients experiences of helpfulness in guided internet-based treatment for depression: Qualitative study of integrated therapeutic dimensions. *Journal of Medical Internet Research*, *15*(6), e126. doi:10.2196/jmir.2531 PMID:23786763

Lim, J., & Dinges, D. F. (2008). Sleep deprivation and vigilant attention. *Annals of the New York Academy of Sciences*, *1129*(1), 305–322. doi:10.1196/annals.1417.002 PMID:18591490

Lockton, D., Harrison, D., & Stanton, N. (2008, June 4-6). Design with intent: Persuasive technology in a wider context. *Proceedings of the 3rd International Conference on Persuasive Technology Persuasive '08*, Oulu, Finland, LNCS (V*ol. 5033*, pp. 274-278). Springer-Verlag, Berlin, Heidelberg. doi:10.1007/978-3-540-68504-3_30

Locock, L., & Brown, J. B. (2010, October). All in the same boat? Patient and carer attitudes to peer support and social comparison in Motor Neurone Disease (MND). *Social Science & Medicine*, *71*(8), 1498–1505. doi:10.1016/j.socscimed.2010.06.043 PMID:20719422

Lone, J. A., Bjørklund, R. A., Østerud, K. B., Anderssen, L. A., Hoff, T., & Bjørkli, C. A. (2014). Assessing knowledge-intensive work environment: General versus situation-specific instruments. *European Journal of Work and Organizational Psychology*, *23*(3), 469–482. doi:10.1080/1359432X.2012.750449

Lorber, J. (1978, January). Is Your Brain Really Necessary. Disease in Childhood, 53(10), 834-834.

Ludwig, A. (1966). Altered states of consciousness. *Archives of General Psychiatry*, *15*(3), 225–234. doi:10.1001/archpsyc.1966.01730150001001 PMID:5330058

Ludwig, A. (1972). Altered states of consciousness. In C. T. Tart (Ed.), *Altered states of consciousness* (pp. 11–24). New York: Doubleday.

Lynch-Jordan, A. M., Sil, S., Peugh, J., Cunningham, N., Kashikar-Zuck, S., & Goldschneider, K. R. (2014). Differential changes in functional disability and pain intensity over the course of psychological treatment for children with chronic pain. *Pain*, *155*(10), 1955–1961. doi:10.1016/j.pain.2014.06.008 PMID:24954165

Magnus, O., & Van der Holst, M. (1987). Zeta waves: A special type of slow delta waves. *Electroencephalography and Clinical Neurophysiology*, *67*(2), 140–146. doi:10.1016/0013-4694(87)90036-8 PMID:2439290

Makai, P., Perry, M., Robben, S. H., Schers, H. J., Heinen, M. M., Rikkert, M. G. O., & Melis, R. F. (2014). Evaluation of an eHealth intervention in chronic care for frail older people: Why adherence is the first target. *Journal of Medical Internet Research*, *16*(6), e156. doi:10.2196/jmir.3057 PMID:24966146

Manber, R., Edinger, J. D., Gress, J. L., San Pedro-Salcedo, M. G., Kuo, T. F., & Kalista, T. (2008). Cognitive behavioral therapy for insomnia enhances depression outcome in patients with comorbid major depressive disorder and insomnia. *sleep*, *31*(4), 489.

Marcus, M., Yasamy, M. T., van Ommeren, M., Chisholm, D., & Saxena, S. (2012). *Depression: A global public health concern*. Geneva, Switzerland: World Health Organization.

Marks, I. M., Cavanagh, K., & Gega, L. (2007). *Hands-on help: Computer-aided psychotherapy*. Psychology Press.

Marks, M., & Bowers, C. (2015). Technology and mental health. In M. Khosrow-Pour (Ed.), *Encyclopedia of information science and technology* (3rd ed., pp. 6455–6465). Hershey, PA: IGI Global. doi:10.4018/978-1-4666-5888-2.ch634

Marshall, I. N., & Zohar, D. (1997). *Who's Afraid of Schrödinger's Cat?* (p. 402). All the New Science Ideas You Need to Keep Up with the New Thinking.

Marsh, S., & Dibben, M. (2003). The role of trust in information science and technology. In B. Cronin (Ed.), *Annual Review of Information Science and Technology, 37* (pp. 465–498). Medford, NJ: Learned Information. doi:10.1002/aris.1440370111

Martin, J., & McKay, E. (2014). Mental health, post-secondary education, and information communications technology. In *Assistive technologies: Concepts, methodologies, tools, and applications* (pp. 1209–1226). Hershey, PA: IGI Global. doi:10.4018/978-1-4666-4422-9.ch063

Masters, R., & Houston, J. (1966). *The Varieties of Psychedelic Experience*. New York: Delta Books.

Masthoff, J., Langrial, S., & van Deemter, K. (2013, April). Personalizing triggers for charity actions. In *Proceedings of the International Conference on Persuasive Technology* (pp. 125-136). Springer Berlin Heidelberg. doi:10.1007/978-3-642-37157-8_16

Matthews, M., Doherty, G., Coyle, D., & Sharry, J. (2008). Designing mobile applications to support mental health interventions. In J. Lumsden (Ed.), *Handbook of research on user interface design and evaluation for mobile technology* (pp. 635–656). Hershey, PA: IGI Global. doi:10.4018/978-1-59904-871-0.ch038

Mazanderani, F., ONeill, B., & Powell, J. (2013). People power or pester power? YouTube as a forum for the generation of evidence and patient advocacy. *Patient Education and Counseling*, *93*(3), 420–425. doi:10.1016/j.pec.2013.06.006 PMID:23830239

McCloughen, A., Foster, K., Huws-Thomas, M., & Delgado, C. (2012). Physical health and wellbeing of emerging and young adults with mental illness: An integrative review of international literature. *International Journal of Mental Health Nursing*, *21*(3), 274–288. doi:10.1111/j.1447-0349.2011.00796.x PMID:22533335

McDaid, D., Knapp, M., & Raja, S. (2008). Barriers in the mind: Promoting an economic case for mental health in low- and middle-income countries. *World Psychiatry; Official Journal of the World Psychiatric Association (WPA)*, *7*(2), 79–86. doi:10.1002/j.2051-5545.2008.tb00160.x PMID:18560485

McKie, A., & Naysmith, S. (2014). Promoting critical perspectives in mental health nursing education. *Journal of Psychiatric and Mental Health Nursing*, *21*(2), 128–137. doi:10.1111/jpm.12061 PMID:23552221

McKinlay, E., Garrett, S., McBain, L., Dowell, T., Collings, S., & Stanley, J. (2011). New Zealand general practice nurses' roles in mental health care. *International Nursing Review*, *58*(2), 225–233. doi:10.1111/j.1466-7657.2010.00859.x PMID:21554297

McKnight, D. H., & Chervany, N. L. (2001). Trust and Distrust Definitions: One Bite at a Time. In R. Falcone, M. Singh, & Y.-H. Tan (Eds.), *Trust in Cybersocieties Berlin*. Springer-Verlag.

Mendenhall, A. N., & Frauenholtz, S. (2015). Predictors of mental health literacy among parents of youth diagnosed with mood disorders. *Child & Family Social Work*, *20*(3), 300–309. doi:10.1111/cfs.12078

Messer, S. B., & Wampold, B. E. (2002). Let's face facts: Common factors are more potent than specific therapy ingredients. *Clinical Psychology: Science and Practice*, *9*(1), 21–25. doi:10.1093/clipsy.9.1.21

Meyer, B., Berger, T., Caspar, F., Beevers, C., Andersson, G., & Weiss, M. (2009). Effectiveness of a novel integrative online treatment for depression (Deprexis): Randomized controlled trial. *Journal of Medical Internet Research*, *11*(2), e15. doi:10.2196/jmir.1151 PMID:19632969

Miller, N. E. (1978). Biofeedback and visceral learning. *Annual Review of Psychology*, *29*(1), 373–404. doi:10.1146/annurev.ps.29.020178.002105 PMID:341785

Miller, W. R., & Rollnick, S. (2002). *Motivational interviewing: Preparing people for change* (2nd ed.). New York: Guilford Press.

Mitrovic, A., Ohlsson, S., & Barrow, D. K. (2013). The effect of positive feedback in a constraint-based intelligent tutoring system. *Computers & Education*, *60*(1), 264–272. doi:10.1016/j.compedu.2012.07.002

Mohr, D. C., Burns, M. N., Schueller, S. M., Clarke, G., & Klinkman, M. (2013). Behavioral intervention technologies: Evidence review and recommendations for future research in mental health. *General Hospital Psychiatry*, *35*(4), 332–338. doi:10.1016/j.genhosppsych.2013.03.008 PMID:23664503

Mohr, D. C., Duffecy, J., Jin, L., Ludman, E. J., Lewis, A., Begale, M., & McCarthy, M. Jr. (2010). Multimodal e-mental health treatment for depression: A feasibility trial. *Journal of Medical Internet Research, 12*(5), e48. doi:10.2196/jmir.1370 PMID:21169164

Mohr, D. C., Schueller, S. M., Montague, E., Burns, M. N., & Rashidi, P. (2014). The behavioral intervention technology model: An integrated conceptual and technological framework for eHealth and mHealth interventions. *Journal of Medical Internet Research, 16*(6), e146. doi:10.2196/jmir.3077 PMID:24905070

Mohr, D., Cuijpers, P., & Lehman, K. (2011). Supportive accountability: A model for providing human support to enhance adherence to eHealth interventions. *Journal of Medical Internet Research, 13*(1), e30. doi:10.2196/jmir.1602 PMID:21393123

Monroe, R. (1982). *The Hemi-Sync process. Monroe Institute Bulletin.* VA: Nellysford.

Monroe, R. A. (1977). *Journeys out of the body* (Vol. 79). Main Street Books.

Mo, P. K. H., & Coulson, N. S. (2008). Exploring the communication of social support within virtual communities: A content analysis of messages posted to an online HIV/AIDS support group. *Cyberpsychology & Behavior, 11*(3), 371–374. doi:10.1089/cpb.2007.0118 PMID:18537512

Morin, C. M., Beaulieu-Bonneau, S., LeBlanc, S., & Savard, M. (2005). Self-help Treatment for Insomnia: A Randomized Controlled Trial. *Sleep*, 28. PMID:16295218

Morin, C. M., LeBlanc, M., Daley, M., Gregoire, J. P., & Merette, C. (2006). Epidemiology of insomnia: Prevalence, self-help treatments, consultations, and determinants of help-seeking behaviors. *Sleep Medicine, 7*(2), 123–130. doi:10.1016/j.sleep.2005.08.008 PMID:16459140

Morris, J., Belfer, M., Daniels, A., Flisher, A., Villé, L., Lora, A., & Saxena, S. (2011). Treated prevalence of and mental health services received by children and adolescents in 42 low-and-middle-income countries. *Journal of Child Psychology and Psychiatry, and Allied Disciplines, 52*(12), 1239–1246. doi:10.1111/j.1469-7610.2011.02409.x PMID:21554305

Moser, D., Dracup, K., Evangelista, L., Zambroski, C., Lennie, T., Chung, M., & Heo, S. et al. (2010). Comparison of prevalence of symptoms of depression, anxiety, and hostility in elderly patients with heart failure, myocardial infarction, and a coronary artery bypass graft. *Heart & Lung, 39*(5), 378–385. doi:10.1016/j.hrtlng.2009.10.017 PMID:20561849

Moul, D. E., Hall, M., Pilkonis, P. A., & Buysse, D. J. (2004). Self-report measures of insomnia in adults: Rationales, choices, and needs. *Sleep Medicine Reviews, 8*(3), 177–198. doi:10.1016/S1087-0792(03)00060-1 PMID:15144961

Murray, E. (2012). Web-based interventions for behavior change and self-management: potential, pitfalls, and progress. *Medicine 2.0, 1*(2), e3.

Murray, E., May, C., & Mair, F. (2010). Development and formative evaluation of the e-Health Implementation Toolkit (e-HIT). *BMC Medical Informatics and Decision Making, 10*(1), 61. doi:10.1186/1472-6947-10-61 PMID:20955594

Mykletun, A., Knudsen, A. K., & Mathiesen, K. S. (2009). *Psykiske lidelser i Norge: Et folkehelseperspektiv* [Mental disorders in Norway: A public health perspective]. Oslo, Norway: Norwegian Institute of Public Health.

Nagel, D. M., & Anthony, K. (2009). *Ethical Framework for the Use of Technology in Mental Health.* Retrieved from http://www.onlinetherapyinstitute.com/id43.html

Nakagawa, K. (1976). Magnetic field deficiency syndrome and magnetic treatment. *Japanese Medical Journal, 2745*, 24–32.

Nakanishi, H., Shimizu, S., & Isbister, K. (2005). Sensitizing social agents for virtual training. *Applied Artificial Intelligence, 19*(3-4), 341–361. doi:10.1080/08839510590910192

Namle, S., Ghapanchi, A. H., & Amrollahi, A. (2016). Information and communication technology for mental health: A systematic literature review. In M. Cruz-Cunha, I. Miranda, R. Martinho, & R. Rijo (Eds.), *Encyclopedia of e-health and telemedicine* (pp. 606–618). Hershey, PA: IGI Global. doi:10.4018/978-1-4666-9978-6.ch047

NBCC. (1999). Standards for the Ethical Practice of Web Counseling. Retrieved from http://www.nbcc.org/AssetManagerFiles/ethics/internetCounseling.pdf

Neuendorf, K. A. (2002). *The content analysis guidebook.* Thousand Oaks, CA: Sage Publications Inc.

Newby, J. M., Twomey, C., Li, S. S. Y., & Andrews, G. (2016). Transdiagnostic computerised cognitive behavioural therapy for depression and anxiety: A systematic review and meta-analysis. *Journal of Affective Disorders, 199*, 30–41. doi:10.1016/j.jad.2016.03.018 PMID:27060430

Newman, D., O'Reilly, P., Lee, S. H., & Kennedy, C. (2015). Mental health service users' experiences of mental health care: An integrative literature review. *Journal of Psychiatric and Mental Health Nursing, 22*(3), 171–182. doi:10.1111/jpm.12202 PMID:25707898

Niemi, H., Nevgi, A., & Virtanen, P. I. (2003). Towards self-regulation in web-based learning. *Journal of Educational Media, 28*(1), 49–71. doi:10.1080/1358165032000156437

Norwegian Directorate of Health. (2004). *Kommunenes helsefremmende og forebyggende arbeid i helsestasjons- og skolehelsetjenesten: Veileder til forskrift av 3. april 2003 nr. 450* [Municipalities health promotion and prevention in well-baby clinics and schools: Guidelines to regulations April 3, no. 450]. Oslo: Norwegian Directorate of Health.

Norwegian Directorate of Health. (2005). *Retningslinjer for svangerskapsomsorgen* [Guidelines for prenatal care]. Oslo: Norwegian Directorate of Health.

Norwegian Directorate of Health. (2009). *Nasjonale retningslinjer for diagnostisering og behandling av voksne med depresjon i primær- og spesialisthelsetjenesten* [National guidelines for diagnosis and treatment of adults with depression in primary and secondary care]. Oslo, Norway: Norwegian Directorate of Health.

Norwegian Directorate of Health. (2013). *Nytt liv og trygg barseltid for familien. Retningslinje for barselomsorgen* [A new life and a safe puerperium for the family. Guidelines for postnatal care]. Oslo: Norwegian Directorate of Health.

O'Donnell, H., & Gormley, K. (2013). Service user involvement in nurse education: Perceptions of mental health nursing students. *Journal of Psychiatric and Mental Health Nursing*, *20*(3), 193–202. doi:10.1111/j.1365-2850.2012.01917.x PMID:22533371

O'Mahen, H. A., Grieve, H., Jones, J., McGinley, J., Woodford, J., & Wilkinson, E. L. (2015). Womens experiences of factors affecting treatment engagement and adherence in internet delivered behavioural activation for postnatal depression. *Internet Interventions*, *2*(1), 84–90. doi:10.1016/j.invent.2014.11.003

OBrien, H. L. (2010). The influence of hedonic and utilitarian motivations on user engagement: The case of online shopping experiences. *Interacting with Computers*, *22*(5), 344–352. doi:10.1016/j.intcom.2010.04.001

Ohayon, M. M. (2002). Epidemiology of insomnia: What we know and what we still need to learn. *Sleep Medicine Reviews*, *6*(2), 97–111. doi:10.1053/smrv.2002.0186 PMID:12531146

Oh, H., Rizo, C., Enkin, M., Jadad, A., Powell, J., & Pagliari, C. (2005). What is eHealth (3): A systematic review of published definitions. *Journal of Medical Internet Research*, *7*(1), e1. doi:10.2196/jmir.7.1.e1 PMID:15829471

Oinas-Kukkonen, H., & Harjumaa, M. (2008, June 4-6). A Systematic Framework for Designing and Evaluating Persuasive Systems. *Proceedings of the 3rd International Conference on Persuasive Technology Persuasive '08*, Oulu, Finland, LNCS (V*ol. 5033*, pp. 164-176). Springer-Verlag, Berlin, Heidelberg. doi:10.1007/978-3-540-68504-3_15

Oinas-Kukkonen, H., & Harjumaa, M. (2009). Persuasive systems design: Key issues, process model, and system features. *Comm. Assoc. Inform. Sys.,* 24(1). Retrieved from http://aisel.aisnet.org/cais/vol24/iss1/28

Oinas-Kukkonen, H. (2010, June 7-10). Behaviour change support systems: A research model and agenda. In *Proceedings of the 5th International Conference on Persuasive Technology,* Copenhagen, Denmark, LNCS (Vol. 6137, pp. 4-14). Springer-Verlag, Berlin, Heidelberg. doi:10.1007/978-3-642-13226-1_3

Oinas-Kukkonen, H., & Harjumaa, M. (2009). Persuasive systems design: Key issues, process model, and system features. *Communications of the Association for Information Systems*, *24*(1), 28.

Okajima, I., Komada, Y., & Inoue, Y. (2011). A meta-analysis on the treatment effectiveness of cognitive behavioral therapy for primary insomnia. *Sleep and Biological Rhythms*, *9*(1), 24–34. doi:10.1111/j.1479-8425.2010.00481.x

ONeill, B., Ziebland, S., Valderas, J., & Lupiáñez-Villanueva, F. (2014). User-Generated Online Health Content: A Survey of Internet Users in the United Kingdom J Med. *Internet Research*, *16*(4), e118. doi:10.2196/jmir.3187 PMID:24784798

Ong, J. C., Ulmer, C. S., & Manber, R. (2012). Improving sleep with mindfulness and acceptance: A metacognitive model of insomnia. *Behaviour Research and Therapy*, *50*(11), 651–660. doi:10.1016/j.brat.2012.08.001 PMID:22975073

Onwuegbuzie, A. J., & Leech, N. L. (2005). On becoming a pragmatic researcher: The importance of combining quantitative and qualitative research methodologies. *International Journal of Social Research Methodology*, *8*(5), 375–387. doi:10.1080/13645570500402447

Or, C. K., Karsh, B. T., Severtson, D. J., Burke, L. J., Brown, R. L., & Brennan, P. F. (2011). Factors affecting home care patients acceptance of a web-based interactive self-management technology. *Journal of the American Medical Informatics Association*, *18*(1), 51–59. doi:10.1136/jamia.2010.007336 PMID:21131605

Ornstein, R. E. (1972). *The psychology of consciousness*. New York: WH Freeman.

Orzeł-Gryglewska, J. (2010). Consequences of sleep deprivation. *International Journal of Occupational Medicine and Environmental Health*, *23*(1), 95–114. doi:10.2478/v10001-010-0004-9 PMID:20442067

Östlund, U., Kidd, L., Wengström, Y., & Rowa-Dewar, N. (2011). Combining qualitative and quantitative research within mixed method research designs: A methodological review. *International Journal of Nursing Studies*, *48*(3), 369–383. doi:10.1016/j.ijnurstu.2010.10.005 PMID:21084086

Overland, S., Glozier, N., Krokstad, S., & Mykletun, A. (2007). Undertreatment before the award of a disability pension for mental illness: The HUNT Study. *Psychiatric Services*, *58*(11), 1479–1482. doi:10.1176/ps.2007.58.11.1479 PMID:17978260

Palagini, L., Bruno, R. M., Gemignani, A., Baglioni, C., Ghiadoni, L., & Riemann, D. (2013). Sleep loss and hypertension: A systematic review. *Current Pharmaceutical Design*, *19*(13), 2409–2419. doi:10.2174/1381612811319130009 PMID:23173590

Patel, S. R., & Hu, F. B. (2008). Sleep deprivation and obesity. *Obesity epidemiology*, 320.

Patel, S. R., Malhotra, A., Gao, X., Hu, F. B., Neuman, M. I., & Fawzi, W. W. (2012). A prospective study of sleep duration and pneumonia risk in women. *Sleep*, *35*(1), 97–101. doi:10.5665/sleep.1594 PMID:22215923

Patrick, K., Raab, F., Adams, M., Dillon, L., Zabinski, M., Rock, C., & Norman, G. et al. (2009). A text message-based intervention for weight loss: Randomized controlled trial. *Journal of Medical Internet Research*, *11*(1), e1. doi:10.2196/jmir.1100 PMID:19141433

Penfield, W., & Perot, P. (1963). The brains record of auditory and visual experience a final summary and discussion. *Brain*, *86*(4), 595–696. doi:10.1093/brain/86.4.595 PMID:14090522

Penrose, R. (1994). *Shadows of the Mind* (Vol. 4). Oxford: Oxford University Press.

Perils, M. L., & Smith, M. T. (2008). How can we make CBT-I and other BSM services widely available? *Journal of Clinical Sleep Medicine*, *4*(1), 11–13. PMID:18350955

Perkins, M. B., Jensen, P. S., Jaccard, J., Gollwitzer, P., Oettingen, G., Pappadopulos, E., & Hoagwood, K. E. (2007). Applying theory-driven approaches to understanding and modifying clinicians behavior: What do we know? *Psychiatric Services (Washington, D.C.)*, *58*(3), 342–348. doi:10.1176/ps.2007.58.3.342 PMID:17325107

Persinger, M. A. (1983). Religious and mystical experiences as artifacts of temporal lobe function: A general hypothesis. *Perceptual and Motor Skills*, *57*(3f), 1255–1262. doi:10.2466/pms.1983.57.3f.1255 PMID:6664802

Persinger, M. A., Tiller, S. G., & Koren, S. A. (2000). Experimental simulation of experience and a elicitation haunt of activity by paroxysmal electroencephalographic transcerebral complex magnetic fields: Induction of a synthetic ghost. *Perceptual and Motor Skills*, *90*(2), 659–674. doi:10.2466/pms.2000.90.2.659 PMID:10833767

Peterson, G., Aslani, P., & Williams, K. A. (2003). How do Consumers Search for and Appraise Information on Medicines On the Internet? A Qualitative Study Using Focus Groups. *Journal of Medical Internet Research*, *5*(4), e33. doi:10.2196/jmir.5.4.e33 PMID:14713661

Phua, J. (2014). The effects of similarity, parasocial identification, and source credibility in obesity public service announcements on diet and exercise self-efficacy. *J. Health Psych.*

Plaistow, J., Masson, K., Koch, D., Wilson, J., Stark, R. M., Jones, P. B., & Lennox, B. R. (2014). Young people's views of UK mental health services. *Early Intervention in Psychiatry*, *8*(1), 12–23. doi:10.1111/eip.12060 PMID:23773401

Ploderer, B., Reitberger, W., Oinas-Kukkonen, H., & van Gemert-Pijnen, J. (2014). Social interaction and reflection for behaviour change. *Personal and Ubiquitous Computing*, *18*(7), 1667–1676. doi:10.1007/s00779-014-0779-y

Pop-Eleches, C., Thirumurthy, H., Habyarimana, J. P., Zivin, J. G., Goldstein, M. P., De Walque, D., & Ngare, D. et al. (2011). Mobile phone technologies improve adherence to antiretroviral treatment in a resource-limited setting: A randomized controlled trial of text message reminders. *AIDS (London, England)*, *25*(6), 825–834. doi:10.1097/QAD.0b013e32834380c1 PMID:21252632

Portnoy, D. B., Scott-Sheldon, L. A. J., Johnson, B. T., & Carey, M. P. (2010). Computer delivered interventions for health promotion and Behavioral risk reduction: A meta-analysis of 75 randomized controlled trials. *Preventive Medicine*, *47*(1), 3–16. doi:10.1016/j.ypmed.2008.02.014 PMID:18403003

Powell, J., & Clarke, A. (2006, September). Internet information-seeking in mental health. *The British Journal of Psychiatry*, *189*(3), 273–277. doi:10.1192/bjp.bp.105.017319 PMID:16946364

Powers, M. B., Zum Vörde Sive Vörding, M. B., & Emmelkamp, P. M. (2009). Acceptance and commitment therapy: A meta-analytic review. *Psychotherapy and Psychosomatics*, *78*(2), 73–80. doi:10.1159/000190790 PMID:19142046

Prasad, B. V. (2017). *Chronic mental illness and the changing scope of intervention strategies, diagnosis, and treatment* (pp. 1–303). Hershey, PA: IGI Global. doi:10.4018/978-1-5225-0519-8

Proctor, E. K., & Rosen, A. (2007). From knowledge production to implementation: Research challenges and imperatives. *Research on Social Work Practice, 18*(4), 285–291. doi:10.1177/1049731507302263 PMID:24089591

Pugh, N. E., Hadjistavropoulos, H. D., & Fuchs, C. M. (2014). Internet therapy for postpartum depression: A case illustration of emailed therapeutic assistance. *Archives of Women's Mental Health, 17*(4), 327–337. doi:10.1007/s00737-014-0439-2 PMID:24965602

Pugh, N. E., Hadjistavropoulos, H. D., Hampton, A. J. D., Bowen, A., & Williams, J. (2015). Client experiences of guided internet cognitive behavior therapy for postpartum depression: A qualitative study. *Archives of Women's Mental Health, 18*(2), 209–219. doi:10.1007/s00737-014-0449-0 PMID:25109484

Pugh, N. E., Hadjistavropoulos, H. D., Klein, B., & Austin, D. W. (2014). A case study illustrating therapist-assisted internet cognitive behavior therapy for depression. *Cognitive and Behavioral Practice, 21*(1), 64–77. doi:10.1016/j.cbpra.2013.08.002

Purpura, S., Schwanda, V., Williams, K., Stubler, W., & Sengers, P. (2011, May). Fit4life: the design of a persuasive technology promoting healthy behavior and ideal weight. *Proceedings of the SIGCHI Conference on Human Factors in Computing Systems* (pp. 423-432). ACM. doi:10.1145/1978942.1979003

Räisänen, T., Lehto, T., & Oinas-Kukkonen, H. (2010). Practical findings from applying the PSD model for evaluating software design specifications. In *Persuasive Technology* (pp. 185–192). Springer Berlin Heidelberg. doi:10.1007/978-3-642-13226-1_19

Räsänen, P., Lappalainen, P., Muotka, J., Tolvanen, A., & Lappalainen, R. (2016). An online guided ACT intervention for enhancing the psychological wellbeing of university students: A randomized controlled clinical trial. *Behaviour Research and Therapy, 78*, 30–42. doi:10.1016/j.brat.2016.01.001 PMID:26848517

Reason, P. (1994). Co-operative inquiry, participatory action research, and action inquiry: Three approaches to participative inquiry. In N. K. Denzin & Y. S. Lincoln (Eds.), *Handbook of qualitative research* (pp. 324–339). Thousand Oaks, CA: Sage.

Reeves, B., & Nass, C. (1996). *The media equation: How people treat computers, television and new media like real people and places*. Stanford, CA: Cambridge University Press.

Reich, W. (1951). *Cosmic Superimposition: Man's Orgonotic Roots in Nature*. Wilhelm Reich Foundation.

Revere, D., & Dunbar, P. J. (2001). Review of Computer-generated Outpatient Health Behavior Interventions Clinical Encounters in Absentia. *Journal of the American Medical Informatics Association, 8*(1), 62–79. doi:10.1136/jamia.2001.0080062 PMID:11141513

Reynolds, P., & Morris, T. (2002). Intimacy as we know it? *Counselling and Psychotherapy Journal, 13*(3), 11.

Riegelsberger, J., Sasse, M. A., & McCarthy, J. (2003). Shiny happy people building trust? Photos on e-commerce websites and consumer trust. *Proceedings CHI '03*. ACM Press.

Ritterband, L. M., & Tate, D. F. (2009). The science of internet interventions.

Ritterband, L. M., & Tate, D. F. (2009). The science of internet interventions. *Annals of Behavioral Medicine*, *38*(1), 1–3. doi:10.1007/s12160-009-9132-5 PMID:19816750

Ritterband, L. M., Thorndike, F. P., Cox, D. J., Kovatchev, B. P., & Gonder-Frederick, L. A. (2009). A behavior change model for internet interventions. *Annals of Behavioral Medicine*, *38*(1), 18–27. doi:10.1007/s12160-009-9133-4 PMID:19802647

Ritterband, L. M., Thorndike, F. P., Gonder-Frederick, L. A., Magee, J. C., Bailey, E. T., Saylor, D. K., & Morin, C. M. (2009). Efficacy of an Internet-based behavioral intervention for adults with insomnia. *Archives of General Psychiatry*, *66*(7), 692. doi:10.1001/archgenpsychiatry.2009.66 PMID:19581560

Robson, D., Haddad, M., Gray, R., & Gournay, K. (2013). Mental health nursing and physical health care: A cross-sectional study of nurses' attitudes, practice, and perceived training needs for the physical health care of people with severe mental illness. *International Journal of Mental Health Nursing*, *22*(5), 409–417. doi:10.1111/j.1447-0349.2012.00883.x PMID:23066812

Robson, D., & Robson, M. (1998). Intimacy and computer communication. *British Journal of Guidance & Counselling*, *26*(1), 33–41. doi:10.1080/03069889808253836

Rogers, C. (1942). The use of electronically recorded interviews in improving psychotherapeutic techniques. *The American Journal of Orthopsychiatry*, *12*(12), 429–434. doi:10.1111/j.1939-0025.1942.tb05930.x

Rogers, E. M. (2003). *Diffusion of innovations*. New York: Free Press.

Rosenberg, S., & McDermott, F. (2016). More than pills and beds: Contemporary challenges in social work practice and mental healthcare. In *Psychology and mental health: Concepts, methodologies, tools, and applications* (pp. 1111–1128). Hershey, PA: IGI Global. doi:10.4018/978-1-5225-0159-6.ch047

Rosenthal, M. (1998). Elaborations and Digressions on Histories of the Book. Retrieved from http://www.mtbs.com/bkhist1.html

Rothschild, E. (1997). E-mail therapy [letter]. *The American Journal of Psychiatry*, *154*(10), 1476–1477. doi:10.1176/ajp.154.10.1476b PMID:9326843

Rozental, A., Boettcher, J., Andersson, G., Schmidt, B., & Carlbring, P. (2015). Negative effects of internet interventions: A qualitative content analysis of patients experiences with treatments delivered online. *Cognitive Behaviour Therapy*, *44*(3), 223–236. doi:10.1080/16506073.2015.1008033 PMID:25705924

Rozmovits, L., & Ziebland, S. (2004). What do patients with prostate or breast cancer want from an internet site? A qualitative study of information needs. *Patient Education and Counseling*, *53*(1), 57–64. doi:10.1016/S0738-3991(03)00116-2 PMID:15062905

Russell, R. J., Murphy, N., & Isham, C. J. (1993). Quantum cosmology and the laws of nature: scientific perspectives on divine action.

Sadah, S. A., Shahbazi, M., Wiley, M. T., & Hristidis, V. (2015). A Study of the Demographics of Web-Based Health-Related Social Media Users. *Journal of Medical Internet Research*, *17*(8), e194. doi:10.2196/jmir.4308 PMID:26250986

Samartzis, L., Dimopoulos, S., Tziongourou, M., & Nanas, S. (2013). Effect of psychosocial interventions on quality of life in patients with chronic heart failure: A meta-analysis of randomized controlled trials. *Journal of Cardiac Failure*, *19*(2), 125–134. doi:10.1016/j.cardfail.2012.12.004 PMID:23384638

Sanders, P. (1998). *Paper presented at the British Association for the Person Centred Approach Annual Conference.*

Schmelter-Davis, H., Anthony, K. & Nagel, D.M. (2009b). Using technology to deliver career and School Guidance services: Establishing a global and inclusive ethical framework. *Student Assistance Journal,* Winter.

Schmelter-Davis, H., Anthony, K., & Nagel, D. M. (2009a). Ethical Framework for the Use of Technology in Career and School Guidance. Retrieved from http://www.onlinetherapyinstitute.com/id51.html

Schneider, F., de Vries, H., Candel, M., van de Kar, A., & van Osch, L. (2013). Periodic email prompts to re-use an internet-delivered computer-tailored lifestyle program: Influence of prompt content and timing. *Journal of Medical Internet Research*, *15*(1), e23. doi:10.2196/jmir.2151 PMID:23363466

Schubart, J. R., Stuckey, H. L., Ganeshamoorthy, A., & Sciamanna, C. N. (2011). Chronic health conditions and internet behavioral interventions: A review of factors to enhance user engagement. *Computers, Informatics, Nursing*, *29*(2), 81–92. doi:10.1097/NCN.0b013e3182065eed PMID:21164337

Selene, G. C., Omar, C. I. F., & Silvia, A. P. (2016). Palliative care, impact of cognitive behavioral therapy to cancer patients. *Procedia: Social and Behavioral Sciences*, *217*, 1063–1070. doi:10.1016/j.sbspro.2016.02.110

Seligman, L. D., & Ollendick, T. H. (2011). Cognitive behavioral therapy for anxiety disorders in youth. *Child and Adolescent Psychiatric Clinics of North America*, *20*(2), 217–238. doi:10.1016/j.chc.2011.01.003 PMID:21440852

Shaffer, V. A., & Zikmund-Fisher, B. J. (2013). All Stories Are Not Alike A Purpose-, Content-, and Valence-Based Taxonomy of Patient Narratives in Decision Aids. *Medical Decision Making*, *33*(1), 4–13. doi:10.1177/0272989X12463266 PMID:23065418

Shakti. (2016). Shakti-Neuromagnetic signal generator. Retrieved from https://www.shaktitechnology.com/winshakti/rotating/

Sharma, D., Clune, S., & Blair, L. (2015). Radicalising the designer: Combating age-related loneliness through radical-digital interventions.

Shea, C. M., Jacobs, S. R., Esserman, D. A., Bruce, K., & Weiner, B. J. (2014). Organizational readiness for implementing change: A psychometric assessment of a new measure. *Implementation Science, 9*, 7. doi:; 10.1186/1748-5908-9-7

Sillence, E., Briggs, P. Herxheimer, A. (2004). Personal experiences matter: What patients think about hypertension information online. *He@lth Information on the Internet, 42*, 3-5.

Sillence, E., Hardy, C., & Briggs, P. (2013, May 2-5). Why don't we trust health websites that help us help each other? *Proceedings of ACM Web Science '13*, Paris. doi:10.1145/2464464.2464488

Sillence, E., Briggs, P., Harris, P. R., & Fishwick, L. (2007). How do patients evaluate and make use of online health information? *Social Science & Medicine, 64*(9), 1853–1862. doi:10.1016/j.socscimed.2007.01.012 PMID:17328998

Sillence, E., Hardy, C., Briggs, P., & Harris, P. R. (2013). How do people with asthma use Internet sites containing patient experiences? *Patient Education and Counseling, 93*(3), 439–443. doi:10.1016/j.pec.2013.01.009 PMID:23415631

Sillence, E., Hardy, C., Briggs, P., & Harris, P. R. (2015). How do carers of people with multiple sclerosis engage with websites containing the personal experiences of other carers and patients? *Health Informatics Journal*. PMID:26460102

Sillence, E., Hardy, C., Harris, P. R., & Briggs, P. (2014). Modelling Patient Engagement in Peer-to-Peer Healthcare. *Proceedings of WWW'14 Proceedings of the companion publication of the 23rd international conference on World wide web companion* (pp. 481-486). doi:10.1145/2567948.2576937

Sillence, E., Hardy, C., Medeiros, L. C., & LeJeune, J. T. (2016). Examining trust factors in online food risk information: The case of unpasteurized or raw milk. *Appetite, 99*, 200–210. doi:10.1016/j.appet.2016.01.010 PMID:26792772

Sillence, E., Harris, P. R., & Briggs, P. (2015, May). Assessing Patient Experience and Patient Preference when Designing Web Support for Smoking Cessation. *Proceedings of the 5th International Conference on Digital Health 2015* (pp. 25-26). ACM. doi:10.1145/2750511.2750516

Simpson, H. B., Foa, E. B., Liebowitz, M. R., Huppert, J. D., Cahill, S., Maher, M. J., & Campeas, R. (2013). Cognitive-behavioral therapy vs risperidone for augmenting serotonin reuptake inhibitors in obsessive-compulsive disorder: A randomized clinical trial. *JAMA Psychiatry, 70*(11), 1190–1199. doi:10.1001/jamapsychiatry.2013.1932 PMID:24026523

Simpson, H. B., Foa, E. B., Liebowitz, M. R., Ledley, D. R., Huppert, J. D., Cahill, S., & Petkova, E. (2008). A randomized, controlled trial of cognitive-behavioral therapy for augmenting pharmacotherapy in obsessive-compulsive disorder. *The American Journal of Psychiatry, 165*(5), 621–630. doi:10.1176/appi.ajp.2007.07091440 PMID:18316422

Sims, H., Sanghara, H., Hayes, D., Wandiembe, S., Finch, M., Jakobsen, H., & Kravariti, E. et al. (2012). Text message reminders of appointments: A pilot intervention at four community mental health clinics in London. *Psychiatric Services (Washington, D.C.), 63*(2), 161–168. doi:10.1176/appi.ps.201100211 PMID:22302334

Singer, J. L., & Streiner, B. F. (1966). Imaginative content in the dreams and fantasy play of blind and sighted children. *Perceptual and Motor Skills, 22*(2), 475–482. doi:10.2466/pms.1966.22.2.475

Sivertsen, B., Omvik, S., Pallesen, S., Bjorvatn, B., Havik, O. E., Kvale, G., & Nordhus, I. H. et al. (2006). Cognitive behavioral therapy vs zopiclone for treatment of chronic primary insomnia in older adults. *Journal of the American Medical Association, 295*(24), 2851–2858. doi:10.1001/jama.295.24.2851 PMID:16804151

Slack, W. V., Porter, D., Balkin, P., Kowaloff, H. B., & Slack, C. W. (1990). Computer assisted soliloquy as an approach to psychotherapy. *M.D. Computing, 7*, 37–42. PMID:2308504

Slack, W. V., & Slack, C. W. (1977). Talking to a computer about emotional problems; a comparative study. *Psychotherapy (Chicago, Ill.), 14*(2), 156–164. doi:10.1037/h0086523

Smart, J. M., & Burling, D. (2001). Radiology and the Internet: A systematic review of patient information resources. *Clinical Radiology, 56*(11), 867–870. doi:10.1053/crad.2001.0738 PMID:11603887

Smith, H. (1964). Have religious import drugs do? *The Journal of Philosophy, 61*(18), 517–530. doi:10.2307/2023494

Smith, M. T., Perlis, M. L., Park, A., Smith, M. S., Pennington, J., Giles, D. E., & Buysse, D. J. (2002). Comparative meta-analysis of pharmacotherapy and behavior therapy for persistent insomnia. *The American Journal of Psychiatry, 159*(1), 5–11. doi:10.1176/appi.ajp.159.1.5 PMID:11772681

Sofaer, S. (1999). Qualitative methods: What are they and why use them? *Health Services Research, 34*(5 Pt 2), 1101. PMID:10591275

Solow. C., Weiss, R.J., Bergen, B., & Sanborn, C.J. (1971). 24-hour psychiatric consultation via TV. *American Journal of Psychiatry, 127*(12), 1684-1687.

Staner, L. (2010). Comorbidity of insomnia and depression. *Sleep Medicine Reviews, 14*(1), 35–46. doi:10.1016/j.smrv.2009.09.003 PMID:19939713

Stanford, J., Tauber, E., Fogg, B. J., & Marable, L. (2002). Experts vs. Online Consumers: A Comparative Credibility Study of Health and Finance Web Sites. Consumer Web Watch Research Report. Retrieved from http://www.consumerwebwatch.org/news/report3_credibility research/slicebread_abstract.htm

Stanton, R., Reaburn, P., & Happell, B. (2015). Barriers to exercise prescription and participation in people with mental illness: The perspectives of nurses working in mental health. *Journal of Psychiatric and Mental Health Nursing*, *22*(6), 440–448. doi:10.1111/jpm.12205 PMID:25855247

Steele, P. (2002). Online Counselling Training. *Counselling and Psychotherapy Journal*, *13*(3), 36–37.

Stibe, A., Oinas-Kukkonen, H., & Lehto, T. (2013, January). Exploring Social Influence on Customer Engagement: A Pilot Study on the Effects of Social Learning, Social Comparison, and Normative Influence. *Proceedings of the 2013 46th Hawaii International Conference on System Sciences (HICSS)* (pp. 2735-2744). IEEE.

Stibe, A., & Oinas-Kukkonen, H. (2012, October). Exploring the Effects of Social Influence on User Behavior Targeted to Feedback Sharing. In B. White (Ed.), *Proceedings of the IADIS WWW/Internet Conference (ICWI), Madrid, Spain.*

Straus, A., & Corbin, J. (1998). Basics of qualitative research: Techniques and procedures for developing grounded theory (2nd ed.).

Strauss, A., & Corbin, J. (1990). *Basics of qualitative research* (Vol. 15). Newbury Park, CA: Sage.

Strecher, V. (2007). Internet methods for delivering behavioral and health-related interventions (eHealth). *Annual Review of Clinical Psychology*, *3*(1), 53–76. doi:10.1146/annurev.clinpsy.3.022806.091428 PMID:17716048

Ström, L., Pettersson, R., & Andersson, G. (2004). Internet-based treatment for insomnia: a controlled evaluation. *Journal of consulting and clinical psychology, 72*(1), 113.

Sutich, A. J. (1969). Some Considerations Regarding transpersonal psychology. *Journal of Transpersonal Psychology*, *1*, 11–20.

Svartvatten, N., Segerlund, M., Dennhag, I., Andersson, G., & Carlbring, P. (2015). A content analysis of client e-mails in guided internet-based cognitive behavior therapy for depression. *Internet Interventions*, *2*(2), 121–127. doi:10.1016/j.invent.2015.02.004

Takacs, B. (2005). Special education and rehabilitation: Teaching and healing with interactive graphics. *Computer Graphics and Applications, 25*(5), 40–48. doi:10.1109/MCG.2005.113 PMID:16209169

Tang, M. F., Liou, T. H., & Lin, C. C. (2010). Improving sleep quality for cancer patients: Benefits of a home-based exercise intervention. *Supportive Care in Cancer*, *18*(10), 1329–1339. doi:10.1007/s00520-009-0757-5 PMID:19834744

Tart, C. T. (1971). Scientific foundations for the study of altered states of consciousness. *Journal of Transpersonal Psychology*, *3*(1), 93–124.

Tart, C. T. (1975). *States of consciousness* (p. 206). New York: EP Dutton.

Tart, C. T. (1976). The basic nature of altered states of consciousness: A systems approach. *Journal of Transpersonal Psychology*, *8*(1), 45–64.

Tart, C. T. (1992). Science, states of consciousness, and spiritual experiences: The need for state-specific sciences. In C. T. Tart (Ed.), *Transpersonal psychologies* (pp. 9–58). New York: Harper.

Tart, C. T. (1992). *Transpersonal psychologies*. Washington, DC: American Psychological Association.

Thabrew, H., Stasiak, K., Hetrick, S. E., Wong, S., Huss, J. H., & Merry, S. N. (2017). eHealth interventions for anxiety and depression in children and adolescents with long-term physical conditions. *The Cochrane Library*.

The Ministry of Health and Care Services. (2003). *Forskrift om kommunens helsefremmende og forebyggende arbeid i helsestasjons- og skolehelsetjenesten* [Regulations to the municipalities health promotion and prevention in well-baby clinics and schools]. Oslo: The Ministry of Health and Care Services.

The National Board of Health and Wellfare. (2010). *Nationella riktlinjer för vård vid depression och ångestsyndrom 2010 - stöd för styrning och ledning* [National guidelines for care in cases of depression and anxiety disorders]. Stockholm, Sweden: The National Board of Health and Wellfare.

Thom, D. H., & Campbell, B. (1997). Patient-physician trust: An exploratory study. *The Journal of Family Practice*, *44*(2), 169–177. PMID:9040520

Thorpe, G. L., Hecker, J. E., Cavallaro, L. A., & Kulberg, G. E. (1987). Insight Versus Rehearsal in Cognitive-Behavior Therapy: A Crossover Study with Sixteen Phobics. *Behavioural Psychotherapy*, *15*(4), 319–336.

Thorpe, G. L., Hecker, J. E., Cavallaro, L. A., & Kulberg, G. E. (1987). Insight versus rehearsal in cognitive-behavior therapy: A crossover study with sixteen phobics. *Behavioural Psychotherapy*, *15*(4), 319–336. doi:10.1017/S0141347300012714

Tornell H. (2001), the quantum man.

Tørning, K., & Oinas-Kukkonen, H. (2009, April). Persuasive system design: state of the art and future directions. *Proceedings of the 4th International Conference on Persuasive Technology* (p. 30). ACM. doi:10.1145/1541948.1541989

Tully, P., Selkow, T., Bengel, J., & Rafanelli, C. (2014). A dynamic view of comorbid depression and generalized anxiety disorder symptom change in chronic heart failure: The discrete effects of cognitive behavioral therapy, exercise, and psychotropic medication. *Disability and Rehabilitation*, *1*, 1–8. PMID:24981015

Turnbull, G. K., & Ritvo, P. G. (1992). Anal sphincter biofeedback relaxation treatment for women with intractable constipation symptoms. *Diseases of the Colon and Rectum*, *35*(6), 530–536. doi:10.1007/BF02050531 PMID:1587169

Vallbona, C., & Richards, T. (1999). Evolution of magnetic therapy from alternative to traditional medicine. *Physical Medicine and Rehabilitation Clinics of North America*, *10*(3), 729–754. PMID:10516987

Valverde, R. (2011). *Principles of Human Computer Interaction Design*. Germany: Lambert Academic Publishing.

Valverde, R. (2015). a. Neurotechnology as a Tool for Inducing and Measuring Altered States of Consciousness in Transpersonal Psychotherapy. *NeuroQuantology*, *13*(4), 502–517. doi:10.14704/nq.2015.13.4.870

Valverde, R. (2015). b. Channeling as an Altered State of Consciousness in Transpersonal Psychology Therapy. *Journal of Consciousness Exploration & Research*, *6*(7), 405–416.

Valverde, R. (2015). Channeling as an Altered State of Consciousness in Transpersonal Psychology Therapy. *Journal of Consciousness Exploration & Research*, *6*(7).

Valverde, R. (2016). Possible Role of Quantum Physics in Transpersonal & Metaphysical Psychology. *Journal of Consciousness Exploration & Research*, *7*(4), 303–309.

van Ballegooijen, W., Cuijpers, P., Van Straten, A., Karyotaki, E., Andersson, G., Smit, J. H., & Riper, H. (2014). Adherence to internet-based and face-to-face cognitive behavioural therapy for depression: A meta-analysis. *PLoS ONE*, *9*(7), e100674. doi:10.1371/journal.pone.0100674 PMID:25029507

Van Der Zanden, R., Curie, K., Van Londen, M., Kramer, J., Steen, G., & Cuijpers, P. (2014). Web-based depression treatment: Associations of clients word use with adherence and outcome. *Journal of Affective Disorders*, *160*, 10–13. doi:10.1016/j.jad.2014.01.005 PMID:24709016

Van der Zee, K., Vos, M., & Luijters, K. (2009). Social identity patterns and trust in demographically diverse work teams. *Social Sciences Information. Information Sur les Sciences Sociales*, *48*(2), 175–198. doi:10.1177/0539018409102406

Van Mierlo, T., Voci, S., Lee, S., Fournier, R., & Selby, P. (2012). Superusers in Social Networks for Smoking Cessation: Analysis of Demographic Characteristics and Posting Behavior From the Canadian Cancer Societys Smokers Helpline Online and StopSmokingCenter.net. *Journal of Medical Internet Research*, *14*(3), e66. doi:10.2196/jmir.1854 PMID:22732103

van Straten, A., & Cuijpers, P. (2009). Self-help therapy for insomnia: A meta-analysis. *Sleep Medicine Reviews*, *13*(1), 61–71. doi:10.1016/j.smrv.2008.04.006 PMID:18952469

Veale, D., Naismith, I., Miles, S., Gledhill, L. J., Stewart, G., & Hodsoll, J. (2016). Outcomes for residential or inpatient intensive treatment of obsessive-compulsive disorder: A systematic review and meta-analysis. *Journal of Obsessive-Compulsive and Related Disorders*, *8*, 38–49. doi:10.1016/j.jocrd.2015.11.005

Vedder, A., Cuijpers, C., Vantsiouri, P., & Ferrari, M. Z. (2014). The law as a 'catalyst and facilitatorfor trust in e-health: Challenges and opportunities. *Law. Innovation and Technology*, *6*(2), 305–325. doi:10.5235/17579961.6.2.305

Veitch, J. A., Gifford, R., & Hine, D. W. (1991). Demand characteristics and full spectrum lighting effects on performance and mood. *Journal of Environmental Psychology*, *11*(1), 87–95. doi:10.1016/S0272-4944(05)80007-6

Vincent, N., & Lewycky, S. (2009). Logging on for better sleep: RCT of the effectiveness of online treatment for insomnia. *Sleep*, *32*(6), 807–815. PMID:19544758

Volpp, K. G., John, L. K., Troxel, A. B., Norton, L., Fassbender, J., & Loewenstein, G. (2008). Financial incentive–based approaches for weight loss: A randomized trial. *Journal of the American Medical Association*, *300*(22), 2631–2637. doi:10.1001/jama.2008.804 PMID:19066383

Wahlbeck, K. (2015). Public mental health: The time is ripe for translation of evidence into practice. *World Psychiatry; Official Journal of the World Psychiatric Association (WPA)*, *14*(1), 36–42. doi:10.1002/wps.20178 PMID:25655149

Walker, E. R., McGee, R. E., & Druss, B. G. (2015). Mortality in mental disorders and global disease burden implications: A systematic review and meta-analysis. *JAMA Psychiatry*, *72*(4), 334–341. doi:10.1001/jamapsychiatry.2014.2502 PMID:25671328

Walker, S., & McAndrew, S. (2015). The same but different: Discussing the literature regarding mental health nurses' difficulty in meeting the physical health needs of service users, regardless of differing education programmes. *Journal of Psychiatric and Mental Health Nursing*, *22*(8), 640–646. doi:10.1111/jpm.12220 PMID:26337595

Wallace, B., & Fisher, L. E. (1991). Consciousness and behavior (3rd ed.). Boston: Allyn & Bacon.

Walsh, J. K. (2004). Clinical and socioeconomic correlates of insomnia. *The Journal of Clinical Psychiatry*, *65*(8), 13–19. PMID:15153063

Walter, V. J., & Walter, W. G. (1949). The central effects of rhythmic sensory stimulation. *Electroencephalography and Clinical Neurophysiology*, *1*(1), 57–86. doi:10.1016/0013-4694(49)90164-9 PMID:18129183

Walter, W. G. (1964). Slow potential waves in the human brain associated with expectancy, attention and decision. *European Archives of Psychiatry and Clinical Neuroscience*, *206*(3), 309–322. PMID:14345314

Walter, W. G. (1964). Slow potential waves in the human brain Associated With expectancy, attention and decision. *European Archives of Psychiatry and Clinical Neuroscience*, *206*(3), 309–322. PMID:14345314

Wand, T. (2011). Real mental health promotion requires a reorientation of nursing education, practice and research. *Journal of Psychiatric and Mental Health Nursing*, *18*(2), 131–138. doi:10.1111/j.1365-2850.2010.01634.x PMID:21299725

Warmerdam, L., van Straten, A., Twisk, J., Riper, H., & Cuijpers, P. (2008). Internet-based treatment for adults with depressive symptoms: Randomized controlled trial. *Journal of Medical Internet Research*, *10*(4), e44. doi:10.2196/jmir.1094 PMID:19033149

Wartella, E., Rideout, V., Montague, H., Beaudoin-Ryan, L., & Lauricella, A. (2016). Teens, health and technology: A national survey. *Media and Communication*, *4*(3).

Waters, F., & Bucks, R. S. (2011). Neuropsychological effects of sleep loss: Implication for neuropsychologists. *Journal of the International Neuropsychological Society*, *17*(04), 571–586. doi:10.1017/S1355617711000610 PMID:21554786

Watson, D., Clark, L. A., & Tellegen, A. (1988). Development and validation of brief measures of positive and negative affect: The PANAS Scales. *Journal of Personality and Social Psychology*, *54*(6), 1063–1070. doi:10.1037/0022-3514.54.6.1063 PMID:3397865

Watson, J. B. (1916). The place of the conditioned reflex in psychology. *Psychological Review*, *23*(2), 89–116. doi:10.1037/h0070003

Webb, T. L., Joseph, J., Yardley, L., & Michie, S. (2010). Using the internet to promote health behavior change: A systematic review and meta-analysis of the impact of theoretical basis, use of behavior change techniques, and mode of delivery on efficacy. *Journal of Medical Internet Research*, *12*(1), e4. doi:10.2196/jmir.1376 PMID:20164043

Webster, J., & Ahuja, J. S. (2006). Enhancing the design of web navigation systems: The influence of user disorientation on engagement and performance. *Management Information Systems Quarterly*, *30*(3), 661–678.

Weist, M. D., Mellin, E. A., Chambers, K. L., Lever, N. A., Haber, D., & Blaber, C. (2012). Challenges to collaboration in school mental health and strategies for overcoming them. *The Journal of School Health*, *82*(2), 97–105. doi:10.1111/j.1746-1561.2011.00672.x PMID:22239135

Weizenbaum, J. (1966). ELIZA – A computer program for the study of natural language communication between man and machine. *Proceedings of Conference of Association for Computer Machinery,* New York. doi:10.1145/365153.365168

Whiteford, H. A., Degenhardt, L., Rehm, J., Baxter, A. J., Ferrari, A. J., Erskine, H. E., & Vos, T. et al. (2013). Global burden of disease attributable to mental and substance use disorders: Findings from the Global Burden of Disease Study 2010. *Lancet*, *382*(9904), 1575–1586. doi:10.1016/S0140-6736(13)61611-6 PMID:23993280

White, M. H., & Dorman, S. M. (2000). Online support for caregivers. Analysis of an Internet Alzheimer mailgroup. *Computers in Nursing*, *18*, 168–176. PMID:10939186

Wiafe, I., Nakata, K., Moran, S., & Gulliver, S. (2011). Considering user attitude and behaviour in persuasive systems design: The 3D-RAB MODEL. Proceedings of ECIS '11. Retrieved from http://aisel.aisnet.org/ecis2011/186

Wiederhold, B. K., & Wiederhold, M. D. (2004). The future of Cybertherapy: Improved options with advanced technologies.

Wilber, K. (1980). Psychologia Perennis: The Spectrum of Consciousness. Walsh and Vaughan.

Wilber, K. (1975). Psychologia Perennis: The Spectrum of Consciousness. *Journal of Transpersonal Psychology*, *7*(2), 105–132.

Wilhelmsen, M., Lillevoll, K. R., Risør, M. B., Høifødt, R. S., Johansen, M.-L., Waterloo, K., & Kolstrup, N. et al. (2013). Motivation to persist with internet-based cognitive behavioural treatment using blended care: A qualitative study. *BMC Psychiatry*, *13*(1), 296. doi:10.1186/1471-244X-13-296 PMID:24199672

Wilson, R. L., & Usher, K. (2015). Rural nurses: A convenient co-location strategy for the rural mental health care of young people. *Journal of Clinical Nursing*, *24*(17/18), 2638–2648. doi:10.1111/jocn.12882 PMID:26098196

Wisner, K. L., Sit, D. K. Y., Mcshea, M. C., Rizzo, D. M., Zoretich, R. A., Hughes, C. L., & Hanusa, B. H. et al. (2013). Onset timing, thoughts of self-harm, and diagnoses in postpartum women with screen-positive depression findings. *Journal of American Medical Association Psychiatry*, *70*(5), 490–498. doi:10.1001/jamapsychiatry.2013.87.Onset

Wood, M., Daly, J., Miller, J., & Roper, M. (1999). Multi-method research: An empirical investigation of object-oriented technology. *Journal of Systems and Software*, *48*(1), 13–26. doi:10.1016/S0164-1212(99)00042-4

World Health Organization. (2009). *Global health risks: Mortality and burden of disease attributable to selected major risks*. Geneva, Switzerland: World Health Organization; doi:10.2471/BLT.09.070565

World Health Organization. (2010). Depression. Retrieved February 19, 2016, from http://www.who.int/mental_health/management/depression/en/

Wyatt Kaminski, J., Valle, L. A., Filene, J. H., & Boyle, C. L. (2008). A meta-analytic review of components associated with parent training program effectiveness. *Journal of Abnormal Child Psychology*, *36*(4), 567–589. doi:10.1007/s10802-007-9201-9 PMID:18205039

Wyatt, J. C. (1997). Measuring quality and impact of the World Wide Web. *British Medical Journal*, *314*(7098), 1879–1881. doi:10.1136/bmj.314.7098.1879 PMID:9224133

Wynaden, D. (2010). There is no health without mental health: Are we educating Australian nurses to care for the health consumer of the 21st century? *International Journal of Mental Health Nursing*, *19*(3), 203–209. doi:10.1111/j.1447-0349.2010.00671.x PMID:20550644

Yazici, E., Kirkan, T. S., Aslan, P. A., Aydin, N., & Yazici, A. B. (2015). Untreated depression in the first trimester of pregnancy leads to postpartum depression : High rates from a natural follow-up study. *Neuropsychiatric Disease and Treatment*, *11*, 405–411. doi:10.2147/NDT.S77194 PMID:25737636

Ybarra, M. L., & Eaton, W. W. (2005). Internet-based mental health interventions. *Mental Health Services Research*, *7*(2), 75–87. doi:10.1007/s11020-005-3779-8 PMID:15974154

Yetim, F. (2011). A set of critical heuristics for value sensitive designers and users of persuasive systems.

Zachariae, R., Lyby, M. S., Ritterband, L. M., & O'Toole, M. S. (2016). Efficacy of Internet-delivered cognitive-behavioral therapy for insomnia: A systematic review and meta-analysis of randomized controlled trials. *Sleep Medicine Reviews*, *30*, 1–10. doi:10.1016/j.smrv.2015.10.004 PMID:26615572

Ziebland S, Powell J, Briggs P, Jenkinson C, Wyke S, Sillence E, et al. (2016). Examining the role of patient's experiences as a resource for choice and decision-making in health care: a creative, interdisciplinary mixed-method study in digital health. *Programme Grants Appl. Res.*, *4*(17).

Ziebland, S., Chapple, A., Dumelow, C., Evans, J., Prinjha, S., & Rozmovits, L. (2004). How the internet affects patients experience of cancer: A qualitative study. *British Medical Journal*, *328*(7439), 564. doi:10.1136/bmj.328.7439.564 PMID:15001506

Ziebland, S., & Wyke, S. (2012). Health and illness in a connected world: How might sharing experiences on the Internet affect people's health? *The Milbank Quarterly*, *90*(2), 219–249. doi:10.1111/j.1468-0009.2012.00662.x PMID:22709387

Ziller, E. C., Anderson, N. J., & Coburn, A. F. (2010). Access to rural mental health services: Service use and out-of-pocket costs. *The Journal of Rural Health*, *26*(3), 214–224. doi:10.1111/j.1748-0361.2010.00291.x PMID:20633089

About the Contributors

Sitwat Usman Langrial, Ph. D in Health Information Systems, is currently working as the Assistant Dean for Academic & Research Affairs at Sur University College, Sultanate of Oman. He has authored over 20 peer reviewed scientific articles and book chapters. His primary research interests include Behavior Change Interventions, Persuasive Information Systems, Acceptance & Commitment Therapy, eHealth Interventions and Information Systems for Mental Health Care.

* * *

Caroline Emilie Andersen, MPhil, graduated from the University of Oslo with a master's degree in health and social psychology. In her thesis, she interviewed Mamma Mia users about their experiences with the program. She is currently working as an environmental therapist, but aspires towards a career in research. Her main interests include early intervention for women and families at risk.

Kate Anthony, MSc, FBACP is a psychotherapist, consultant and international expert regarding online therapy and the impact of technology on mental health. She is co-founder of The Online Therapy Institute, She is widely published on such topics as the use of email, bulletin boards, IRC, videoconferencing, stand-alone software and more radical innovative use of technology within therapeutic practice, such as virtual reality. She co-edited *Technology in Counselling and Psychotherapy: A Practitioner's Guide* with Stephen Goss in 2003, co-authored *Therapy Online [a practical guide]* with DeeAnna Merz Nagel in 2010, co-edited 2 editions of *The Use of Technology in Mental Health: Applications, Ethics and Practice* with both Goss and Nagel, and co-authored all three editions of the British Association for Counselling and Psychotherapy's *Guidelines for Online Counselling and Psychotherapy*. Her doctorate on technology and therapy with Metanoia Institute was completed in 2010.

Cato Alexander Bjørkli, PhD, is an Associate Professor at the Department of Psychology, University of Oslo with specialization in human factors and man-machine interaction. He has published a number of articles in man-machine interaction and has contributed to the development of new methods for intervention research and organizational development (i.e., modified-SWOT).

Pam Briggs holds a Research Chair at Northumbria University, where she explores identity, trust, privacy, and security and inclusion issues in social media. Her current projects address trust issues in peer-to-peer health care, the influence of social media in message dissemination during pandemics, location-based services and technologies, and cybersecurity identity management and digital personhood.

Filip Drozd, PhD, is a researcher at the National Centre for Infant Mental Health. In the last decade, he has developed and studied web-based interventions and is interested in the youngest children and their parents' mental health. In his research, he is concerned with the implementation of interventions for sustainable changes in practice, and is involved in several research projects (e.g., Mamma Mia, Newborn Behavioral Observation, and Marte Meo).

Stephen Goss, PhD, MBACP, BA (Hons) began working in mental health care over 25 years ago and carried out some of the first developmental work on the use of technology in counselling in the UK in the early 1990s. He is Principal Lecturer on the DPsych (Professional Studies) programme at the Metanoia Institute, Middlesex University, London and also works as an independent consultant in counselling and support service development, mental health technology, research and evaluation in the UK and worldwide. Author of over 70 public items, including the BACP guidelines on the ethics of online counselling and psychotherapy, his books include *The Use of Technology in Mental Health: Applications, Ethics and Practice*, edited with Kate Anthony and DeeAnna Merz Nagel and published by CC Thomas in 2010 as well as *Technology in Counselling and Psychotherapy A Practitioner's Guide*, edited with Kate Anthony and published by Palgrave MacMillan in 2003 and *Evidence Based Practice in Counselling and Psychotherapy*, edited with Nancy Rowland and published by Routledge in 2000.

Silje Marie Haga, PhD, is a researcher at the National Network for Infant Mental Health. She is the Principal Investigator of the intervention trial on Mamma Mia and is involved in several projects such as Newborn Behavioral Observation and Assessment tools in primary care. Her main interests include preventive interventions and how these may be implemented to promote mental health in children, women, and their partners.

Peter Harris holds a Research chair at Sussex University. He is a social and health psychologist and his principal research interests lie in the cognitive, emotional and behavioural response to risk, especially health risks. Recent projects focus on using self-affirming to encourage less defensive responding to risk information and the impact of this on subsequent behavior.

Kijpokin Kasemsap received his BEng degree in Mechanical Engineering from King Mongkut's University of Technology, Thonburi, his MBA degree from Ramkhamhaeng University, and his DBA degree in Human Resource Management from Suan Sunandha Rajabhat University. Dr. Kasemsap is a Special Lecturer in the Faculty of Management Sciences, Suan Sunandha Rajabhat University, based in Bangkok, Thailand. Dr. Kasemsap is a Member of the International Economics Development and Research Center (IEDRC), the International Foundation for Research and Development (IFRD), and the International Innovative Scientific and Research Organization (IISRO). Dr. Kasemsap serves on an International Advisory Board for International Journal of Productivity Management and Assessment Technologies (IJPMAT), International Journal of ICT Research in Africa and the Middle East (IJICTRAME), International Journal of Knowledge Society Research (IJKSR), International Journal of Virtual and Personal Learning Environments (IJVPLE), Journal of Cases on Information Technology (JCIT), International Journal of Virtual Communities and Social Networking (IJVCSN), International Journal of Handheld Computing Research (IJHCR), and International Journal of Knowledge Management (IJKM). Dr. Kasemsap is the sole author of over 250 peer-reviewed international publications and book chapters on business, education, and information technology. Dr. Kasemsap is included in the TOP 100 Professionals–2016 and in the 10th edition of 2000 Outstanding Intellectuals of the 21st Century by the International Biographical Centre, Cambridge, England.

Päivi Lappalainen, Ph.D. in Clinical Psychology, is currently working as a Post Doctoral Researcher at the Department of Psychology at the University of Jyväskylä, Finland. She is authored over 20 scientific articles and books. Her primary research interests include Acceptance and Commitment Therapy, in particular web and mobile interventions for depression, sleep and general well-being. She also has several years of experience in the field of Higher Education and web-based learning.

Raimo Lappalainen, Ph.D. in Clinical Psychology, professor in Clinical Psychology and Psychotherapy at the Department of Psychology, University of Jyväskylä, Finland. He is a licensed psychologist and psychotherapist. He has over 25 years of experience of Cognitive Behavioral Therapies (CBT) with expertise especially in the third wave CBT, Acceptance and Commitment Therapy (ACT). He has authored more than 100 scientific articles and books. His current research interests include Acceptance and Commitment Therapy, *Web/Mobile-based interventions* and brief psychological interventions.

Harri Oinas-Kukkonen, Ph. D is a professor in Information Systems at the Faculty of Information and Electrical Engineering at Oulu University, Finland. His research interests include Human Computer Interaction, User Behavior, Behavior Change, Persuasive Design and the next generation of the Web. More recently, he has co-authored a book titled, "Humanizing the Web: Change and Social Innovation"(Palgrave MacMillan, 2013).

Elizabeth Sillence is a Senior Lecturer in Psychology at Northumbria University, UK, and a founding member of the PaCT Lab (http://www.pactlab.org.uk/). Her research investigates trust, social exchange, and decision making within e-health environments https://www.northumbria.ac.uk/about-us/our-staff/s/liz-sillence/.

Kari Slinning, PhD, is the Director of Research at the National Centre for Infant Mental Health. She has an active role in several projects, some of which include Mamma Mia, Circle of Security, and Assessment tools in primary care. Her main interests are early intervention, attachment, and the importance of early risk factors for child development. She also has a longstanding clinical experience working with infants and at-risk families.

Raul Valverde is a Senior Lecturer in Supply Chain and Business Technology Management at Concordia University. He holds a Doctorate in Information Systems from the University of Southern Queensland, PhD in Counseling from Open International University, Post MBA from McGill University, MSc in Accounting & Financial Management from the University of the West of England, Master of Logistics and Supply Chain Management from Camilos Jose Cela University, MEng in Electrical & Computer Engineering from Concordia University and a BSc in Management Mathematics and Computer Technologies from Excelsior College of the University of the State of New York. Dr Valverde's main research interests include IT and Finance in Supply Chain, IT in Finance, Project Cost Management, Risk in IT and Supply Chain, NeuroQuantology and NeuroIS.

Index

A

Acceptance and Commitment Therapy 53, 57, 111, 114, 116-117, 128, 137
act 9, 53, 57-58, 60, 114, 116-117, 128, 137, 151, 156, 162, 189, 195, 221, 246-247
adherence 6-7, 28-31, 33-34, 42-44, 56-57, 59, 112, 117-119, 220
Adolescence 4
adulthood 1, 3
altered states of consciousness 139-142, 144, 159-161, 164-165, 168, 172-173, 185, 187, 192-195, 200-203, 205, 207
and treatment 3
anxiety 1, 3, 6-7, 9, 25, 29, 55, 58, 112, 115, 117, 154, 188, 221-222

B

behavior 2-3, 5, 10, 25, 28-29, 40, 51, 53, 55-58, 61-62, 80, 84, 91, 102, 112-114, 117-118, 150, 161-162, 194, 196
Behavior Change Support Systems 112
biofeedback 139-142, 144, 149-150, 160, 168, 172-173, 186-188, 191, 193, 201, 206-207

C

CBT 1-3, 6-10, 29-30, 33, 45, 114-117, 128, 137
clinical guidelines 79, 81, 90, 96
Cognition 25
Cognitive Behavioral Therapy 1, 3, 6-8, 25, 51, 56, 114
Core Component 110
counselling 212-225, 227, 231, 234
credibility 39, 44, 46, 61, 247-249

D

depression 1, 3, 6-7, 9, 26-29, 31-34, 36-37, 39, 41-43, 45-46, 51, 54-56, 63-64, 79-83, 97, 105, 110-112, 114-118, 120, 122, 127-128, 137, 154-155, 188, 203
digital interventions 113

E

e-health 69, 118, 241-242, 245, 247-248, 251-252
eHealth interventions 53-59, 61, 63, 69, 111-117, 119, 125, 127-129, 137-138
ethics 212, 216, 219-220, 225, 233

G

guidance 29-30, 83-84, 90, 119, 212-221, 223-226, 231-234, 251
guided intervention 33, 82, 110
guidelines 28, 58, 79-85, 90-91, 96, 110, 212-213, 216-234, 241-242, 251

I

implementation 79-88, 90-91, 93, 95-96, 110
insomnia 1, 3, 7-9, 26, 54-55, 67, 115, 117,

156, 188
integration 3, 61, 101, 147, 199, 251-252
internet 2, 5, 27-34, 38, 42-45, 51-52, 57, 59, 62, 68, 79-82, 85, 95, 97-100, 110, 116, 120, 139-142, 152, 158, 168, 173, 186-187, 205, 207, 213-217, 220, 223, 225-227, 230-234, 241-246, 248
internet interventions 27-33, 42, 45, 79-80, 82, 85, 95
Internet-Based Cognitive Behavioral Therapy (iCBT) 51

L

LITERATURE REVIEW 2, 29, 33, 142

M

Mamma Mia 35-39, 41-46, 51, 82-84, 86-87, 89-91, 93, 95-106, 110
mental health 1-6, 9-10, 26, 36, 39, 41, 43, 45-46, 51, 55, 57, 59, 80-84, 86, 97, 106, 111-119, 125, 127-129, 212, 214-215, 218, 220, 233
mental illness 1-6, 9, 25-26, 81
mobile health applications 241-242, 247, 249
moderate depression 63, 111-112, 114-115, 118, 122, 127-128

N

Neurotechnology 139-142, 144-145, 147, 155, 164, 172-173, 185-187, 191, 198-201, 203-207

O

online 31, 38-39, 55-56, 97-98, 112, 116, 141, 212-213, 217-221, 223-234, 241-248, 251

P

peer resources 234, 241, 244, 247-248
perinatal depression 34, 36, 42-43, 45-46, 51, 80-81, 97
personal experiences 55, 243, 247-249, 251
Persuasive Technology 61, 138
practitioner 85, 89, 91, 93, 110, 154, 191, 213-214, 217-221, 223-224, 226-230, 233
pregnancy 34, 36-43, 45, 51, 81-83, 89, 99, 110
prevention 1, 4, 8, 42-43, 45-46, 80, 83, 86
primary care 4, 79, 83
process 3, 6, 9, 28, 30, 33, 37, 45, 58, 62, 67, 79, 81, 84, 87, 110, 113-114, 117-118, 120, 129, 147-151, 153-156, 160, 162, 187, 191, 194-195, 199-200, 203, 215, 222, 228, 249, 251
psychotherapy 1, 6, 10, 28, 32, 139-142, 168, 173, 185-186, 200-202, 207, 212-214, 216-217, 219, 221, 224, 231

Q

qualitative research 27, 33, 63, 119

R

rehearsal 56, 58, 60, 62-63, 66, 68-69, 111-112, 114-115, 117-118, 121-124, 127-128, 138
reminders 41, 56, 58-60, 62-63, 66, 68-69, 111-112, 114-115, 117-118, 120-124, 127-128, 138

S

self-help 30, 44, 82, 110, 112
sleep disorders 53-57, 59-60, 63-64, 69, 120
sleeplessness 54, 56-57, 64, 111-112, 114-116, 118, 124, 127-128, 138
staged model of trust 246
Strengths, Weaknesses, Opportunities, and Threats (SWOT) 34-35, 52
subjective well-being 36-37, 45, 51-52, 82, 110
SWOT 34-35, 37-38, 52

T

technology 1-5, 9, 57, 61, 69, 129, 138,

140-141, 144-149, 153-158, 164, 172-173, 186, 191, 198-199, 203, 206-207, 213-216, 219-220, 223, 232, 234, 241-243, 248, 251
therapy 1, 3, 6-8, 25-26, 28-29, 32, 45, 51, 53, 55-57, 59, 69, 80, 111, 114-117, 120, 128, 137, 141-142, 144, 151-152, 171, 173, 186-187, 213, 215, 220, 222-228, 230, 232-233
transpersonal therapy 141, 171, 173, 186-187
tunneled design 36, 41, 44, 52

U

unguided intervention 27-28, 42, 45, 52

W

well-baby clinics 44, 80-84, 93
women 27-29, 32, 34, 36-46, 51, 81-84, 86, 89-91, 93, 95, 97-101, 106, 110

Purchase Print, E-Book, or Print + E-Book

IGI Global books can now be purchased from three unique pricing formats: Print Only, E-Book Only, or Print + E-Book. Shipping fees apply.

www.igi-global.com

Recommended Reference Books

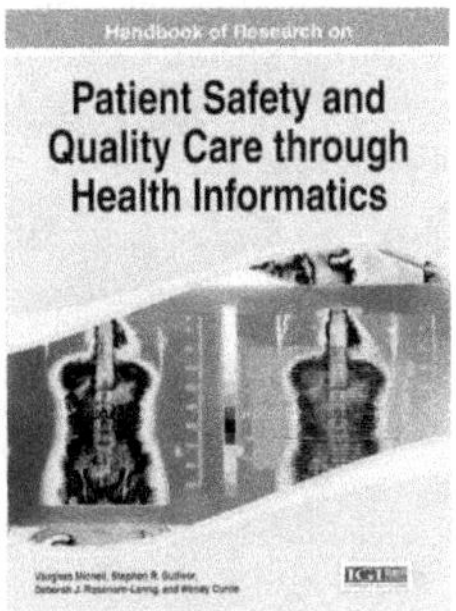

ISBN: 978-1-4666-4546-2
© 2014; 486 pp.
List Price: $292

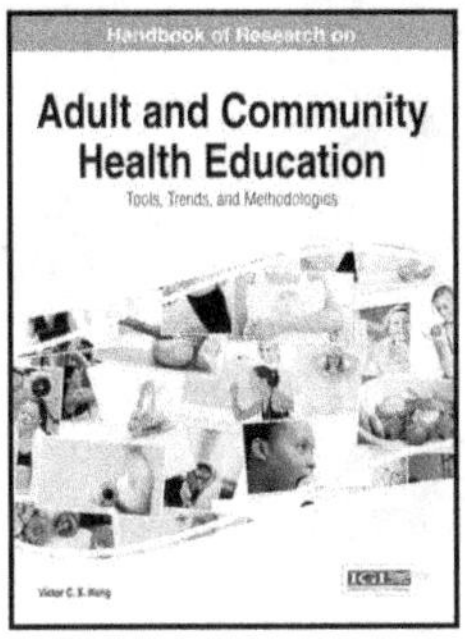

ISBN: 978-1-4666-6260-5
© 2014; 485 pp.
List Price: $260

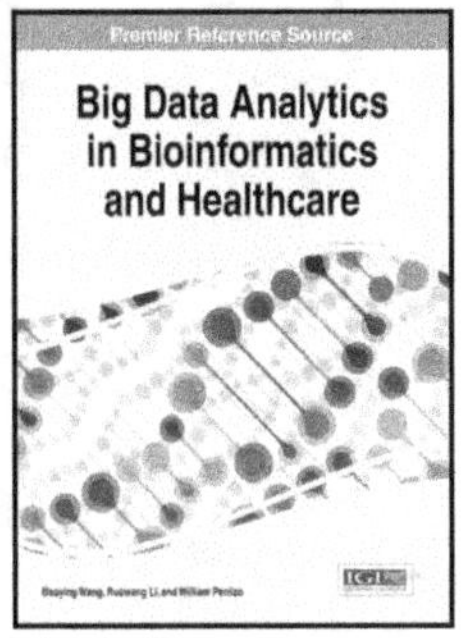

ISBN: 978-1-4666-6611-5
© 2015; 528 pp.
List Price: $204

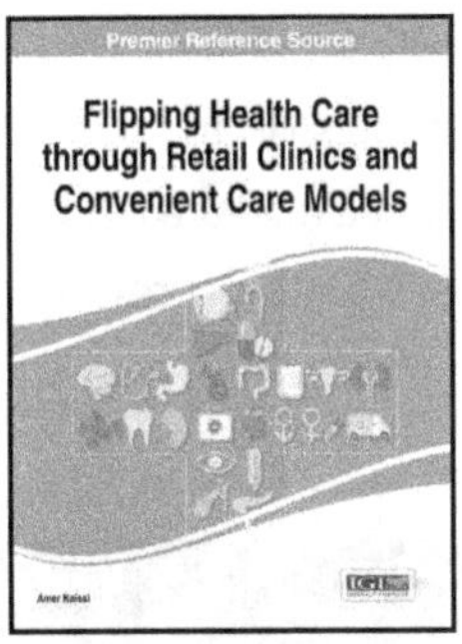

ISBN: 978-1-4666-6355-8
© 2015; 306 pp.
List Price: $196

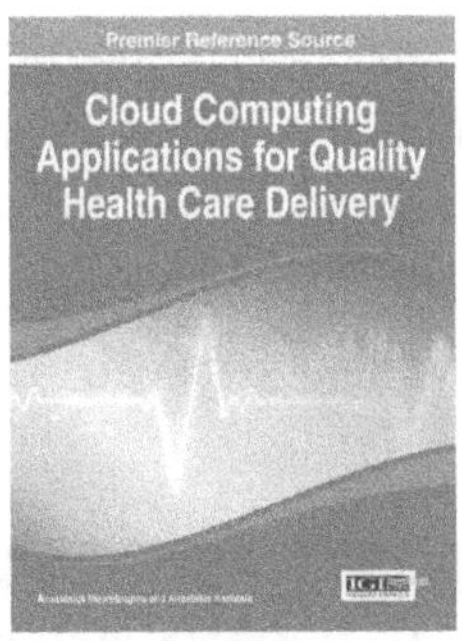

ISBN: 978-1-4666-6118-9
© 2014; 342 pp.
List Price: $196

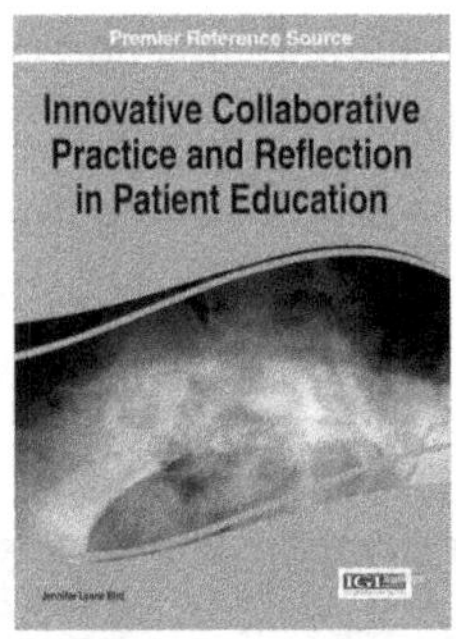

ISBN: 978-1-4666-7524-7
© 2015; 308 pp.
List Price: $180

Looking for free content, product updates, news, and special offers?
Join IGI Global's mailing list today and start enjoying exclusive perks sent only to IGI Global members.
Add your name to the list at **www.igi-global.com/newsletters.**

Publishing Information Science and Technology Research Since 1988

IGI Global
DISSEMINATOR OF KNOWLEDGE

www.igi-global.com Sign up at www.igi-global.com/newsletters facebook.com/igiglobal twitter.com/igiglobal

www.ingramcontent.com/pod-product-compliance
Lightning Source LLC
LaVergne TN
LVHW081337300926
849161LV00008B/1995